Visual Problems in Childhood

Edited by

Terry Buckingham BSc MSc PhD FBCO DCLP
Department of Optometry, University of Bradford

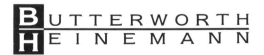

BUTTERWORTH
HEINEMANN

Butterworth-Heinemann Ltd
Linacre House, Jordan Hill, Oxford OX2 8DP

A member of the Reed Elsevier group

OXFORD LONDON BOSTON
MUNICH NEW DELHI SINGAPORE SYDNEY
TOKYO TORONTO WELLINGTON

First published 1993

British Library Cataloguing in Publication Data

Visual Problems in Childhood
  I. Buckingham, Terry
  618.92

ISBN 0 7506 1061 1

Library of Congress Cataloguing in Publication Data

Visual problems in childhood/edited by Terry Buckingham.
  p. cm.
  Includes bibliographical references and index.
  ISBN 0 7506 1061 1
  1. Vision disorders in children. I. Buckingham, Terry.
  [DNLM: 1. Eye Diseases – in infancy & childhood. WW 600b V834 1993]
  RE48.2.C5U54 1993   92–48430
  618.92'0977–dc20   CIP

Typeset by EJS Chemical Composition, Midsomer Norton, Bath
Printed in Great Britain at the University Press, Cambridge

Contents

Contributors

T.G. Baker BSc PhD DSc CBiol FIBiol FIMLS FRSA FRCPath FRSE
Head of Department of Biomedical Sciences, University of Bradford

Terry Buckingham BSc MSc PhD FBCO DCLP
Senior Lecturer, Department of Optometry, University of Bradford

A. Jane Dickinson MCChB MRCP FCOphth
Senior Registrar in Ophthalmology, General Infirmary at Leeds, Leeds

Alistair R. Fielder MRCP FRCS FCOphth
Department of Ophthalmology, University of Birmingham Medical School, Birmingham

Elizabeth Gould BSc FBCO
Senior Optometrist, Moorfields Eye Hospital, London
The Wolfson Centre, London

Jill Grose-Fifer PhD MBCO
Research Fellow, Infant Study Center, Department of Psychology, Brooklyn College of the City University of New York, New York

David Haigh DCH FRCP
Consultant Paediatrician, Paediatric Unit, St Luke's Hospital, Bradford

J.A.M. Jennings PhD MSc FBCO
Senior Lecturer, Department of Optometry and Vision Sciences, University of Manchester Institute of Science and Technology, Manchester

A.J. Kempster PhD MSc FBCO DCLP
Principal Optometrist, Birmingham and Midland Eye Hospital, Birmingham

John Muldoon BSc MEd
Deputy Headmaster, Roundthorn Special School, Bradford

Suman C. Patel MSc (Tech) FBCO
Lecturer, Department of Optometry, University of Bradford

David Pickwell MSc FBCO FBOA:HD DOrth
formerly Head of Department and Professor of Optometry, Department of Optometry, University of Bradford

A.G. Sabell MSc FBCO DCLP
University of Birmingham, The Health Centre, Birmingham

A.R. Shakespeare FBCO
Lecturer, Department of Optometry, University of Bradford

Michael Sheridan MSc FBCO FBOA:HD DCLP
formerly Senior Lecturer, Department of Optometry, University of Bradford

Derek R. Sherwood FRCS FCOphth
Consultant Ophthalmologist, Whangerei, New Zealand

Janet Silver MPhil FBCO
Principal Optometrist, Moorfields Eye Hospital, London

Alan Slater BSc PhD
Senior Lecturer, Department of Psychology, University of Exeter, Exeter

Caroline Thompson PhD MBCO
Research Fellow, Department of Vision Sciences, University of Aston, Birmingham

W.S. Topliss FBDO
Dispensing Optician, Private Practice

Preface

There is, clearly, a relationship between a child's visual performance and other aspects of pre-natal and childhood development. When considering this it will be recalled that of 37 cell divisions which take place as the fetus develops into the man, 34 take place before birth.

Some years ago Professor David Pickwell invited me to develop a post-graduate course for those interested in the clinical assessment of infants' vision. Surprisingly, this proved to be extremely popular and I was subsequently asked by the publishers to edit a text for practitioners who wished to develop their work in this area.

This has been no mean feat. It has been difficult not to imagine oneself as an ageing sheepdog shepherding a flock of independent, not to say wayward, sheep toward pastures which appear decidedly less pleasant. None the less we have journeyed together and, in doing so, I have been privileged to gain a great many new friends. In such a work it is inevitably the case that, in the time taken to draw everything together, the subject moves on as it continues to develop. If the contributors have anything in common, it has been their kindness, generosity and patience.

It was the aim of this book to consider the development of vision in infants, their management as patients, as well as reviewing the theoretical and practical aspects of assessing visual performance. It is always difficult to break new ground and I hope that the book goes at least some way toward achieving its aim. It has been a particular pleasure working with those from other disciplines and I hope that their perspective brings valuable insight into the visual problems of childhood.

I am deeply grateful for the support of my friends and colleagues in the Department of Optometry at the University of Bradford. My thanks go to Joan Marston for her secretarial assistance and to Elizabeth Buckingham for her enduring encouragement and proof reading. Tom Jenkins, Russell Watkins, John Nicholls, Mark Howes, as well as many of the contributors, provided wise council and advice. The staff of Butterworth-Heinemann have always been helpful, witty and entertaining. Surprisingly, a number who have been associated with the book have embarked upon the perilous path of parenthood – I have assumed this to be purely co-incidental.

The University of Bradford
May 1993

Embryology of the eye: normal and abnormal development

T.G. Baker

Introduction

The development of the eye is a complex process and requires an understanding of genetics, reproductive biology and embryology. Consequently the early sections of this chapter consist of a brief account of the genetic basis of life, gametogenesis, cellular differentiation and the early development of the human embryo. Subsequent sections deal with the development of the components of the eye from the brain and surrounding tissues, and the structure of the mature eye. In the final section anomalies of eye development and the influence of certain genes provide an understanding of some of the pathological conditions encountered in clinical practice.

The genetic basis of life

Each of the somatic cells of the body contains two sets of *haploid* chromosomes; one set derived from the mother (maternal) and the other set from the father (paternal). These *diploid* structures, consisting of thousands of genes contain the blue-print for the development of an individual of that species. Somatic cells are all produced by mitotic divisions from a few stem cells in the early embryo and are thus identical (clones) unless a mutation or a chromosomal aberration occurs in one of the divisions, in which case two clones will exist in the same individual (mosaic).

Somatic cells in the adult are said to be *differentiated*; that is only selected genes are 'switched on' at any time and thus the range of cell types that somatic stem cells can form is limited. Thus we speak of *unipotent cells*, which theoretically can only form one type of cell in the body, and *pluripotent cells* which can form a variety of cell types. By contrast the fertilized egg or *zygote* has the potential to switch on any combination of genes, and is therefore *totipotent* (i.e. has the potential to form any differentiated cell in the embryo).

In plants and some lowly types of animals a new individual can develop from one or more somatic cells (asexual reproduction), but such progeny are identical (clones) to the individual from whom the cells were obtained. The principle of sexual reproduction, however, is to ensure that individuals are not identical clones but receive a unique set of genes, unless the individual has an identical twin derived from one half of the original zygote.

Each gene is present in two forms (alleles), one of which (*dominant*) is usually more powerful in its influence than its homologue (the *recessive* allele). Where each chromosome of an homologous pair has the same gene present (homozygous for either dominant or recessive genes) the character will be expressed but when one homologous chromosome has the dominant gene while the other partner has the recessive gene only the dominant trait will be seen. In practice the end result (e.g. coat colour in mice or eye colour in man) may depend on the interaction of many genes, and each gene consists of one or more *codons* (triplets of base pairs in the deoxyribonucleic acid, or DNA, of a chromosome: see Alberts *et al.*, 1989).

Gametogenesis

Genetic diversity is initially brought about in the ovaries and testes of the parents by the process of *meiosis*. Before entering meiosis the gonadal stem cells (*oogonia* and *spermatogonia* in females and males respectively) divide mitotically to ensure that sufficient stem cells are present: this occurs before birth in the female but largely after puberty in the male (*Figure 1.1*).

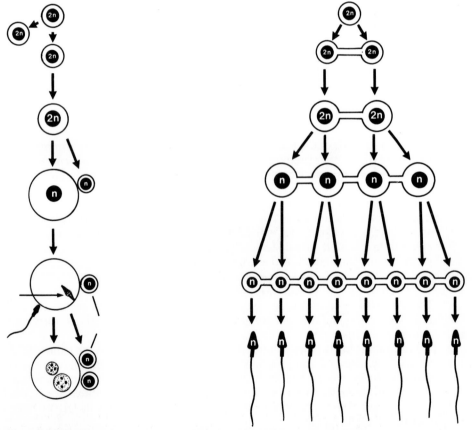

Figure 1.1. Diagrammatic representation of the processes of gametogenesis. Meiotic divisions in oocytes produce a single large ovum while similar divisions in spermatocytes produce four spermatozoa

Meiosis consists of two cell divisions. During the prophase of the first division the homologous maternal and paternal chromosomes undergo pairing (or *synapsis*; each gene pairing with its homologue) until the pairs are 'zippered' together (the *pachytene* stage of first meiotic prophase). During the ensuing diplotene stage, parts of the maternal and paternal chromosomes are exchanged and hence four sets of gene sequences for each homologous chromosome are laid down (*Figures 1.2, 1.3*). The completion of the first meiotic division results in two *haploid* cells, containing half the number of chromosomes, each of which is potentially different from that derived from the parent. The second meiotic division separates the individual

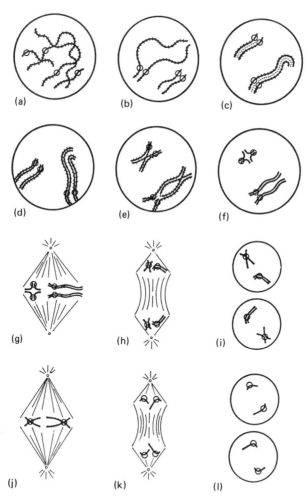

Figure 1.2. Diagram showing the behaviour of chromosomes during meiosis. For simplicity only two pairs of chromosomes are depicted, a short pair with terminal pairing, and a long pair with intermediate synapsis. Only the nuclei are shown; the cytoplasm of the cells has been disregarded. (a) Leptotene; (b) zygotene; (c) pachytene; (d) late pachytene, showing tetrads (two pairs of bivalents); (e) diplotene; (f) diakinesis; (g) metaphase I; (h) late anaphase I; (i) telophase I (egg and polar body); (j) metaphase II; (k) anaphase II; (l) telophase II. (From Baker, 1982)

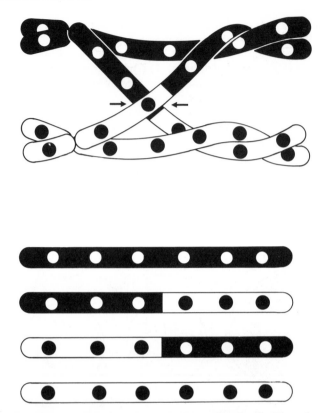

Figure 1.3. Diagram showing crossing over between the chromatids of a pair of homologous chromosomes at the diplotene stage of first meiotic prophase. The chromatids break ($\rightarrow$ $\leftarrow$) and rejoin to ensure genetic diversity

chromatids of each chromosome (*Figures 1.1, 1.4*) to produce four gametes (spermatozoa) in the male but only one large secondary oocyte in the female, together with the abortive polar body (*Figures 1.1, 1.4*). The secondary oocyte is 'blocked' in meiosis at metaphase II and is ovulated at around the 14th day of the menstrual cycle in response to the mid-cycle 'surge' of gonadotrophins. The penetration of this ovulated egg by a spermatozoon induces the completion of meiosis and the release of another polar body (*Figure 1.4;* Baker, 1972, 1982).

Sex determination

In man the haploid number of chromosomes is 23 and this is only found in eggs and spermatozoa. The normal diploid number of 46 is restored during fertilization (*Figure 1.5*), which is thus the antithesis of meiosis.

Each diploid cell contains 22 pairs of autosomes and one pair of sex chromosomes – XX in the female and XY in the male. One set of 22 autosomes and an X chromosome is provided by the egg cell while the spermatozoon provides the other set of autosomes and either an X or a Y: thus half the progeny will be female and the

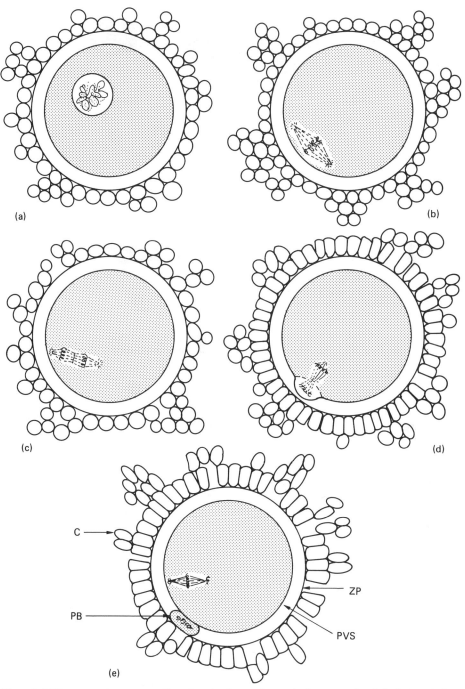

Figure 1.4. Diagrammatic representation of pre-ovulatory changes in the oocyte shortly before ovulation from the Graafian follicle. These changes are brought about by the midcycle surge of gonadotrophins. (a) Diplotene stage; (b) metaphase I; (c) rotation of spindle; (d) extrusion of first polar body; (e) metaphase II. C, cumulus cells; PB, 1st polar body; ZP, zona pellucida; PVS, perivitelline space. (From Baker, 1982)

other half male. It is now well established that the Y chromosome contains testis-determining sequences (TDY) that cause the early gonad to differentiate into a testis (Burgoyne and Baker, 1984). It is the absence of these genes which fails to induce testis formation and hence the production of an ovary. An occasional transfer of the testis-determining sequences from a Y to an X chromosome during crossing over in meiosis I accounts for the rare cases of sex reversal (XX males and XY females). For a fuller account of the processes of gametogenesis, ovulation and fertilization the interested reader is referred to standard books on the subject (Baker, 1972; Monesi, 1972; Austin, 1968; Baker, 1982; Philipp and Setchell, 1992); while for accounts of the genetic basis of life the reader is referred to Alberts *et al.* (1989) and Connor and Ferguson-Smith (1987).

Early human development

The head of the spermatozoon swells within the egg to form a male pro-nucleus which lies close to the female pro-nucleus. The nuclear envelopes of these two structures break down to liberate the two haploid sets of chromosomes (*Figure 1.5*(a)). The homologues pair to restore the diploid condition and arrange themselves on a metaphase spindle. Thus the cell divides mitotically into two identical daughter cells (*Figure 1.5*(b)). Should these cells separate, identical twins will be produced. Further mitotic divisions occur to produce four, then eight cells (*Figure 1.5*(c)), and so on until a ball of cells is produced (the morulla; *Figure 1.5*(d)). An ingress of fluid into the morulla produces a cavity (blastocele) and the early embryo is then a *blastocyst* which, once liberated from its mucopolysaccharide 'shell' (zona pellucida), will implant in the wall of the uterus (*Figures 1.5*(e, f)). The blastocyst consists of a cluster of cells (the inner cell mass) which will form the embryo and fetal membranes (amnion, chorion), and a shell of trophoblast cells which will form the fetal component of the placenta (*Figures 1.5*(f), *1.6*(a, b)). A more detailed account of these processes is to be found in textbooks of embryology (Hamilton, Boyd and Mossman, 1962; Moore, 1973).

The trophoblast invades the wall of the uterine endometrium to expose the maternal blood, thus obtaining a source of nutrients, while the inner cell mass rearranges itself to form a bilaminar embryonic disc which represents two of the three primary cell types of the early embryo (embryonic ectoderm and endoderm; *Figure 1.6*(b–d)).

The embryo is now aged about 9 days *post conception* (p.c) and at this stage the mother will not yet know that she is pregnant. Soon thereafter the trophoblast cells will produce *human chorionic gonadotrophin* (hCG) which mimics pituitary luteinizing hormone and thus prevents the mother's next menstrual period from occurring. This is the first indication that pregnancy has occurred and already the embryo is about 15 days old. At this time a thickened band of embryonic ectoderm (the primitive streak) is formed caudally in the midline of the embryonic disc. Concurrently a groove appears above the primitive streak and the third primary germ layer, the *embryonic mesoderm,* forms from the embryonic ectoderm and primitive streak (*Figure 1.7*(a–d)). The cranial end of the primitive streak forms Hensen's node: the latter gives rise to the notochord which is subsequently important in the formation of the vertebrae (*Figure 1.7*(b–d)).

At about this time (3rd week p.c.) part of the ectoderm becomes arranged into a pear-shaped plate (the neural plate) which rolls up to eventually form the neural

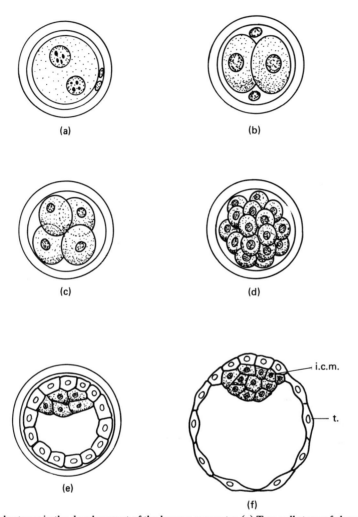

Figure 1.5. Early stages in the development of the human conceptus (a) Two-cell stage of cleavage;
(b) four-cell cell stage; (c) eight-cell stage; (d) morulla (or ball of cells); (e) early blastocyst in zona
pellucida; (f) 'hatched; blastocyst 5 days after ovulation. i.c.m. Inner cell mass; t., trophoblast

tube (*Figure 1.7*(e, f)), while its remnants form the posterior root ganglia on either
side of the spinal cord. The rest of the ectoderm closes over the neural tube to form
the skin and integument of the adult. At the same time the mesoderm thickens and
will eventually form the *somites* (segmented muscles and vertebral bones). Part of
the anterior mesoderm forms the heart and primitive blood vessels to provide a
circulatory system into the maternal (uterine) blood lacunae within the developing
placenta by around the 22nd day after fertilization (i.e. about 36 days after the last
menstrual period experienced by the mother). The early blood cells seem to be
formed from the endothelia of the primitive blood vessels and at this stage the
erythrocytes have nuclei. The derivatives of the three primary germ layers are shown
in *Figure 1.8*.

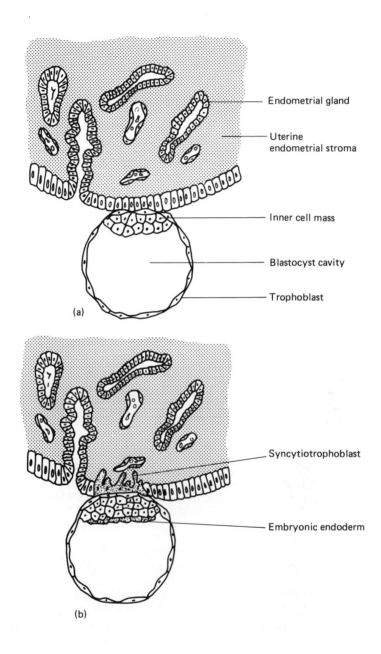

(a)

(b)

Endometrial gland

Uterine
endometrial stroma

Inner cell mass

Blastocyst cavity

Trophoblast

Syncytiotrophoblast

Embryonic endoderm

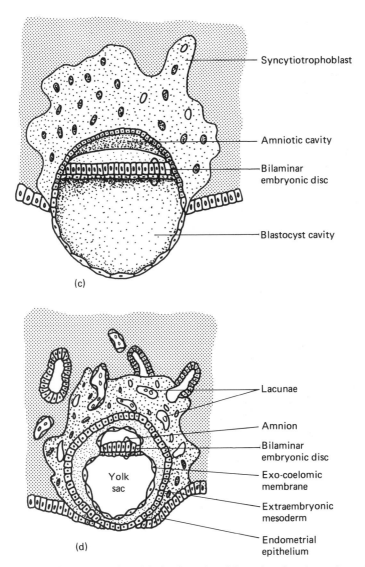

Syncytiotrophoblast

Amniotic cavity

Bilaminar
embryonic disc

Blastocyst cavity

(c)

Lacunae

Amnion

Bilaminar
embryonic disc

Exo-coelomic
membrane

Extraembryonic
mesoderm

Endometrial
epithelium

Yolk
sac

(d)

Figure 1.6. Diagrammatic representation of the implantation of the embryo into the uterine endometrium and the formation of the early embryonic disc. (a) Attachment of blastocyst to uterine endometrium; (b) proliferation of trophoblast (syncytiotrophoblast) which invades endometrial stroma; (c) further invasion of endometrium by trophoblast and formation of bilaminar embryonic disc; (d) invasion of embryo completed and endometrium has healed at surface (note amniotic sac and yolk sac on either side of bilaminar disc)

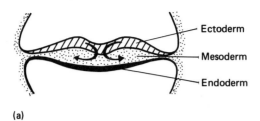

(a)

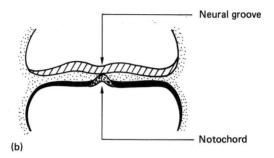

(b)

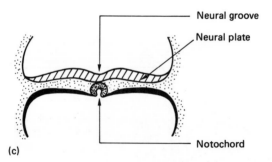

(c)

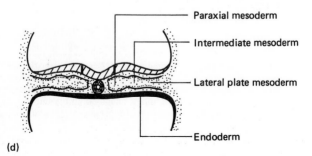

(d)

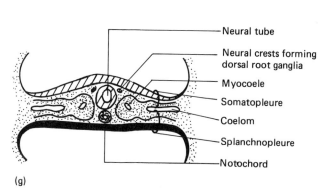

Figure 1.7. Transverse section through embryonic disc to depict formation of neural tube, notochord and mesoderm. (a), Cells of the 'ectoderm' roll inwards to form mesoderm and thus trilaminar disc; (b) grooves form above and below the disc (neural and notochordal grooves respectively); (c) notochord now forming a tube; (d) mesenchyme developing as somites. (e), (f) neural tube about to part from ectoderm; remnants of neural folds will form dorsal (posterior) root ganglia; (g) neural tube complete and ectoderm continuous over it; neural crests will form dorsal (posterior) root ganglia. (Redrawn after Moore, 1988)

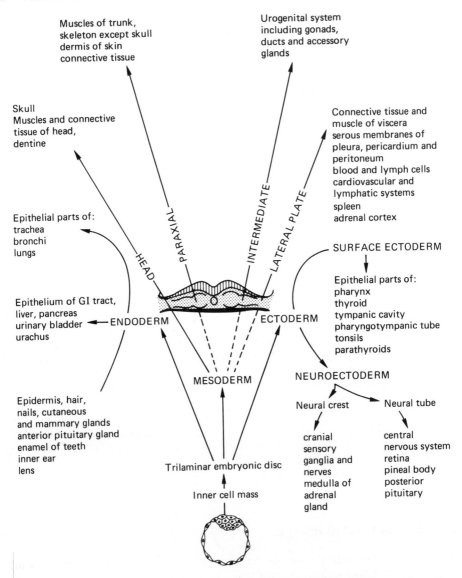

Figure 1.8. Scheme illustrating the origins and derivatives of the three primary germ layers. (From Moore, 1988, with permission)

Subsequent development of the neural tube

Figure 1.9 depicts the neural tube with its swollen anterior end consisting of the three early chambers of the brain and its subsequent rearrangement into five areas. The rest of the neural tube will form the spinal cord.

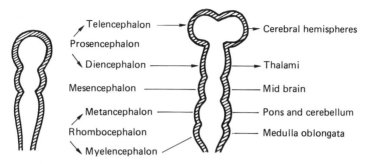

Figure 1.9. Development of front end of neural tube to form initially three chambers and subsequently five chambers that contribute to the brain. (After Hamilton, Boyd and Mossman, 1962)

Estimation of embryonic/fetal age

By definition, an embryo becomes a fetus when bone formation commences at the centres of the long bones (*c.* 7 weeks p.c.; Streeter, 1951). This event clearly marks the end of the embryonic period and the onset of fetal life.

In an idealized menstrual period of 28 days duration, ovulation occurs on day 14. However, the variability in the duration of the menstrual cycle means that ovulation can only be detected by assays for gonadotrophins and this information is rarely available in routine pregnancies. It is for this reason that pregnancy is often dated from the day of the mother's last menstrual period (LMP) and conceptional or gestational age is obtained by substracting 13 ± 1 days from the LMP age of the pregnancy. Unfortunately, however, few women keep precise records of their menstrual periods and thus errors in LMP (and hence conception age) are fairly common. Embryologists must, therefore, check the data provided against certain reliable morphometric parameters including *greatest length* of early embryos, *sitting height* or crown–rump length for later (curved) embryos and even by measurements of the head, to produce idealized gestational age (i.e. the age p.c.; see Streeter, 1920).

Early development of the eye

The eyes develop from three sources in the embryo; the neural tube (neurectoderm), the surface ectoderm and the mesoderm. Around day 22 p.c. two optic grooves (*sulci; Figure 1.10*(a)) develop on either side of the swollen cranial end of the neural tube. Should the sulci develop too close together only one eye will develop to produce a cyclops (with or without a proboscis; see Hamilton, Boyd and Mossman, 1962). The optic sulci subsequently invaginate to form bulbous *optic vesicles* on either side of the forebrain (*Figure 1.10*(b–f)). As the optic vesicles approach the outer ectoderm a process of induction occurs that causes the ectoderm to thicken to form the *lens placodes*, which then invaginate to form pits on either side (*Figure 1.10*(g–i). Simultaneously, the optic vesicles invaginate to form double-layered optic cups ready to receive the lens placodes (now lens vesicles; *Figure 1.10*(g–i)), which become separated from the surface ectoderm.

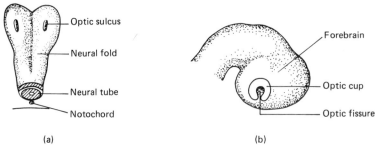

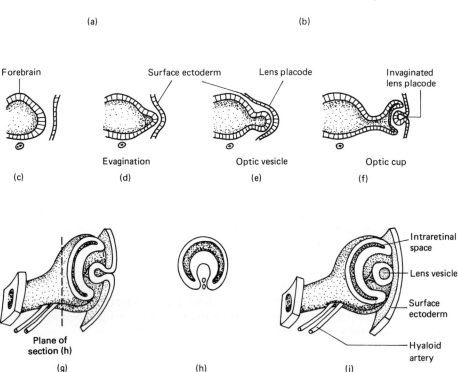

Figure 1.10. Diagrammatic representation of formation of eye from brain and lens from surface ectoderm. (a) Optic sulci developing in neural folds; (b) optic cup and fissure in later embryo; (c) – (f) cross-section through brain showing formation of optic vesicle (which invaginates to form optic cup) and of lens placode; (g), (i) ingrowth of hyaloid vessels in optic fissure and separation of lens from surface ectoderm; (h) cross-section of optic stalk to show fissure and ingrowth of hyaloid vessels closes around the blood vessels. (Redrawn after Moore, 1988 and Hamilton *et al.*, 1962)

A fissure develops in the lower area of the optic cup and optic stalk (the choroidal fissure *Figure 1.10*(g)) and blood vessels grow along this to supply the inner layer of the optic cup, the intervening mesenchyme and the lens: soon thereafter this fissure closes around the blood vessels. The non-fusion of the fissure results in a condition known as coloboma (*Figure 1.11*) where the iris (and sometimes the choroid) is absent inferomedially.

Histogenesis of the retina

The process of invagination of the optic vesicle results in a double-layered optic cup

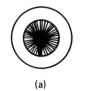 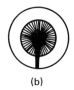

(a)   (b)

Figure 1.11. Failure of the optic fissure to close can result in coloboma of the iris, (a) and of both iris and choroid (b)

(*Figures 1.10*(d–g), *1.12*(a–d), the outer layer of which consists of cells that acquire pigment (*pigmented layer*) while the inner layer develops into the visual receptive (nervous) part of the retina (*Figure 1.13*). The gap between these two layers is continuous with the ventricular system of the brain. This gap becomes virtually eliminated by the fusion of the two layers, but a potential connection to the ventricles persists as the intraretinal space which can result in cases of detached retinae in older patients.

It should be remembered that the optic cups are outgrowths of the forebrain. It is believed that the developing lens placodes produce inductor substances which cause the inner layer of the optic cup to develop two regions, a thicker *pars optica retina* (developing rods and cones: see *Figure 1.12*(c, d)) towards the back of the eye and a more anterior and thinner zone, the *pars caeca retina*; where the two zones meet, a fine line can be detected. The pars caecae contain neither rods nor cones.

Since the inner layer of the optic cup is formed by a process of invagination the retina can be said to be 'inverted' with the tips of the cones and rods resting on the pigmented cells and the neurones passing over the inner surface of the eye. As a result, incoming light must pass through the retina to reach the photoreceptive cells at the boundary with the pigment cells. The light must, therefore, pass through a layer of nerve fibres radiating towards the optic nerve, a layer of bipolar cells, and the light-sensitive rods and cones (*Figure 1.13*).

The lens

It was seen earlier that the lens is formed as a pouch of the ectoderm which subsequently becomes detached to form the lens vesicle consisting of a thin outer (cuboidal) layer of cells and a thicker inner (columnar) layer of cells. The cavity between the two layers becomes obliterated as the inner columnar cells increase in height and eventually lose their nuclei to become lens fibres. Surrounding mesoderm cells form the lens capsule which is vascularized by the hyaloid artery and by the annular artery, but this blood supply retrogresses around the time of birth (*Figure 1.12*(c–d)).

The coverings of the eye and the anterior chamber

Since the eye forms as an outgrowth of the brain it is not surprising that its coverings are analogous to the coverings of the brain (meninges). Beneath the pigment cell layer of the eye is the *choroid* which is continuous with the *pia-arachnoid* of the brain. The *sclera* of the eye is formed from a condensation of mesenchyme and is continuous with the fibrous *dura mater* of the brain via the sheath around the optic

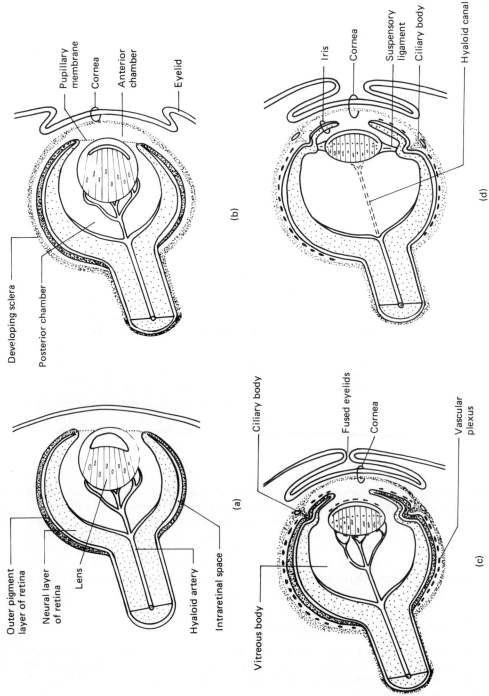

Figure 1.12. Development of the anterior chamber, lids, sclera, choroid, iris, etc., of the eye

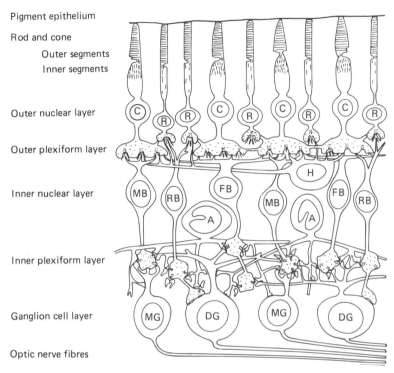

Pigment epithelium

Rod and cone

Outer segments
Inner segments

Outer nuclear layer

Outer plexiform layer

Inner nuclear layer

Inner plexiform layer

Ganglion cell layer

Optic nerve fibres

Figure 1.13. Neural components of the retina. C, cone; R, rod; MB, RB and FB, midget, rod and flat bipolar cells; DG and MG, diffuse and midget ganglion cells; H, horizontal cells; A, amacrine cells. (Reproduced from Dowling and Boycott, 1966, with permission)

nerve. The *cornea* probably has a similar origin, but consists of a characteristic meshwork of collagen fibres to ensure its transparency: it is lined with Descemet's mesothelium. The outer membrane of the cornea, and also the *conjunctiva*, form from the surface ectoderm. The *anterior (aqueous) chamber* of the eye is homologous to the subarachnoid space in the coverings of the brain. Hence the fluid in the anterior chamber is analogous to cerebrospinal fluid.

Ciliary body

This is formed from the outer layer of the optic cup as a ring around the developing lens. Therefore, part of it is pigmented while the non-pigmented part forms from adjacent (non-neural) inner cup tissue. An ingrowth of mesenchyme cells leads to the formation of muscle and fibrous connective tissue in the ciliary body (*Figure 1.12*(d)).

Around the 10th week of development a ring of 70–75 radial folds develops between the ciliary body and the lens. These folds become the ciliary processes that subsequently anchor the lens and provide the mechanism for altering the focus of the lens (accommodation).

The iris

Both layers of the optic cup and mesenchyme cells contribute to the formation of the iris immediately anterior to the lens. The double-layered epithelium of the iris contains blood capillaries and pigment to give the characteristic (and inherited) colour to the eyes, while dilator and sphincter muscles form from the neuroectoderm. Should pigment not be induced in the iris the characteristic red eyes of the albino will form where the only colour is that of the blood within the capillaries derived from the mesenchyme.

The extraocular muscles

These form between the orbit (bone) and the sclera in characteristic positions – probably from mesenchyme cells around the prochordal plate, although their precise origin remains unclear. The myoblasts forming each group of eye muscles are supplied by cranial nerves III, IV and VI (for example, see Warwick and Williams, 1973).

There are seven muscles associated with each eye, one of which (levator palpebrae superioris) raises the upper eyelids while the other six provide rotation of the eye in any direction (four *recti* – *superior, inferior, medialis* and *lateralis*, and the two *obliqui* – *superior* and *inferior*; see Warwick and Williams, 1973).

Eyelids (or palpebrae) and lacrimal glands

These arise as ectodermal folds above and below the cornea which grow rapidly to fuse in the midline by around the 10th week. During the 26th week the eyelids separate and develop eyelashes (*Figure 1.12*(c, d)).

The lacrimal glands develop in the superior fornix (upper outer angles) part of each conjunctival sac. The latter covers the cornea and lines the eyelids. The lacrimal glands are initially small solid epithelial buds which increase in number and become branched to form an acinous gland. Since these glands provide copious lubrication to the surface of the eye (conjunctiva) drainage is needed in the form of the carunculus and plica semilunaris (inner lower aspect of each eye) leading to the nasolacrimal duct which drains into the inferior meatus of the nose.

Optic nerve

The axons of the retinal ganglion cells converge on the optic disc where they leave the eye on their course to the optic chiasmata below the brain. The optic nerve contains blood vessels and glial cells (derived from mesoderm and neuroectoderm respectively).

Myelination of axons within the optic nerve begins during the 7th month: it can sometimes continue into the nerve fibre layer of the retina where it produces characteristic white patches near the optic nerve.

Vitreous (posterior chamber)

The space in the optic cup between the back of the lens and the developing retina becomes occupied by ectodermal and mesodermal cells (probably from the retina and blood vessels respectively). Around the 6th week of development the ectodermal and/or mesodermal cells secrete a viscous material – the primary vitreous humour or hyaloid substance. At this time the hyaloid vascular channels begin to atrophy (*Figure 1.12*(d)). Subsequently a secondary vitreous forms around the primary vitreous which becomes limited to a cone-shaped region with its wide axis adjacent to the lens and its pointed end near to the retina.

The orbit

The orbit is developed early in the 2nd month from bony tissue derived from the frontal, sphenoid, ethmoid and zygomatic bones with a small process from the palatine bone (Warwick and Williams, 1973).

Postnatal development of the eye

By the time of birth the eye is almost fully developed and is a functional sensory organ of near-adult proportions. The iris becomes pigmented shortly after birth, but the adult colouration may not initially be displayed.

Abnormalities of eye development

Genetic factors

Many genetic disorders have been implicated in defective vision, especially genes associated with inborn errors of metabolism, but these are outside the scope of the present chapter (but see Scheie and Albert, 1977).

In this chapter selected examples will be provided to indicate both the range of developmental defects and the mechanism of the genetic defect. More detailed accounts can be found elsewhere (e.g. Sheie and Albert, 1977).

Genetic errors affecting eye development can be due to mutations involving individual genes or those that exert control over them (e.g. retinoblastoma, see pp. 20–1). They can also be caused by chromosomal disorders in which parts (or whole) chromosomes are present in excess, where parts of chromosomes are deleted, or where structural rearrangements occur (translocations, inversions, etc.; see Connor and Ferguson-Smith, 1987).

Mutations

Genes for colour vision and night blindness are on the X chromosome and are thus sex-linked. A female will only have defective colour vision if both her X chromosomes have the defective alleles, while males who inherit defective genes on their mother's X chromosomes will not be able to detect some or all colours and/or be night blind, depending on which gene is defective.

Another X-linked condition is ocular albinism in which eye pigmentation is reduced or absent. This should not be confused with complete albinism in which pigment is absent from hair, eyelashes and the iris (but not the retina) since this is an autosomal recessive condition which thus can affect either sex. Incomplete albinism, where the iris is paler than usual, is also caused by an autosomal recessive gene.

A further example of an autosomal recessive condition is found in Tay–Sachs disease: a cherry red spot develops in the foveal area of the retina and this subsequently changes to a grey colour before death of the child. The condition is most commonly seen in Ashkenazi Jews but can be found in other races and is caused by an autosomal recessive trait.

Autosomal dominant genes will affect a minimum of 25% of progeny (where only one parent is heterozygous for the defective gene) and this will reach 50% if both parents are heterozygous. Should both parents be homozygous for the allele in question, all the children of the union will be affected. Examples of autosomal dominant traits include aniridia, cataracts (both acquired and congenital), corneal dystrophies, glaucoma, macula degeneration, microphthalmia, myopia, detached retinae, retinitis pigmentosa and absence of tears. Coloboma, ptosis and retinoblastoma (see below) show irregular dominant autosomal inheritance.

It should be noted, however, that many of the conditions listed above can have more than one mode of inheritance and thus can also be caused by autosomal recessive genes.

Chromosomal disorders

The absence of an autosome is always lethal owing to the loss of so many genes but the deletion of part of a chromosome (or of the Y chromosome or one of a pair of X chromosomes) is sometimes compatible with life. Such conditions can lead to severe developmental abnormalities which can influence the development of the eye.

Perhaps the most common autosomal trisomy is Down's syndrome where three copies of chromosome 21 are found instead of the usual two, or where a translocation has resulted in an extra copy of part of this chromosome (see Connor and Ferguson-Smith, 1987). As well as the common anatomical features of this condition (short stature, protruding tongue, reduced IQ), individuals exhibit some eye defects including cataracts, oblique fissures that are slanted upwards and outwards (so-called mongoloid eyes), epicanthus and changes in the iris.

Trisomy 18 (Edward's syndrome) is associated with microphthalmia, ptosis, epicanthus, corneal opacities, cataracts and optic atrophy. Since this syndrome is fatal at an early age treatment is not necessary.

Trisomy 13 (Patau's syndrome) is very rare but eye defects can be detected in a large proportion of affected children, particularly those with an embryological origin. Thus Patau's syndrome is associated with microphthalmos, coloboma, cataract and retinal dysplasia: the anterior chamber may be absent and cyclopia has been reported.

Deletions of parts of chromosomes can also cause abnormalities of the eye. Thus absence of all or part of the short arm of chromosome 5 (cri-du-chat syndrome) is associated with anti-mongoloid slants to the eyelids, epicanthus, myopia and optic atrophy, while a similar deletion to chromosome 4 (Wolf's syndrome) can lead to exophthalmos, epicanthus, strabismus and coloboma of the iris.

Retinoblastoma

This condition is associated with a gene on chromosome 13 (probably in band 21). It is fairly certain that the gene has a normal role to play in development (possibly as a growth or cell-division promoter) but can also cause a particularly nasty cancer of retinal tissue. It is thus said to be an *oncogene* and problems occur when the gene is altered (mutation), absent from one or both chromoses, or translocated to a site on another chromosome where it is placed next to a particularly active gene sequence.

The parents of an affected child (especially where the tumour is present in both eyes) have a 40–45% chance of having further affected children and thus genetic counselling is necessary (Connor and Ferguson-Smith, 1987).

Treatment of an affected child consists of the complete and immediate removal of the affected eye(s) since otherwise the tumour will spread via the optic nerve to the brain, as well as by rapid metastasis to various organs.

Recent research has shown that the retinoblastoma oncogene, when 'activated' in other organs, is implicated in a range of other tumours including those of the breast, bone (osteosarcoma) and lung (small-cell carcinoma). In these cases, as with the eye tumours, mutations, deletions or translocations of the gene on chromosome 13 in appropriate cell lines may be caused by some viruses (especially the retroviruses) or by ionizing radiations.

Embryological abnormalities of the eye

Most of the anomalies in eye development can be deduced from first principles if one has a basic understanding of embryology. These anomalies arise from abnormal development of the components of embryonic tissue that contribute to the eye or the orbit. The underlying causes may be genetic, environmental (ionizing radiations, cytotoxic chemicals or certain teratogenic drugs) or result from some transplacental infections at critical stages in development.

Anencephalus

This severe condition is more common in females than males (*c.* 5 : 1) and its incidence is high in Scotland and Ireland but low in Scandinavia and Japan. The vault of the skull fails to develop and most of the brain above the medulla oblongata is subsequently destroyed (possibly due to contractions of the uterus). Cyclops is occasionally observed and the eyes protrude and thus appear to be enlarged. It is claimed that the nerve fibre layer of the retina, and its ganglion layer, are absent or imperfectly developed. The condition is related to spina bifida (indeed, infants may exhibit both conditions), is almost certainly of genetic origin, and infants usually live for only a few hours.

Abnormalities of the orbit

The orbit may fail to develop or be too small to accommodate the eyes which, therefore, protrude such that the lids are difficult to close.

In patients with 'tower skull' (oxycephaly) premature fusion of the coronary and lamboidal sutures results in arrested growth both laterally and in the anteroposterior planes. This autosomal dominant condition is more common in males and may be associated with exophthalmia and optic atrophy as the result of increased intracranial pressure.

Exophthalmia also occurs in Crouzon's disease and Apert's syndrome, both of which are probably caused by dominant autosomal traits.

Hypertelorism is characterized by an excessive distance between the orbits: it seems to be inherited and may be associated with glaucoma, ptosis and optic atrophy.

Defective development of the optic cup

In its extremes this can result in anophthalmia or (if the optic sulci develop too close together) in cyclops where the single eye is placed below the proboscis-like nose.

Cyclopia is caused by an autosomal gene and the associated abnormalities are so severe as to be lethal.

In microphthalmia the eye is normal in structure but only about two-thirds of normal size. The condition is usually bilateral and is associated with a number of ocular conditions including a marked disposition to glaucoma.

Coloboma (*Figure 1.11*) is the result of a failure of all or part of the optic fissure to close (see p. 14). This may result in bilaterial slots in the iris, ciliary body, choroid, retina, optic nerve or any combination of these in the same patient.

Corneal defects

These range from microcornea, where the diameter of the cornea is markedly reduced, to the opposite condition – megalocornea. The cornea may be flattened with opacification (cornea plana).

Abnormalities of the iris and lens

The iris may be greatly reduced but never truly absent (aniridia) and the condition is usually bilateral.

In early development, blood vessels from the iris cover the surface of the lens. These should atrophy in early development but sometimes they may persist as pupillary membranes.

The pupils may vary in size and the irides in colour within the same patient.

The lens may be defective in size, shape and position and may be (or become) opaque (cataract formation; see Scheie and Albert, 1977).

Vitreous anomalies

The hyaloid artery may fail to regress such that parts of it may be attached to the rear of the lens (Mittendorf dot). Hyaloid remnants usually appear as white strands but if the vessel remains patent blood may impart a pinkish colour. The primary vitreous may persist in a hyperplastic condition and is diagnosed as a white pupil (leukokoria).

The above examples serve to show that complex developmental processes can often be defective and that many of these defects are related to specific genes. It is thus perhaps surprising that the abnormalities do not occur more often. By its very nature, a short chapter covering a wide range of topics can only provide the mechanisms and selected examples of abnormalities. A fuller account of defects in eye development can be found elsewhere (e.g. Scheie and Albert, 1977).

References

ALBERTS, B., BRAY, D, LEWIS, J, RAFF, M, ROBERTS, K. and WATSON, J.D. (1989). *Molecular Biology of the Cell*. Garland Publishing, New York.

AUSTIN, C.R. (1968). *Ultrastructure of Fertilization*. Holt, Rinehart & Winston, New York.

BAKER, T.G. (1972). Oogenesis and ovarian development. In *Reproductive Biology*, edited by H. Balin and S.R. Glasser. Excerpta Medica, Amsterdam, pp. 398–437.

BAKER, T.G. (1982). Oogenesis and ovulation. In *Reproduction in Mammals*, vol. 1, *Germ Cells and Fertilization*, edited by C.R. Austin and R.V. Short, Cambridge University Press, Cambridge, pp. 17–45.

BURGOYNE, P.S. and BAKER, T.G. (1984). Meiotic pairing and gametogenic failure. In *Controlling Events in Meiosis*, edited by C.W. Evans and H.G. Dickinson. Company of Biologists Ltd, Cambridge, pp. 349–362.

CONNOR, J.M. and FERGUSON-SMITH, M.A. (1987). *Essential Medical Genetics*, 2nd edn. Blackwell Scientific, Oxford.

DOWLING, J. E. and BOYCOTT, B.B. (1966). Organisation of the primate retina: electron microscopy. *Proceedings of the Royal Society of London. Series B: Biological Sciences,* **166**, 80–111.

HAMILTON, W.J., BOYD, J.D. and MOSSMAN, H.W. (1962). *Human Embryology*. W. Heffer, Cambridge.

MONESI, V. (1972). Spermatogenesis and spermatozoa. In *Reproduction in Mammals*, vol. 1, *Germ Cells and Fertilization*, edited by C.R. Austin and R.V. Short. Cambridge University Press, Cambridge, pp. 46–84.

MOORE, K.L. (1988). *The Developing Human: Clinically Oriented Embryology*, 4th edn. W.B. Saunders, Philadelphia.

PHILIPP, E.E. and SETCHELL, M.E. (eds) (1991). *Scientific Foundations in Obstetrics and Gynaecology*, 4th edn. Butterworth-Heinemann, Oxford.

SCHEIE, H.G. and ALBERT, D.M. (eds) (1977). *Textbook of Ophthalmology*. W.B. Saunders, Philadelphia.

STREETER, G.L. (1920). Weight, sitting height, foot length and menstrual age of the human embryo. *Contributions to Embryology,* **11**, 143–170.

STREETER, G.L. (1951). Developmental horizons in human embryos. Description of age groups XIX, XX, XXI, XXII and XXIII, being a fifth issue of a survey of the Carnegie Insitution. *Contributions to Embryology,* **34**, 167–196.

WARWICK, R. and WILLIAMS, P.L. (eds) (1973). *Gray's Anatomy*, 35th edn. Longman, Edinburgh.

2

Human growth and development

David Haigh

Pregnancy and its complications

The development of the human fetus from a single cell is a complex process and it is perhaps not surprising that it commonly goes wrong. It is suggested that up to half of all fertilized ova result in an abnormal embryo which either fails to implant or is aborted in the first weeks of pregnancy. The 2% of newborns with a major congenital anomaly are thus the ones who have escaped nature's weeding out process.

About 10% of malformations are the result of a chromosomal abnormality. The presence of an extra chromosome 21, so-called trisomy 21, gives rise to Down's syndrome, a condition with a characteristic facial appearance, mental retardation and malformations of various organ systems especially the heart. Less commonly, trisomy 18 and trisomy 13 produce syndromes of mental retardation, growth failure and congenital heart disease. Other trisomies of the autosomes occur much more rarely in liveborn infants, probably because the abnormalities they produce are usually lethal to the embryo. A deletion of the short arm of chromosome 5 produces an infant with a low birth weight, a small head with mental retardation and a characteristic cry which gives the syndrome its name, cri du chat.

Between 6% and 9% of anomalies are due to environmental influences on a previously normal embryo. Inflammation from viral infections may interfere with cell division and lead to abnormality. Rubella, cytomegalovirus, herpes and the protozoon toxoplasma are known examples. Drugs taken by the mother may cross the placenta and interfere with embryogenesis. Thalidomide when given to women in early pregnancy commonly affected growth of the limb buds so that affected individuals have dramatically short and deformed limbs. Anticonvulsants sometimes cause abnormality such as cleft palate and it is likely that many drugs, even aspirin, trigger fetal abnormality occasionally.

Heavy alcohol consumption, several measures of alcohol per day, in early pregnancy results in a specific syndrome with low birth weight, a small brain, facial, cardiac and renal abnormalities. The effect of more modest alcohol consumption is not known. Nicotine is a powerful constrictor of blood vessels and smoking is known to interfere with placental blood flow. Smoking also leads to raised fetal concentrations of carbon monoxide causing tissues to be short of oxygen. The combination of these two effects means that maternal smoking causes fetal growth retardation, 12 cigarettes a day decreasing birth weight by an average of 180 g (6 oz).

The average term newborn weighs around 3500 g (7.5 lb), but about 8% of neonates in the UK are of low birth weight, weighing less than 2500 g (5.5 lb). The majority are small because they are born prematurely, but around one third have intrauterine growth retardation, i.e. they have grown poorly in the uterus. At its worst, the problem may lead to intrauterine death and fetal growth retardation is a leading cause of perinatal mortality. The fetus may grow poorly because it is abnormal, because the placenta is abnormal or because of maternal disease. The fetus who is intrinsically small will usually have poor long-term growth potential. Chromosomal abnormalities and viral infections have already been described, but there are also various dysmorphic syndromes – those characterised by abnormalities of physical structure, form and size – in which poor growth plays an important part. Russel–Silver dwarfism, for example, is characterized by low birth weight, short stature and asymmetry.

Placental function is poor in pre-eclamptic toxaemia, a common disease of pregnancy whose features are high blood pressure, protein loss in the urine and generalized swelling. Similarly in twin pregnancies the nutritional needs of the twins eventually exceed the capacity of the placental blood supply and fetal growth slows. In such situations, brain growth is often spared so that the babies have a relatively large head. The potential for growth is normal and after birth the infants show rapid 'catch-up' growth.

Mothers who are malnourished will have small babies and maternal diseases such as cyanotic heart disease, hypertension and anaemia interfere with fetal nutrition. Again, such babies often display catch-up growth after birth.

In extreme cases, abnormal placental function through poor fetal nutrition and hypoxia will cause death of the fetus or serious brain damage. Much of the work of obstetricians and midwives is dedicated to preventing these deaths by monitoring the health of the pregnant woman and the growth of her fetus. The fetus who is showing evidence of poor placental function may then be delivered early to allow it to escape the constraints of its abnormal placent.

Women normally gain weight throughout pregnancy and weight gain of say less than 0.5 kg (1 lb) per week in the last third of pregnancy suggests that the fetus may not be growing adequately. Regular weighings are therefore part of traditional antenatal care although their value is controversial. The size of the uterus may be assessed clinically by measuring its height from the pubic symphysis. Between 28 and 36 weeks of pregnancy, this distance in centimetres should equal the gestational age.

Many women cannot give enough information to fix the length of pregnancy but this can be accurately estimated by ultrasound measurement of the fetal head at around 16 weeks. This method loses accuracy after 20 weeks as normal fetuses diverge in size. Once the length of pregnancy is known, however, serial ultrasound estimations plotted on standard curves enable the obstetrician to pick up abnormally slow growth and to intervene where necessary.

The fetus who is hypoxic may well fail to move normally and this forms the rationale for so-called kick charts. Mothers are asked to record the number of fetal movements felt in a standard period each day. A fall in the number of kicks will indicate the need for more sophisticated assessment of fetal well-being such as cardiotocography in which ultrasound is used to pick up the fetal heart rate. The unhealthy fetus responds to movement or to uterine contractions with a deceleration in heart rate.

Measurement of various chemicals in the mother's blood or urine, particularly oestriol and human placental lactogen, gives some indication of placental function and size respectively. A downward trend in serial estimations may point to a failing placenta.

The fetus with a major congenital abnormality or serious genetic disease may sometimes be detected early in pregnancy and therapeutic abortion performed. Detailed ultrasound examination may reveal abnormalities of the nervous system, the heart and the kidneys. Chorion villus biopsy, a technique by which fetal cells are obtained from the placenta, usually by a needle through the mother's abdominal wall, allows chromosome analysis or genetic probing for diseases such as cystic fibrosis. Such a technique carries its own risks and can only be offered in selected pregnancies. Thus the risk of Down's syndrome rises with increasing maternal age and in Britain amniocentesis, taking fluid from around the fetus, is offered to women over the age of 35. With this system, 7.5% of pregnancies are tested but only 35% of cases are detected. Recently a composite risk system has been developed in which the mother's age and serum levels of various chemicals, oestriol, chorionic gonado-trophin and alphafetoprotein, are combined to give a much more accurate idea of risk. Sixty per cent of cases may then be detected with only 5% of pregnancies requiring amniocentesis.

Abnormalities of labour

From the fetal point of view the two most important abnormalities of labour are early or preterm labour and asphyxia. Together these play a major part in perinatal mortality and morbidity.

Babies born before 37 weeks are said to be preterm infants. Clearly the earlier the birth, the more immature the infant and the more likely it is that there will be problems, particularly problems of maintaining body temperature, adequate respiration and nutrition. Until recently infants of less than 28 weeks gestation were legally non-viable in the UK, and did not need to be registered if born dead, the implication being that they could not possibly have survived. In fact, infants of only 24 weeks and weighing no more than 500 g (18 oz) do sometimes survive, albeit with a need for prolonged intensive care. Legislation has caught up with practice, and infants are now legally viable from 24 weeks.

Babies may be born abnormally early for a variety of reasons including maternal hypertension, incompetence of the neck of the uterus, multiple pregnancy and haemorrhage behind the placenta. In 30% of cases there is no obvious cause.

Perinatal asphyxia may be defined as a shortage of oxygen occurring during the birth process which leads to significant damage to the fetus or even to death. This is usually due to a pre-existing placental abnormality with labour exacerbating a chronic situation of insufficiency. The normal fetus has the reserves to withstand moderate hypoxia, but the fetus who has suffered intrauterine growth retardation due to an abnormal placenta may be unable to withstand the extra stress of labour. Occasionally acute episodes of anoxia, due for example to a prolapsed cord, may kill or damage a previously normal fetus.

One of the principal aims of the active management of labour practised in our hospitals is to identify the asphyxiated fetus and to expedite delivery, by forceps if the uterine cervix is fully dilated or otherwise by caesarean section. Maternal ill-health and poor fetal growth will point to the high-risk fetus, but increasingly all labours in hospital are being monitored.

Cardiotocography is now widely used during labour, replacing the traditional method of auscultating the fetal heart. The heart rate of the healthy fetus varies between contractions and accelerates during them and with movement. The attendant looks for flattening of the heart rate trace and for decelerations in response to contractions, particularly those occurring late, the so-called type II dips (*Figure 2.1*). These are likely to be due to fetal hypoxia and acidosis. The logical next step is to measure the pH of blood taken from the fetal scalp and if this is below 7.2, to deliver the infant.

The condition of the infant may then be assessed by estimating the Apgar score at 1 and 5 minutes after delivery (Table 2.1). A low score at 1 minute indicates the need

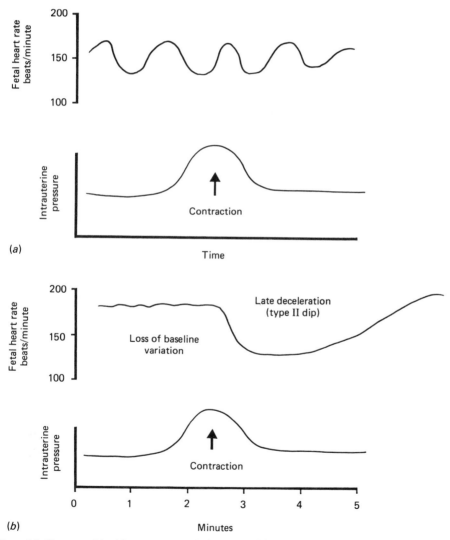

Figure 2.1. The normal fetal heart rate trace during labour (*a*) is shown compared to that for an asphyxiated fetus (*b*)

TABLE 2.1. The Apgar scoring system, developed by Virginia Apgar, may be used to evaluate an infant's physical condition at birth. Apgar 9/10 would indicate a score of 9 at 1 minute and 10 at 5 minutes

	Score		
	0	*1*	*2*
Heart rate	Absent	<100	>100
Respiration	Nil	Weak	Regular
Muscle tone	Limp	Some tone	Good tone
Reflex irritability	Nil	Grimace	Cry
Colour	Pallor or cyanosis	Centrally pink	Pink

for resuscitation, whilst that at 5 minutes shows some correlation with eventual neurodevelopmental outcome. Although the principle of the system is simple, the practice is more difficult and increasingly paediatricians are recording the time from birth to the first breath as a more objective measure of the amount of resuscitation needed. Shortage of oxygen in labour depresses the infant's attempts at respiration and hence the amount of resuscitation needed is an indication of the degree of pre-existing asphyxia.

In the days following delivery the asphyxiated infant may show the effects of tissue hypoxia. Damage to the cortex of the kidney may present with acute renal failure, or to the heart muscle with heart failure. Most importantly, brain damage may lead to neurological complications or even death. The infant may be comatose with irregular respirations, fixed dilated pupils and fits. Less severely affected infants may be irritable with a high-pitched cry.

After the first few days there is often a quiet period when the infant appears to behave normally but feeding difficulties may herald the onset of developmental problems. The severity of long-term handicap will depend on the degree of asphyxia. One series of neonates who had not taken their first spontaneous breath by 20 minutes, showed a 44% mortality. A further 31% were severely handicapped with fits, cerebral palsy and mental retardation. In the survivors of asphyxia, more subtle handicaps such as specific learning difficulties and behavioural problems may not present until the child goes to school.

Birth weight

Several factors influence birth weight, the most important of which is gestational age. At 28 weeks, the average fetus weighs around 1100 g (2 lb 7 oz). It then gains at a rate of 200 g (7 oz) per week so that at 40 weeks, the usual time of birth, it weighs 3500 g (7.5 lb). After a short interruption whilst the baby adjusts to extrauterine life, growth continues at the same rate for a further 3 months.

Boys are heavier than girls at birth by an average of 150 g (5 oz). First babies are lighter than subsequent infants, again by an average of 150 g. A woman with previous pregnancies who has a new mate, will, as it were, go back to the beginning and produce a baby with birth weight similar to her firstborn.

Genetic factors play a part, but the mother's size is a more important constraint than the father's. This is well seen in animal experiments. When a Shetland mare is crossed with a Shire stallion, the foal is larger than the average Shetland foal, but much nearer to it than to a Shire foal.

Racial influence is illustrated by the fact that the heaviest babies are born to Russian Eskimos in the Arctic, whereas eastern races tend to have the lightest newborns.

These genetic and racial factors may be obscured by nutritional factors. Mean birth weight has been used as an indicator of the nutritional health of a population because malnutrition in the last third of pregnancy will substantially lower it. Birth weight is positively related to prepregnancy weight and to weight gain in pregnancy. The influence of placental factors and maternal disease has already been discussed, most diseases having a negative effect on fetal growth. Poorly controlled maternal diabetes mellitus, however, will usually cause excessive fetal growth although some 20% of such fetuses suffer intrauterine growth retardation.

For some reason, seasonal factors play a part and babies born between June and August are the lightest with those born between March and May the heaviest.

Birth weight has a long term influence on height and weight, although the fetus whose growth has been severely constrained by placental or uterine factors may display catch-up growth postnatally.

Sensory and motor abilities of the newborn

It is traditionally held that the human newborn is no more than a gastrointestinal tract with no sense of responsibility at either end. Research by developmental psychologists and paediatricians over the past 30 years, however, has demonstrated that the newborn is in fact a perceptive individual with substantial auditory and visual skills.

Within the first hour the baby can appreciate moving stimuli and demonstrates this by turning head and eyes. The newborn can differentiate between an organized picture of a face and a scrambled one; between black and white patterns and a grey card; and between stripes and a single patch of colour. The baby perceives the difference between vertical and oblique lines; and between straight and curved ones.

Within the first week of life, the human baby shows boredom when looking at pictures, demonstrating a renewed interest when shown a fresh picture. It is able to track objects which move horizontally and can focus on the mother's face, following it through an angle of 180 degrees.

The demonstration of optokinetic nystagmus is a useful indication that vision is present in a particular newborn, but visual acuity is best measured by the 'acuity card' procedure which uses paired cards of plain and patterned stimuli. This is a development of the preferential looking technique, based on the finding that patterned objects are visually interesting to newborn infants. After the age of 2 months, visual evoked responses to patterns become a useful tool in the assessment of function.

The ability to hear is demonstrated, not only by stilling to noise, by recognizing the direction from which it comes and by turning the eyes towards it, but by more sophisticated audioperceptual skills. The human voice is preferred to pure tones of similar frequency and female voices to male. Sudden noise produces a startle response but rhythmical low frequency sound is soothing.

By 2 weeks the baby recognizes the mother's face and has some perception of distance, pulling back from an object moving towards its face. The baby turns away from unpleasant smells but responds to pleasant ones by turning to the mother's breast. The difference between human and cow's milk is appreciated and the baby's own mother's face, voice and smell are preferred. When presented with two pads, one soaked in its own mother's milk and the other in milk from another mother, the newborn will turn towards its own mother's smell.

Motor abilities are less sophisticated and take the form of the primitive reflexes. Many have been described but the following will serve to illustrate the level of ability of the newborn. The Moro reflex is elicited by supporting the baby's head above the bed and then allowing it to drop back a short way. The arms move apart and extend with open palms. The arms then come together as if to catch hold of the mother. The grasp reflex occurs when an object stimulates the baby's palm and is then grasped by the fingers. Touching the back of the hand will cause it to open. Similar responses can be obtained from the feet.

When the newborn is held upright with feet pressing on the table, it shows leg movements which simulate walking. When the cheek is touched the babe 'roots' for the object. This is clearly useful in finding the mother's nipple. When the nipple or a finger is placed in the baby's mouth, it sucks vigorously.

These reflexes disappear as the central nervous system matures, so that just as an absent Moro response at birth suggests neurological abnormality, its presence after 3 months is equally of concern.

Problems of the newborn

Currently about 1% of babies born in Britain are either stillborn or die in the first week of life. Between 10% and 20% of those born alive have a problem serious enough to warrant admission to a special care baby unit. Three main factors contribute to this mortality and morbidity: asphyxia, which has already been discussed, congenital abnormalities and the effects of low birth weight.

The central nervous and the cardiovascular systems are commonly affected by life-threatening anomalies. The nervous system forms from a plate of tissue which curls on itself to form a tube. If this tube fails to close at the lower end, an event which normally occurs about 4 weeks after conception, the infant is left with spina bifida, one form of neural tube defect. The nerves within the spinal cord are open to the outside and sensation and power in the lower limbs, bladder and bowels is impaired. The infant is likely to develop hydrocephalus with brain damage due to an associated abnormality of cerebrospinal fluid drainage. In severe cases the infant is likely to be both physically and mentally handicapped and the paediatrician is faced with an ethical dilemma concerning the provision of life-saving care where the quality of life is likely to be poor.

In transposition of the great vessels, the aorta and the main pulmonary artery are reversed so that there are in effect two separate circulations. This condition is incompatible with life but is eminently treatable by surgery. The condition of hypoplastic left heart syndrome, in which the left ventricle is poorly formed, is also incompatible with life but is not correctable by surgery.

Perhaps 6% of infants weigh less than 2500 g (5.5 lb) because they are preterm – they are born before 37 weeks. Their problems are those of size and immaturity. They have difficulty in maintaining their body temperature, they need help with nutrition and they develop problems because of their immature enzyme systems, for example jaundice. Most importantly, many of them have difficulty in breathing due to a condition called respiratory distress syndrome (RDS). In the normal lung a detergent-like substance called surfactant reduces the surface tension in the lung fluid and helps to maintain the patency of the lung spaces, the alveoli. In many small preterm infants, the enzyme systems which produce surfactant are immature and absence of the substance leads to collapse of the alveoli. The heart continues to supply blood to these alveoli and this blood therefore returns to the heart without having been oxygenated. If enough alveoli are collapsed the infant will become profoundly hypoxic and may suffer brain damage or die. In milder cases the symptoms reach a peak by 3 days and then, as the enzyme systems within the alveoli begin to produce surfactant, the symptoms settle and the infant recovers. Even in severe cases recovery may be complete before 2 weeks of age. The basal metabolic defect in RDS is hypoxia, and treatment is designed to correct this. The earlier forms of treatment involved nursing the infant in high concentrations of oxygen. More recently two forms of respiratory support have been used. Continuous positive airways pressure (CPAP) is produced by blowing air or oxygen across the infant's airway whilst allowing him to breathe spontaneously. The pressure inside his lungs is then maintained at a higher level than atmospheric pressure throughout the phases of respiration. This helps to prevent collapse of the alveoli and hence to maintain oxygenation. More severely affected infants, who are unable to maintain satisfactory blood gases whilst breathing spontaneously, will need artificial ventilation.

There is no doubt that the mortality from RDS falls substantially with treatment. Babies weighing less than 1000 g (2 lb 3 oz), at least 70% of whom develop the condition, now have a 50% chance of survival. Larger infants have a much better chance of recovery. Unfortunately, as the treated babies began to survive their RDS, it became clear that the high oxygen levels used were toxic to tissues, particularly to those of the developing retina and many survived their RDS only to become blind as a result of retrolental fibroplasia. For a time the concentration of oxygen given to premature infants was restricted to 30%, but this resulted in an increased mortality and morbidity from brain damage. The management of RDS then became a matter of balancing the risks of death or brain damage against the risks of treatment and, to some extent, even now, there is a trade-off between these two sorts of risk.

Vascularization of the retina occurs from the disc outwards, the vanguard of blood vessels reaching the ora serrata nasally by 36 weeks and temporally by 40 weeks. In small preterm infants the peripheries, especially in the temporal region, are incompletely vascularized and are susceptible. One of the most potent toxins is an arterial oxygen tension greater than the relatively low intrauterine levels.

Oxygen produces constriction of the small arteries leading to ischaemia or inadequate blood supply, followed by proliferation of capillaries, scarring and retinal detachment. In mild cases the changes are confined to the peripheries but the entire retina may sometimes be involved. A cicatricial stage may begin at around 3 months with proliferation of retrolental fibrous tissue leading to severe visual impairment. This may vary in degree from myopia to complete blindness.

Milder cases with proliferation of blood vessels only in the periphery of the retina would usually be classified as retinopathy of prematurity. Cases in which the whole retina has undergone neovascularization, and the cicatricial stage has begun, would warrant the term retrolental fibroplasia. To a large extent the two terms are used interchangeably and classification varies from one centre to another and in different countries.

The severity of the condition is largely related to the duration and level of abnormal arterial oxygen tension, but no level is safe. Preterm infants who have never received supplemental oxygen have developed the condition, probably because the arterial oxygen tension of the fetus in the uterus is around 3 kPa, whereas a healthy newborn breathing air will probably achieve a tension greater than 8 kPa. The role of other toxins, for example, low carbon dioxide levels which are known to produce vasoconstriction in the brain, and vitamin E deficiency, are not yet clear.

The neonatal paediatrician approaches the task of preventing both brain damage and retrolental fibroplasia by monitoring the oxygen tension within the baby's arteries. That oxygen concentration is then carefully controlled to keep the arterial oxygen at levels associated with minimal risk (7–10 kPa). Monitoring of oxygen tensions is achieved in several ways. Specimens of blood are taken at least every 3 or 4 hours for blood gas estimation, either from an indwelling catheter in the umbilical artery or from the radial artery. Because of the anatomy of the arterial circulation in the sick neonate, specimens obtained from the radial artery more truly reflect the state of blood reaching the brain and eyes. Sophisticated indwelling arterial catheters with a built-in oxygen electrode, and transcutaneous electrodes which measure oxygen tensions in the skin, enable a continuous record of arterial oxygen to be obtained. Blood gas measurements are then performed to calibrate these devices.

The success of this form of management may be judged from the fact that in hospitals offering intensive neonatal care, the mortality of RDS is between 5% and 10% compared to an untreated mortality of greater than 50%. Retrolental fibroplasia is relatively uncommon. Only 3% of babies weighing less than 1500 g (3 lb 5 oz) develop the condition in Britain. The fact that in America 40% of babies of similar weight have the condition is probably due to a difference in classification rather than a true increase in incidence.

Psychomotor development in the first five years

A developmental screen is part of the complete examination of the child. It enables the observer to be reassuring to the anxious parents of the great majority and to diagnose abnormality in the few at an early stage when treatment is more likely to be effective. Serious mental retardation and most cases of cerebral palsy may be diagnosed in the first year of life, moderate retardation before school age, and specific learning difficulties at the time of school entry, when extra help may be given by the teaching staff. Problems of the special senses should be picked up early as part of routine regular assessment of all preschool children.

Although development is a continuous process with its many parts interwoven and interdependent, it is helpful for the purpose of assessment, particularly in the early years, to divide it into four facets. These are gross motor performance, vision and fine motor skills, hearing and speech, and social development. It is also helpful to assess development at certain ages and we will describe the normal child at 6 weeks, 7 months, 18 months, 3 and 5 years.

The 6-week infant shows momentary head control when pulled to sitting, and will lift its head when lying prone. The infant fixes on the mother's face and will follow a brightly coloured object to the midline. It will startle to a loud sudden noise and still to soothing ones. The 6 week old smiles when it sees a face.

The 7-month infant has good head control and is able to sit without support for 10 seconds on a firm surface. The infant supports its weight when the feet are in contact with a surface and can roll over. It reaches for objects with either hand and transfers from one to the other. Hand preference is abnormal at this stage. There is a full range of eye movements including convergence on a near object. Squint is abnormal at this stage. The infant will turn to a noise made at ear level. This skill forms the basis of the hearing screening test done at this age. The 7 month old is playful, laughs readily and can babble and produce some consonants.

The 18 month old walks alone and can often climb stairs. The toddler picks up small objects between finger and thumb and releases them and can, therefore, begin to stack bricks. The 18 month old's near vision can be crudely tested by getting the child to pick up hundreds and thousands and distance vision by using Stycar balls. The toddler should follow a 3 mm white ball against a black background at 3 m. Squint can be detected using the cover test. The child responds to simple commands and will point to two parts of the body. Several single words are said with meaning, and two words may be put together into a phrase. The 18 month old is wary of strangers, can drink from a cup and feed with fingers and a spoon. The toddler begins to imitate its mother around the house and to display independence with tantrums.

The 3 year old walks up and down stairs with one foot on each step. The child can run, jump, climb and pedal, and can dress and undress but needs help with buttons and zips. The child holds a pencil, copies a circle, cooperates with tests of vision and is able to match some letters, particularly V, O, X and T. In the Stycar test the 3 year old is shown these single letters at 3 m and picks out the matching letter on a card in front of him. The child should be able to match the letters of size 4 with each eye. The 3 year old has a vocabulary of at least 200 words, speaks in short sentences and uses pronouns and prepositions. Questions are asked and quite complex commands understood. The child is increasingly independent in feeding, washing and dressing and is able to stay clean and dry by day.

The 5 year old is a much more complex individual. It is already clear that some children are clumsy, lacking the precise coordination usual at this age. The normal child holds a pencil between thumb and fingers and can copy a cross, a square and a triangle. By 5 years the child can build a bridge and steps using cubes. Myopia may be present and the school entrant should have his distance vision tested using the Stycar 7 letter comparison test. Five year olds should be tested for squint and for colour vision using the modified Ishihara tests (see Chapter 12). The Stycar picture cards for high and low frequency sounds are used to test hearing, for example, the child may be asked to distinguish between pictures of a tree and a key, between a cat and a cot. If there is real doubt about hearing, one may obtain cooperation with full audiometric testing. At this stage speech should be clearly understood by strangers and should include imaginative, complex ideas using the various tenses appropriately. Substitutions of some consonants, particularly R and L, F and Th, are common at this age. Socially the child manages at school by using independent self-care skills and by separating from the family, sharing toys with others and playing games.

At 5 years the more complex tests of intellect become useful. Two will be discussed. In the Draw-a-Man test described by Goodenough, the child between about 3 and 10 years is asked to draw the best possible man without any time limit being given. The drawing is then scored by giving one point for the presence of each of 51 standard features (Table 2.2).
The number of points is divided by four and added to the baseline age of 3 years to give a so-called mental age (*Figure 2.2*). The result is said to correlate well with more formal intelligence tests.

The Goddard formboard (*Figure 2.3*), a standardized form of the common

TABLE 2.2. The scoring system used in the Draw-a-Man test by Goodenough

1. Head present
2. Legs present
3. Arms present
4. Trunk present
5. Length of trunk greater than breadth
6. Shoulders indicated
7. Both arms and legs attached to trunk
8. Legs attached to trunk; arms attached to trunk at correct point
9. Neck present
10. Neck outline continuous with head, trunk or both
11. Eyes present
12. Nose present
13. Mouth present
14. Nose and mouth in two dimensions; two lips shown
15. Nostrils indicated
16. Hair shown
17. Hair non-transparent, over more than circumference
18. Clothing present
19. Two articles of clothing non-transparent
20. No transparencies, both sleeves and trousers shown
21. Four or more articles of clothing indicated
22. Costume complete without any incongruities
23. Fingers shown
24. Correct number of fingers shown
25. Fingers in two dimensions, length greater than breadth, angle less than 180 degrees
26. Opposition of thumb shown
27. Hand shown distinct from fingers or arms
28. Arm joint shown, elbow, shoulder or both
29. Leg joint shown, knee, hip, or both
30. Head in proportion
31. Arms in proportion
32. Legs in proportion
33. Feet in proportion
34. Both arms and legs in two dimensions
35. Heel shown
36. Firm lines without overlapping at junctions
37. Firm lines with correct joining
38. Head outline greater than a circle
39. Trunk outline greater than a circle
40. Outline of arms and legs without narrowing at junction with body
41. Features symmetrical and in correct position
42. Ears present
43. Ears in correct position and proportion
44. Eyebrows or lashes
45. Pupil of eye
46. Eye length greater than height
47. Eye glance directed to front in profile
48. Both chin and forehead shown
49. Projection of chin shown
50. Profile with not more than one error
51. Correct profile

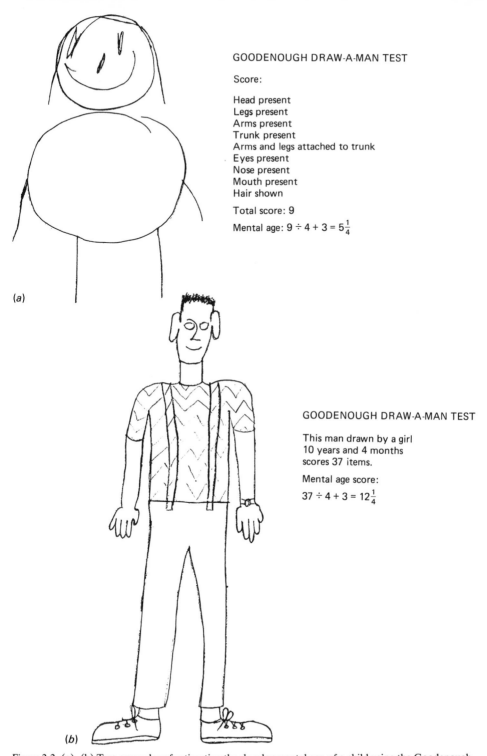

GOODENOUGH DRAW-A-MAN TEST

Score:

Head present
Legs present
Arms present
Trunk present
Arms and legs attached to trunk
Eyes present
Nose present
Mouth present
Hair shown

Total score: 9

Mental age: $9 \div 4 + 3 = 5\frac{1}{4}$

(a)

GOODENOUGH DRAW-A-MAN TEST

This man drawn by a girl
10 years and 4 months
scores 37 items.

Mental age score:

$37 \div 4 + 3 = 12\frac{1}{4}$

(b)

Figure 2.2. (a), (b) Two examples of estimating the developmental age of a child using the Goodenough 'Draw a Man' test

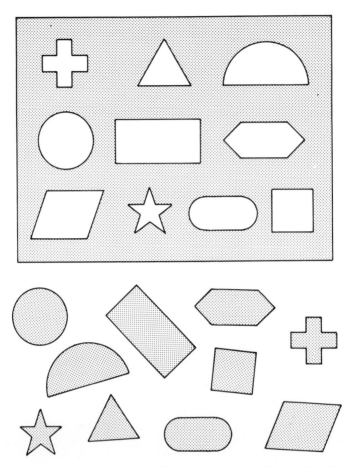

Figure 2.3. The Goddard formboard is a standardized test to assess coordination, intelligence and vision

posting-box toy, tests vision, coordination and intelligence, by requiring the child to place shapes in their appropriate holes in a measured time. The average 5 year old can complete it in 35 seconds, the average 8 year old in 20.

Although the above account presents a didactic picture of child development, there is of course a considerable variation in what is normal and a knowledge of this variation can only be obtained through repeated examination of normal children. Some milestones show a narrow range of normality, other skills a wide spread. Thus smiling usually begins at 6 weeks and the infant who does not smile at 8 weeks needs further assessment, whereas walking may begin at any age from 9 months to 2 years. The typical pattern of child development with age is shown in *Figure 2.4*.

The interpretation of abnormal patterns of development revealed by screening is of importance in the diagnosis of neurodevelopmental disease. Development is usually assessed in four areas, gross motor performance, vision and fine motor skills, hearing and speech, and social abilities. The child who fails to reach his milestones in all four areas is said to have global retardation, and this is most probably due to an

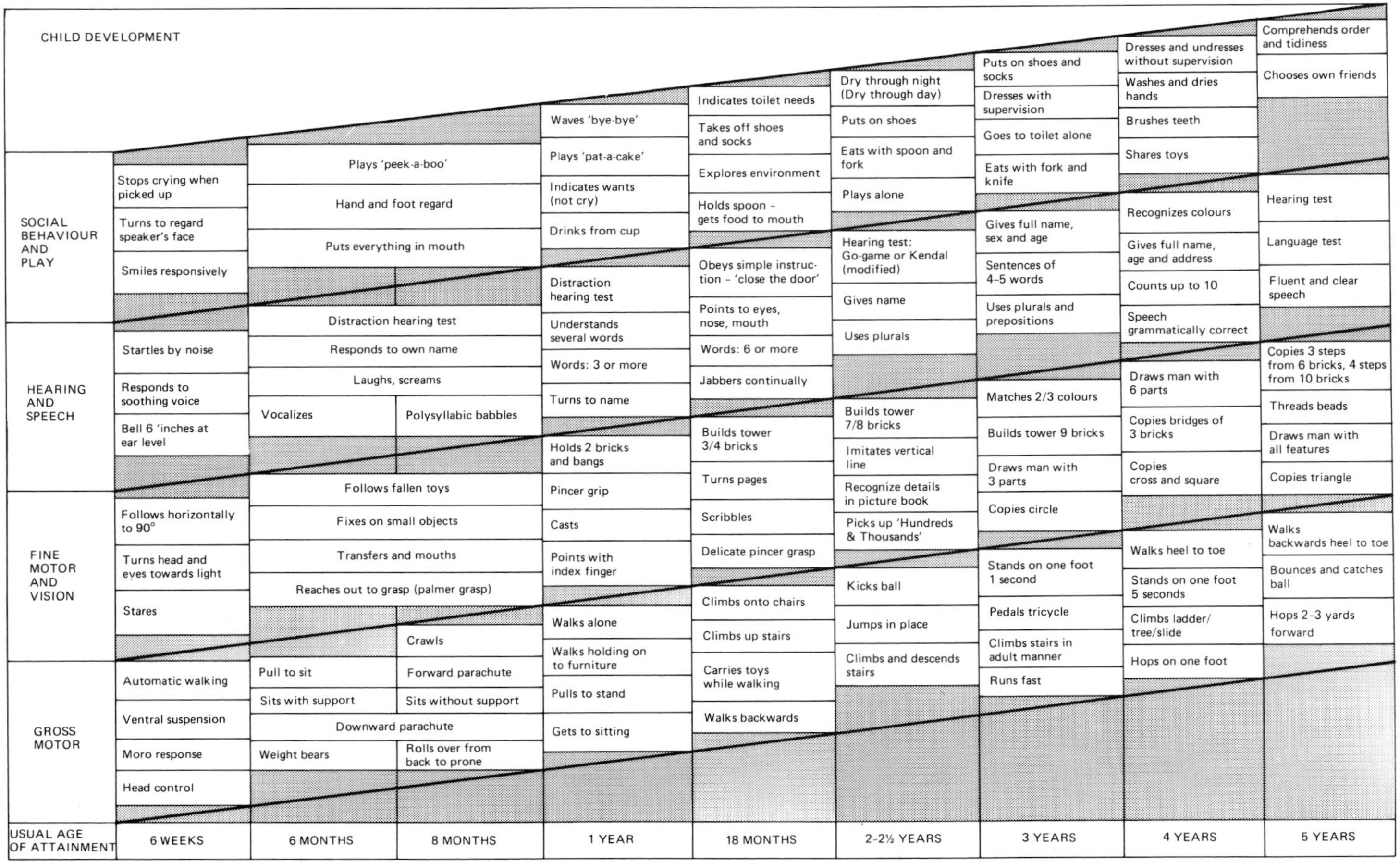

CHILD DEVELOPMENT

Category	6 WEEKS	6 MONTHS	8 MONTHS	1 YEAR	18 MONTHS	2–2½ YEARS	3 YEARS	4 YEARS	5 YEARS
SOCIAL BEHAVIOUR AND PLAY	Stops crying when picked up; Turns to regard speaker's face; Smiles responsively	Plays 'peek-a-boo'; Hand and foot regard; Puts everything in mouth		Waves 'bye-bye'; Plays 'pat-a-cake'; Holds spoon – gets food to mouth; Drinks from cup	Indicates toilet needs; Takes off shoes and socks; Explores environment; Indicates wants (not cry)	Dry through night (Dry through day); Puts on shoes; Eats with spoon and fork; Plays alone	Puts on shoes and socks; Dresses with supervision; Goes to toilet alone; Eats with fork and knife	Dresses and undresses without supervision; Washes and dries hands; Brushes teeth; Shares toys	Comprehends order and tidiness; Chooses own friends
HEARING AND SPEECH	Startles by noise; Responds to soothing voice; Bell 6 inches at ear level	Distraction hearing test; Responds to own name; Laughs, screams; Vocalizes; Polysyllabic babbles		Understands several words; Words: 3 or more; Turns to name; Distraction hearing test	Obeys simple instruction – 'close the door'; Points to eyes, nose, mouth; Words: 6 or more; Jabbers continually	Hearing test: Go-game or Kendal (modified); Gives name; Uses plurals	Gives full name, sex and age; Sentences of 4–5 words; Uses plurals and prepositions	Recognizes colours; Gives full name, age and address; Counts up to 10; Speech grammatically correct	Hearing test; Language test; Fluent and clear speech
FINE MOTOR AND VISION	Follows horizontally to 90°; Turns head and eyes towards light; Stares	Fixes on small objects; Transfers and mouths; Reaches out to grasp (palmer grasp)	Follows fallen toys	Pincer grip; Casts; Points with index finger; Holds 2 bricks and bangs	Turns pages; Scribbles; Delicate pincer grasp; Builds tower 3/4 bricks	Recognize details in picture book; Picks up 'Hundreds & Thousands'; Builds tower 7/8 bricks; Imitates vertical line	Matches 2/3 colours; Builds tower 9 bricks; Draws man with 3 parts; Copies circle	Draws man with 6 parts; Copies bridges of 3 bricks; Copies cross and square	Copies 3 steps from 6 bricks, 4 steps from 10 bricks; Threads beads; Draws man with all features; Copies triangle
GROSS MOTOR	Automatic walking; Ventral suspension; Moro response; Head control	Pull to sit; Sits with support; Downward parachute; Weight bears; Rolls over from back to prone	Crawls; Forward parachute; Sits without support	Walks alone; Walks holding on to furniture; Pulls to stand; Gets to sitting	Climbs onto chairs; Climbs up stairs; Carries toys while walking; Walks backwards	Kicks ball; Jumps in place; Climbs and descends stairs	Stands on one foot 1 second; Pedals tricycle; Climbs stairs in adult manner; Runs fast	Walks heel to toe; Stands on one foot 5 seconds; Climbs ladder/tree/slide; Hops on one foot	Walks backwards heel to toe; Bounces and catches ball; Hops 2–3 yards forward
USUAL AGE OF ATTAINMENT	6 WEEKS	6 MONTHS	8 MONTHS	1 YEAR	18 MONTHS	2–2½ YEARS	3 YEARS	4 YEARS	5 YEARS

Figure 2.4. The typical pattern of child development with age. (Redrawn from a chart by Lingam, 1983)

intellectual defect. When a child fails in only one area, the possibilities are more diverse. The 7 month old who is bright and alert, babbles and turns to noise, reaches for objects and transfers but cannot sit alone, is clearly not globally retarded. The problems of gross motor performance are more probably due to muscle disease, to a form of cerebral palsy without intellectual retardation or even to malnutrition with gross muscle wasting. Further examination will clarify the diagnosis.

The child who is not walking at 18 months but has reached his other milestones, may have one of the above conditions or may simply be following a different pattern of development. Siblings may have been late walkers or the family may be 'bottom-shufflers', a term applied to a group of children who never crawl, preferring to sit and shuffle, and who often do not walk until 2 years. This pattern of development is often familial and the children eventually show completely normal development.

The toddler of 3 years who cannot match letters on a card may have a visual problem but could equally be globally retarded so that the stage of maturation has not been reached where the child is able to tackle the test, even though vision is normal. Similarly the 7 month old who fails a hearing test may be deaf, may be globally retarded, or may have a motor defect which interferes with the ability to turn to noise.

Speech delay may be due to global retardation, to deafness, to a physical problem such as athetoid cerebral palsy, to emotional deprivation or to an isolated speech defect. The child with autism may also present in this way. In all these situations a more comprehensive assessment will reveal the true problem.

Physical growth in childhood

The normal human fetus reaches an average weight of 3500 g (7.5 lb) when it is born at term. In the first few days of extrauterine life, the newborn often loses up to 10% of its birth weight as it adjusts to the new form of nutrition, but then regains this before 10 days and continues to grow at 200 g (7 oz) a week for a further 3 months. Weight gain then slows so that the baby puts on 150 g (5 oz) a week between 3 and 6 months and 100 g (3 oz) a week in the second 6 months of life. The average newborn doubles its birth weight by 5 months and trebles it by a year, reaching 10 kg (22 lb) before the first birthday (*Figure 2.5*). General growth is rapid in the first 2 years as the individual moves towards his genetically determined growth curve, but he then follows this curve, gaining 2 kg (4.4 lb) in weight and 6 cm in height each year until the growth spurt of puberty begins.

Brain growth, as reflected by the changes in head circumference, progresses rapidly in the first 4 years of life but then slows and stops long before the growth of other organs. Lymphoid tissue, including the tonsils and adenoids, grows rapidly at first, reaching its maximum size at around 11 years, and then shrinking, so that the adenoidal 9 year old spontaneously improves. Reproductive tissue grows little in the first few years of life but then increases massively in size with the onset of puberty. Pituitary gonadotrophins triggered by the hypothalamus cause growth of testes and ovaries, whilst the androgens and oestrogens they secrete cause development of the secondary sex characteristics.

The regular assessment of growth is an important part of the health care of children in that variations in growth pattern may well be the first indication of physical disease. In infancy weight and head circumference should be measured about every month, possibly more frequently at first. In the toddler twice yearly measurements of height and weight are useful, and then occasional examinations, checking for normal growth and pubertal development, are performed until the teenager leaves school. More frequent measurements, particularly in the infant, may cause unnecessary anxiety to the parents, particularly as growth occurs not as a smooth process but in a series of spurts.

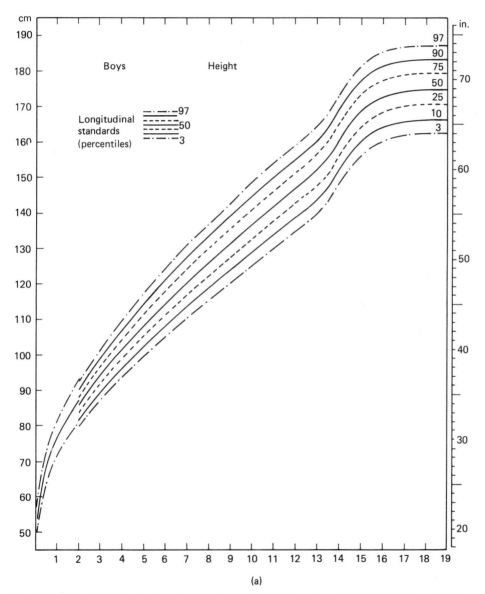

(a)

Figure 2.5. (pages 39–44) Typical growth curves for male ((a)–(c)) and female ((d)–(f)) infants published by Gairdner and Pearson (1988). The curves are based on data of Lucas (1986) and Yudkin *et al.* (1987) for weight and head measurements and of Kitchen *et al.* (1981) for length. Reproduced with permission from Castlemead Publications (chart reference numbers 11A, GPB 3, 12A, GPB 3)

The values obtained by measurement must be properly interpreted by plotting them on a standard chart showing normal growth curves for head circumference, height and weight and the range of normality. Children whose measurements fail to follow these curves or fall outside the normal range should then be referred for a paediatric opinion.

When assessing the height of an older child, it is important to remember that the parents' heights will be a major influence. Mid-parental height is obtained by taking the average of the parent's heights but adding 13 cm (the difference between the average height of men and women) to the mother's height for boys and taking 13 cm away from the father's height for girls. For example, if the

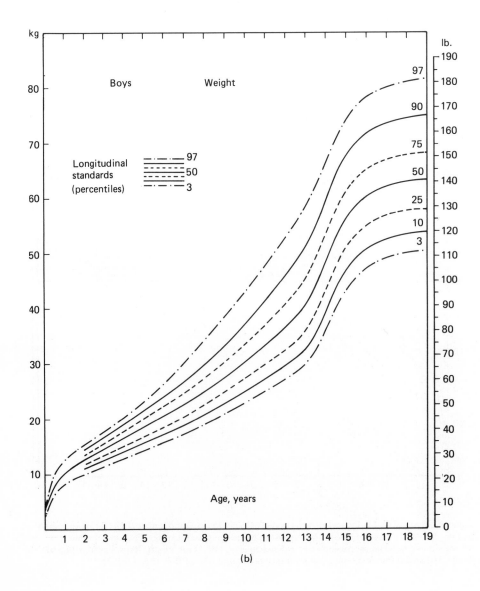

(b)

mother is 153 cm and the father 176 cm tall the expected height for a boy will be (176 + 153 + 13) ÷ 2 = 171 cm and for a girl (176 − 13 + 153) ÷ 2 = 158 cm. Children in the family should reach an eventual height within 8 cm of their predicted value, and the standard charts enable the paediatrician to see whether this is likely.

Once it has been decided that the child does indeed have a growth problem, the paediatrician must work systematically to look at the many possible causes. Optimal intake and absorption of food are clearly crucial to normal growth. The baby whose mother fails, through ignorance or neglect, to give adequate nourishment, will gain weight poorly. The infant or child who is emotionally deprived may well fail to grow, sometimes as a result of poor eating but at others because emotional deprivation interferes with the complex balance of growth factors including growth hormone. Some infants, whether because of a mechanical problem such as cleft palate or a neurological disorder such as cerebral palsy, may be unable to achieve an adequate intake. Others fail to thrive because they vomit what they take. The child who in the first few weeks of life develops a partial obstruction to the outlet of the stomach, so-called pyloric stenosis, or the infant with a serious urinary tract infection, both present in this way.

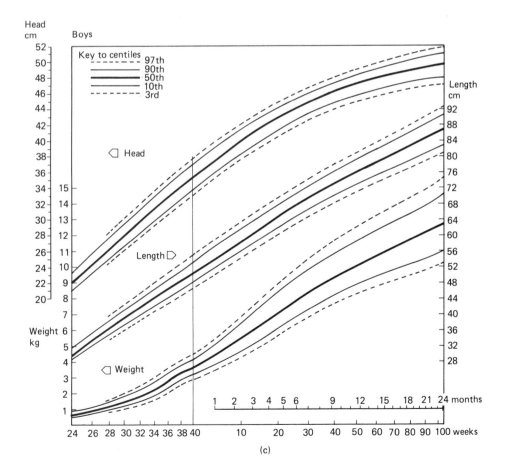

(c)

A child may fail to absorb adequately the food given. Two important childhood diseases cause growth problems in this way. Cystic fibrosis is an inherited disease affecting about 1 in 2500 live births in this country. Sufferers make an abnormal bronchial mucus and fail to produce digestive enzymes. They have frequent chest infections and malabsorb food. These two factors contribute to their failure to thrive. Coeliac disease occurs when the individual becomes sensitized to gluten, a fraction of wheat protein. Ingested gluten then damages the mucosal lining of their small bowel and again they malabsorb and fail to grow.

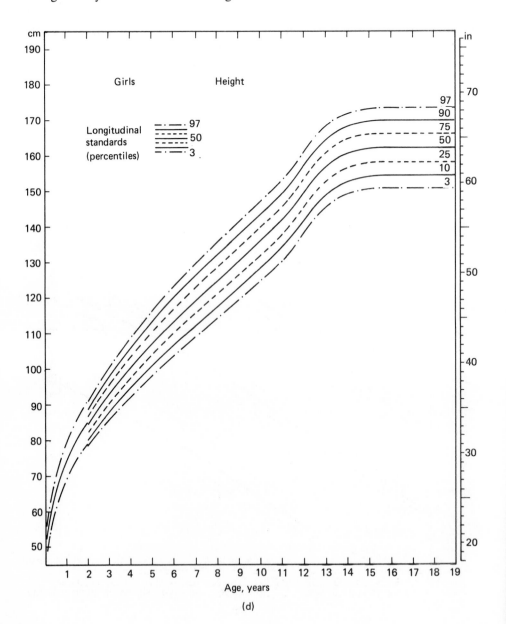

(d)

Major congenital abnormalities, particularly those of the heart, often cause failure to thrive, by one of several mechanisms. The baby with heart failure from a ventriculoseptal defect (a hole in the wall between the two ventricles of the heart) may become breathless with the exertion of sucking and so fail to take adequate milk. The heart may fail to supply the tissues with adequate blood or, in cyanotic heart disease, the blood it does supply may be poorly oxygenated. Lastly, the heart may work so hard to overcome the problems of an abnormal anatomy that it uses up energy which should be going to promote growth.

Finally, metabolic and hormonal disease may present with growth failure. The first sign of chronic renal failure in childhood may be a plotted growth line which falls

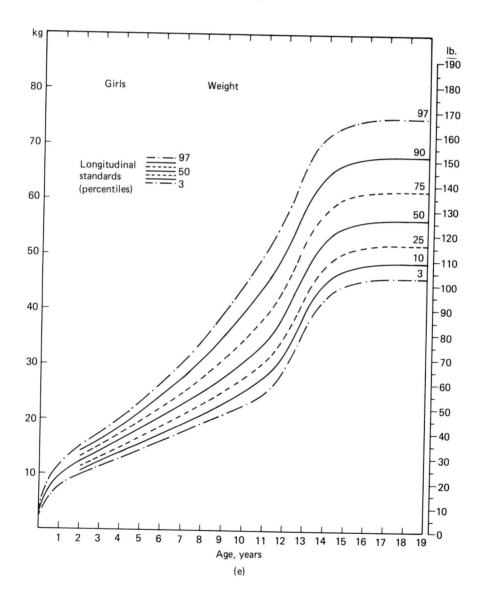

(e)

away from the standard curve. Two hormones are especially important in stimulating growth. Thyroid hormone is especially important in the first year of life but is necessary throughout the growth period, and growth hormone, produced by the anterior pituitary, drives normal growth until it stops in the teens. Thyroid hormone is cheap and can be given by mouth, making the treatment of thyroid deficiency easy and rewarding. Growth hormone, manufactured nowadays by a bioengineering process, is enormously expensive and has to be given by injection, so that the diagnosis of growth hormone deficiency must be accurate before treatment is justified.

Puberty and adolescence

The biological factors which trigger the onset of puberty are unknown, but the first measurable change is the release of luteinizing hormone releasing factor (LHRG) from the hypothalamus. This and other releasing factors stimulate the anterior

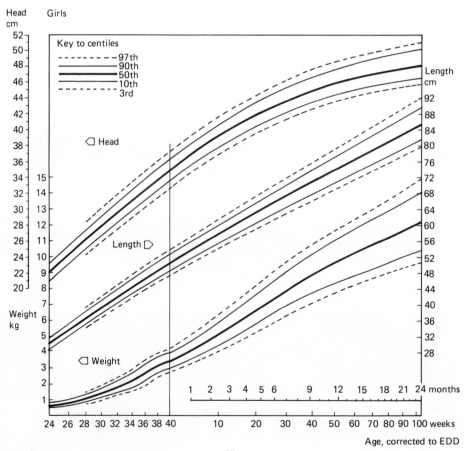

(f)

pituitary gland to produce gonadotrophic hormones which in turn cause the ovaries and testes to grow in size and to secrete oestrogens and androgens respectively. These sex hormones are responsible for the development of the secondary sex characteristics and the distinctive body shape of each sex. Girls acquire wide hips with increased subcutaneous fat giving soft contours. The typical boy has wide shoulders, narrow hips and powerful muscles with relatively little fat. At the same time, androgens from the adrenal cortex cause growth of body hair in girls and oestrogens from the same source are responsible for the temporary breast development which is common and often distressing in pubertal boys.

The first obvious sign of puberty in girls is breast enlargement which begins at an average age of 11 years (range 9–13), and this is followed after 2 years by the menarche (onset of periods). In boys enlargement of the testes begins at 12 years (range 10–14) and 2 years later sexual maturity is reached with emissions of semen. In girls the spurt in height and weight growth occurs before the menarche and slows dramatically once sexual maturity is reached. In boys the growth spurt continues for some time after puberty.

Puberty and adolescence is a time of emotional as well as physical growth. Classical psychoanalytical theory speaks of a time of 'turmoil', when the teenager's search for independence, sexual identity and maturity leads him to rebel against his parents and their values. The theory goes on to suggest that adolescents who do not experience 'turmoil' suffer emotional problems in adult life with inhibition, 'constriction of the personality' and dependency on parents.

More recent studies have shown that the majority of adolescents want the approval of their parents and are satisfied and happy at home. Anxiety and depression are a normal part of growing up, but 'turmoil' is not.

The physical changes of puberty are accompanied by an enormous increase in heterosexual behaviour, with more than half of 15–19 year olds surveyed having experienced sexual intercourse. Failure to use contraception is especially common in teenagers. Girls may use pregnancy as a means of obtaining their independence from from the parental home. Boys with their adolescent bravado see their pregant girlfriend as proof of their sexual maturity. The statistics demonstrate the effect of this behaviour. In England and Wales in 1986 there were 51.6 pregnancies per 1000 girls between 15 and 19 years, with 40% ending in legal abortion. In older women between 20 and 45 years only 18% of pregnancies were legally terminated.

And so the cycle of human growth and development begins again. The fetus survives the hazards of birth, the child learns from and adapts to its environment, growing and maturing into an adult. The survival of the species is assured.

Further reading

BOWER, T.G.R. (1966). The visual world of infants. *Scientific American,* **215**, 80–92.

BOWER, T.G.R. (1979). *The Perceptual World of the Child.* Fontana/Open Books, London.

BOWLBY, J. (1953). *Child Care and the Growth of Love.* Penguin, London.

COHEN, L.B., DELOACHE, J.S. and STRAUSS, M.S. (1979). Infant visual perception. In *Handbook of Infant Development,* edited by J. Osofsky. Wiley, Chichester.

COLEMAN, J.C. (1980). *The Nature of Adolescence.* Methuen, London.

Committee for the Classification of Retinopathy of Prematurity (1984). An international classification of retinopathy of prematurity. *Archives of Ophthalmology,* **102**, 1130–1134.

CURNOCK, D.A. (1989). The senses of the newborn. *British Medical Journal,* **299**, 1478–1479.

DAVIE, R, BUTLER, N.R. and GOLDSTEIN, H. (1972). *From Birth to Seven.* Longman (National Children's Bureau), Edinburgh.

FANTZ, R.L. (1961) The origin of form perception. *Scientific American,* **204**, 66–72.

FIELDER, A.R.(1988). Disorders of vision. In: *Fetal and Neonatal Neurology and Neurosurgery,* edited by M.I. Levene, M.J. Bennett and J. Punt. Churchill Livingstone, Edinburgh, pp. 517–534.

FLYNN, J.T. (1987). Retinopathy of prematurity. *Pediatric Clinics of North America,* 34, 6.

ILLINGWORTH, R.S. (1987). *The Development of The Infant and Young Child,* 9th edn. Churchill Livingstone, Edinburgh.

KAIL, R.V. and PELLEGRINO, J.W. (1985) *Human Intelligence: Perspectives and Prospects.* Freeman, London.

KAYE, K. (1982). *The Mental and Social Life of Babies.* Methuen, London.

KINSEY, V.E., ARNOLD, H.S. and KALINA, R.E. *PaO$_2$* levels and retrolental fibroplasia: a report of the cooperative study. *Pediatrics,* **60**, 655–658.

MCCLURE, G., HALLIDAY, H.L. and THOMPSON (1988). *Perinatal Medicine.* Bailliere Tindall, London.

MEAD, M. (1928). *Coming of Age in Samoa.* Morrow, (republished by Pengin, London, 1943).

MUSHIN, J. (1988) Visual evoked potentials. In: *Fetal and Neonatal Neurology and Neurosurgery,* edited by M.I. Levene, M.J. Bennett and J. Punt. Churchill Livingstone, Edinburgh, pp. 206–212.

PHELPS, D.L. (1981). Vision loss due to retinopathy of prematurity. *Lancet,* i, 606.

ROBERTON, N.R.C. (1986) *Textbook of Neonatology.* Churchill Livingstone, Edinburgh.

ROBSON, K.S. (1968). The role of eye to eye contact in maternal–infant attachment. *Journal of Child Psychology and Psychiatry*, **8**, 13–25.

SAMUELS, C.A. and EWY, R. (1985). Aesthetic perception of faces during infancy. *British Journal of Developmental Psychology,* **3**, 221–228.

SMITH, P.K. and COWIE, H. (1988). *Understanding Children's Development.* Blackwell, London.

TANNER, J.W. (1978) *Fetus into Man, Physical Growth from Conception to Maturity.* Harvard University Press, Harvard.

VAN HOF-VAN DUIN, J. and MOHN, G. (1984). Vision in the preterm infant. In *Continuity of Neural Functions from Prenatal to Postnatal Life,* edited by H.F.R. Prechtl. Spastics International Medical Publications, London, pp. 93–114.

3

Chronic disorders of childhood

David Haigh

Introduction

Most children grow to adulthood without experiencing serious disease or disability. A few, however, are born with or develop a handicapping condition. If the less serious forms of learning difficulty are included, as many as 20% of schoolchildren have a significant handicap. Abnormalities of the special senses are commonly associated. In this chapter we will describe the important handicapping conditions in which disorders of the eye play a part.

Cerebral palsy and mental retardation

Mental retardation

Mental retardation is difficult to define in that there is no clear dividing line between normal and abnormal intelligence. IQ testing is notoriously unreliable at the extremes of intelligence but it does offer some objectivity. An IQ of 70 is two standard deviations below the mean and the 3% of the population with intelligence below this may be said to be moderately handicapped. The 0.4% with a developmental quotient below 50 are severely retarded.

Aetiology

About 75% of cases of mental retardation are thought to be of prenatal origin, caused by the various developmental syndromes (see below). Perinatal problems account for another 15%. The causes and management of asphyxia have been described in Chapter 2. Birth trauma is now rare in developed countries, but occasionally in difficult deliveries such as those by the breech, damage to the venous sinuses of the head during delivery may cause intracranial bleeding and subsequent brain damage. Before the advent of exchange transfusion and phototherapy, severe neonatal jaundice sometimes caused damage particularly to the basal ganglia. Hypoglycaemia, a low blood glucose which happens particularly in growth-retarded neonates whose carbohydrate reserves are low, may compromise the vulnerable brain.

Postnatal events account for another 10% of cases. Injury, particularly non-accidental injury such as shaking the young infant, can produce intracranial trauma. Meningitis and encephalitis are two forms of infection which, particularly in the young infant, interfere with brain development. Hypothyroidism and phenylketonuria are examples of metabolic diseases which cause mental retardation. Newborn population screening now detects these conditions and treatment is offered before brain damage can occur. Blood is taken from the infant between 5 and 10 days after birth. Hypothyroidism is detected by the finding of high serum levels of Thyroid Stimulating Hormone (TSH), a substance which is produced in excess by the pituitary when the thyroid gland functions poorly. Phenylketonuria, which is caused by a genetically determined deficiency of the enzyme phenylalanine hydroxylase leading to high and therefore toxic serum levels of the amino acid phenylalanine, may be found by the Guthrie test, a bioassay of phenylalanine, or by a chromatographic method, the Scriver test.

Cerebral palsy

Cerebral palsy may be defined as a defect of movement or posture due to a non-progressive lesion of the developing brain. For the purposes of this definition, development of the brain occurs in the fetus and in the first 2 or 3 years of extrauterine life, although in practice myelination of the brain continues into the late teens.

Cerebral palsy occurs in about 3 per 1000 live births and is classified into five types. Children with *spasticity* are weak with stiff muscles, brisk tendon reflexes and a tendency to develop contractures. Spastic cerebral palsy may be further divided into spastic quadriplegia where all four limbs are affected, hemiplegia with one side of the body involved, and diplegia where both legs are spastic and the arms are only minimally involved. Quadriplegic children make up about 15% of the total with cerebral palsy, hemiplegic children 30%, and those with a diplegia about 5%.

Athetosis is a slow writhing movement of the limbs or face occurring on intention. The child with athetoid cerebral palsy may have no movements whilst resting but when he tries to walk or talk, abnormal movements of limbs or tongue appear and interfere with his voluntary movements. Children with pure athetosis make up about 20% of the total.

Hypotonia or reduced muscle tone is common in the early stages of cerebral palsy, particularly in athetosis, but it is the predominant long-term problem in only 5% of cases. *Ataxia*, an incoordination of movement particularly affecting fine motor skills and usually due to a lesion in the cerebellum, forms a further 5%. The remaining 20% of children have a *mixed form of cerebral palsy*, usually with spasticity and athetosis.

Aetiology

The aetiology of cerebral palsy is broadly similar to that of mental retardation. Perinatal problems have previously been thought to be of particular importance. Recent work, including an analysis of the two national cohort studies of babies born in 1958 and 1970, has cast doubt on this. It is suggested that babies who show neurological abnormality in the newborn period and who eventually develop cerebral palsy, have in fact been compromised by events in early fetal life rather than damage during labour.

Particular syndromes of cerebral palsy have been associated with certain causative situations. Thus the child with a spastic diplegia was classically of very low birth weight and in the past athetosis was associated with severe neonatal jaundice, although with better treatment of jaundice, the infant with perinatal asphyxia is now the one at risk of athetosis.

Presentation

The presentation of cerebral palsy is diverse, but early feeding difficulties are common, possibly with floppiness. The primitive reflexes may fail to disappear at the correct time and may be hyperactive so that the child has an exaggerated Moro response and shows 'fisting' – tightly clenched fists because of a continuously active grasp reflex. Later in the first year of life, the hypotonia will give way to the spasticity or athetosis which becomes the major long-term problem. One important pattern of presentation is delayed motor milestones. As an example, the child whose legs are spastic may well have difficulty in sitting alone because of his tight thigh muscles which prevent him flexing his hips and abducting (moving apart) his thighs.

The abnormal movements of athetosis or the abnormal posture of spasticity, with 'scissoring', the thighs tightly clenched together and the legs crossed below the knee, appear late in the first year of life. If spasticity is severe, joint contractures may eventually fix the deformity, seriously interfering with function and care. The child with hip contractures and fixed scissoring will be very difficult to dress, for example. The asymmetrical pull of spastic muscles may dislocate joints, particularly the hips, and one of the aims of physiotherapy is to prevent these problems by continuously stretching affected muscles.

Pseudobulbar palsy is the term given to disorders of mouth and tongue movement due to lesions in the cerebral cortex. This condition simulates abnormalities of the 9th 10th, and 12th cranial nerves and is very common in cerebral palsy, resulting in drooling, difficulty in sucking, chewing and swallowing, and later problems with speech production.

Associated problems

Thirty-five per cent of children with cerebral palsy have *epilepsy*. The fits are usually generalized but may be focal. They are unusual in pure athetosis but common in hemiplegia, especially of postnatal origin, and in quadriplegia. Treatment with anticonvulsants is often required, but unfortunately, as with all drug therapies, unwanted effects may occur. Anticonvulsants probably interfere with the metabolism of brain neurotransmitters, but their effect is non-specific so that normal nerve impulses are depressed as well as abnormal ones. This may lead to learning problems, a most unwelcome side-effect in a child who is already handicapped.

Learning difficulties are frequent. Seventy-five per cent of children with cerebral palsy have an IQ below 100 and 50% below 70. Children with cerebral palsy may well have above normal intelligence however, but be unable to express their intellect because of the limitations imposed by poor motor function and perceptual problems. In addition, such children are deprived of normal sensory experience which limits their ability to form concepts which are fundamental to normal perception and communication.

Deafness occurs in 15% of children, especially with athetosis. Again this may be difficult to assess because of motor problems and global delay which themselves interfere with testing. Hearing defects may contribute to *speech problems*. Twenty per cent of the population of children with cerebral palsy have serious speech delay and a further 50% have articulation difficulties. Global retardation, pseudobulbar palsy and specific language problems also contribute.

Severe visual handicap occurs in around 10% of cerebral palsy children but as many as 45% have some form of eye defect. About 30% have strabismus, commonly esotropia, which is sometimes paralytic but often associated with high hypermetropia. High refractive error is commonly found, particularly when low birth weight and perinatal asphyxia are both aetiological factors. Field defects have been found in up to 25% of cases and homonymous hemianopia is frequent in children with a hemiplegia. Optic atrophy, which is common, is dealt with in Chapter 4. Cortical blindness occurs in only a minority but as many as 50% may have a disorder of visual perception. For example, the child may not connect a picture of a mechanical object with the object itself. There is a clear difference between seeing, the reception of visual data by the occipital cortex, and receiving, which involves analysis and understanding of that data. Dysfunction of auditory-visual integration has been described which is independent of intellectual delay. These cortical problems may present with conceptual difficulties of space, shape, direction and body image. They are particularly common in children with a lesion in the right hemisphere. They may become evident when intelligence testing produces a discrepancy between verbal ability and performance in copying shapes or in completing formboards. Visuomotor disorders may cause fine motor incoordination with an inability to tie shoe-laces, for example.

Although the vision of the handicapped child may be assessed using the STYCAR toy matching or Sheridan–Gardiner tests developed by Mary Sheridan, they have obvious limitations in cerebral palsy. Ophthalmoplegia may interfere with the tracking ability of the young child and visuospatial problems with his ability to match toys or letters. Hence the child's intellectual level will determine the suitability of a particular test and must be taken into account.

The eventual outcome in cerebral palsy is largely related to intelligence. The adult with athetoid cerebral palsy, but a normal or above normal intelligence, may well achieve independent living and employment despite grave physical handicap. Yet the individual with a spastic quadriplegia, microcephaly and severe intellectual retardation will be totally dependent on others.

The needs of children with cerebral palsy are complex and an integrated approach to them will be discussed elsewhere. Some of the medical, social and educational services available will however be mentioned. Medical management is designed to limit the handicap due to the disorder of movement and posture. *Physiotherapy* is the mainstay of treatment although scientific evidence of its success is difficult to find. The physiotherapist uses various methods to reduce muscle tone and prevent contractures. Passive exercises will stretch the affected muscles and joints. Stroking, icing or vibration will inhibit spasm. Correct positioning will overcome the effect of persisting primitive reflexes and allow the child to be fed, dressed and toileted. Serial splinting has been shown to lengthen muscles and can correct deformity. The Peto method, developed in Budapest in the 1960s, has recently become fashionable. A single individual takes on the function of nurse, teacher, physiotherapist and speech therapist. This 'conductor', hence the term 'conductive education', supervises all the daily activities in a structured programme. It is claimed that the method increases the acquisition of independence skills and it is said that in Hungary most children with cerebral palsy are able to attend normal school.

Drugs such as baclofen are used to reduce tone and extensor spasms and anticonvulsants are often necessary. L-dopa has been given with limited success in athetosis. *Surgery* is often used. Neurosurgery, including stereotactic surgery to destroy particular areas of the brain, has been disappointing. The orthopaedic surgeon however, can successfully lengthen muscles and their tendons or alter the direction of pull. Lengthening of the Achilles tendon is beneficial in many hemiplegic children but may actually inhibit walking if done bilaterally in the child with a spastic diplegia. Destruction of the obturator nerve in the groin to reduce 'scissoring' is one example of a 'peripheral neurectomy'.

The most important trend in the *education* of the handicapped child is that towards 'integration' into normal schools. In the UK this practice is enshrined in the 1981 Education Act which provides for the comprehensive assessment of the child, the preparation of a Statement of Educational Needs, an appeals procedure, and the statutory provision of education for the handicapped from 2 years. The emphasis has changed from fitting the child into an available special school to providing whatever help the child needs in the most suitable school. The act also imposes a duty on health authorities of informing the education authority of a child with special needs. In the USA this process of 'mainstreaming' has so far had limited success but is moving forwards as more resources are made available.

A seriously handicapped child imposes enormous extra stress on a family but this may be limited to some extent by the provision of help, both financial and actual, in caring for the child. In the UK various allowances are available, particularly the Disability Living Allowance and most local authorities offer short-term facilities ranging from baby-sitting services through holiday play-schemes to short periods of full-time care. In the USA the various charitable bodies try to ensure a high standard of medical and educational care for children with specific handicaps. Such services may help a family to continue to look after their child within the home and avoid the need for long-term residential placement.

Internationally, a lack of facilities has delayed the move of handicapped people out of institutions and special schools into the community.

Hydrocephalus

Interference with the flow of cerebrospinal fluid or its reabsorption leads to a rise in cerebrospinal fluid pressure and enlargement of the ventricular system of the brain, hydrocephalus. The cerebral cortex is stretched over the enlarging ventricles and the head increases in size. Hydrocephalus is often found with spina bifida, when it is due to an associated anomaly, the Arnold–Chiari malformation. It also occurs as a solitary congenital abnormality due to stenosis or atresia of the aqueduct of Sylvius which may be inherited as an autosomal recessive condition. Alternatively, the aqueduct may be compressed by a subdural haemorrhage from birth trauma, or child abuse, or by a posterior fossa tumour. Haemorrhage into the ventricular system, which occurs particularly in the tiny premature infant, may obliterate the cerebrospinal fluid pathways and meningitis produces adhesions which both impede the flow of cerebrospinal fluid and delay its absorption. Thus excessive head growth may be present from fetal life or may appear postnatally. The sutures between the skull bones separate, the fontanelle bulges and the eyes are pushed downwards producing the characteristic 'sunsetting' sign, in which the lower eyelid crosses the pupil and iris and a rim of sclera is visible above the iris. The legs may become spastic and the intellect deteriorates. Reasoning skills may be poor but verbal ability tends to be preserved. The child then displays meaningless chatter, the 'cocktail party' syndrome. Some children with only a thin rim of cortex, however, have normal intellect.

The treatment of choice is a surgical procedure to drain fluid from the ventricles and prevent brain damage. The one-way valve system shunts fluid into either the heart or the peritoneal cavity.

Squint, papilloedema and optic atrophy are all seen in hydrocephalus. About 50% of children with valves have strabismus which is often due to a VIth nerve palsy. Papilloedema occurs particularly in older children because the sutures are fused and the skull cannot increase in size to accommodate the increased amount of cerebrospinal fluid. Optic atrophy happens as a primary phenomenon when changes in skull shape produce compression or traction on the optic nerves and chiasm, or secondary to longstanding papilloedema.

The developmental syndromes

There are many developmental syndromes which include eye abnormalities. These are conveniently classified into nine groups and one or more in each group will be described for the purpose of illustration.

I.   The storage diseases

In these conditions, an abnormal substance, usually a lipid, is stored in the neurones of the central nervous system, resulting in degenerative brain disease. Most of these conditions are due to a single gene defect and are inherited in an autosomal recessive fashion. When two individuals who carry the same abnormal gene mate, each of their offspring has a one in four chance of receiving a double dose of the gene and developing the disease. The parents are said to be heterozygous for the condition, the affected child is homozygous. Tay–Sachs disease, which is due to a deficiency of the enzyme hexosaminidase-A, presents between 2 and 6 months when an apparently normal child begins to show neurological and developmental deterioration. The child loses previously acquired motor skills and visual awareness. He/she typically develops an exaggerated startle reflex and continues to deteriorate until death, usually before 4 years. The classic eye sign in Tay–Sachs is the cherry red spot, a bright red area surrounded by a whitish rim at the fovea. This appearance is caused by the accumulation of the lipid GM2 ganglioside within the retinal ganglion cells. Cherry red spots also occur in Sandhoff disease in which the same ganglioside is stored in the brain and in Niemann–Pick disease caused by the deposition of sphyngomyelin. The clinical picture in these diseases is similar and differentiation is only possible by the measurement of the involved enzymes in white cells or cultured skin fibroblasts. Carrier detection and antenatal detection is available for Tay–Sachs disease. Screening is appropriate in siblings of patients, who have a two in three chance of being carriers, but also in susceptible populations. In Eastern European (Ashkenazi) Jews, for example, the condition is 100 times more common than in the population as a whole, with the carrier rate estimated at 2.7%.

II.   Connective tissue disorders

Marfan's syndrome is inherited as an autosomal dominant, the presence of one abnormal gene being enough to produce the disease. Sufferers therefore either have an affected parent or their disease must be due to a new mutation. Half of all their children will in turn develop the condition, which has characteristic abnormalities of the skeleton, the cardiovascular system and the eyes. Affected individuals are tall with long limbs and long spindly fingers. Their span exceeds their height. They have long ribs which produce thoracic deformities such as 'pigeon breast'. The aortic valve of the heart is incompetent, allowing blood to flow in both directions and this leads to heart failure and eventual death. Eye problems are frequent with upward dislocation of the lens, high axial myopia, strabismus, nystagmus and retinal detachment. The metabolic disease homocystinuria produces similar deformities but in this condition the lens tends to subluxate downwards. There is, however, marked individual variation and the direction in which the lens displaces is not diagnostic.

III.   The neurocutaneous syndromes

These syndromes present with abnormalities of the skin and central nervous system, typically with eye problems.

Ataxia telangiectasia, inherited as an autosomal recessive, is a syndrome consisting of ataxia (disordered movements), immune deficiency with chronic respiratory infection and telangiectasia of the skin, but more particularly of the bulbar conjunctiva. Nystagmus and apraxia of conjugation may also occur.

Tuberous sclerosis is inherited as an autosomal dominant but there is wide variability in the expression of the gene, so that an apparently normal parent may produce more than one severely handicapped child. The skin, brain, eyes and kidneys may all be affected with the typical sclerotic patches or tubers affecting the brain. Adenoma sebaceum is the classic rash which appears in butterfly distribution over the bridge of the nose. Hypopigmented patches, best seen in ultraviolet light, occur on the trunk. About 90% of affected patients have convulsions and 65% have mild to severe mental retardation. In addition, about 50% have eye signs with phacomata, malformations of the nerve fibres of the retina which appear as white or yellow raised areas near the edge of the optic disc. These do not usually interfere with vision. Genetic counselling is especially important and parents of affected children must be carefully examined, both clinically and by cranial computerized tomography (CT scanning).

Neurofibromatosis (Von Recklinghausen's disease), inherited as an autosomal dominant, is a common condition with very variable manifestations. More than six irregular areas of brown pigment greater than 1.5 cm in diameter (café-au-lait spots) are pathognomonic. In childhood soft swellings appear along the course of the peripheral nerves and there is an increased incidence of neural tumours, especially gliomas of the optic nerve and chiasm. Mild intellectual impairment is common but severe retardation is unusual.

IV.   Chromosomal disorders

Chromosomal disorders occur in 0.4% of live births but in as many as half of all spontaneously aborted fetuses. The most common abnormalities are the trisomies in which the fertilized egg has three copies of a particular chromosome instead of two, and deletions of chromosome material including the so-called ring chromosomes.

Down's syndrome, or trisomy 21, occurs about once in every thousand live births. It becomes more common with increasing maternal age, so that in mothers between 41 and 45 years the incidence rises to 1 in 60 births. Affected children are hypotonic with a small flattened head, a flat nose, a small mouth and a darting tongue. The small brain leads to mental retardation of varying degrees. Serious congenital heart disease is common, as is duodenal atresia, an obstruction of the bowel. Eye abnormalities are common. The palpebral fissures are oblique and malformation of the nasolacrimal ducts may lead to chronic blepharoconjunctivitis. Brushfield spots, white spots forming a ring on the iris, occur in about 85% of individuals having trisomy 21 (Brushfield, 1924), although less pronounced spots may be observed in about 24% of normal individuals (Donaldson, 1961). Cataracts are also commonly observed together with high myopia, strabismus and nystagmus.

Trisomy 13, (Patau's syndrome) occurs less commonly and most affected children die within the first few months of life. The babies are microcephalic with deformed ears, a cleft lip and palate, extra digits and serious heart and kidney abnormalities. Ocular abnormalities, often bilateral, occur so frequently in this syndrome that they are described as a principal feature (Keith, 1966). Microphthalmos is often encountered, sometimes anophthalmos and, rarely, the cyclops deformity. Other abnormalities include colobomas, cataracts, corneal opacities, retinal dysplasia and optic atrophy. Sometimes defective development of the angle can result in glaucoma.

Absence or deletions of small pieces of chromosome material may cause abnormality including eye anomalies or even tumours. Deletion of the long arm of chromosome 13 (13q−) produces a syndrome of mental retardation with the development of retinoblastomas. It is now thought that all forms of hereditary retinoblastomas are due to an abnormality of chromosome 13, with at least two abnormal genes being needed to trigger tumour development (see Chapter 4). Deletion of part of chromosome 11 results in congenital aniridia with a high risk of Wilm's tumour of the kidney. Most cases of congenital aniridia, however, are inherited as an autosomal dominant and carry no extra risk of tumour formation.

V. Craniostenosis

In fetal life and early childhood, growth of the skull occurs at the edges of the plates of bone of which it is formed. These plates of bone join at the suture lines which are very mobile in the newborn baby, allowing substantial moulding of the skull to occur during the birth process. The sutures fuse completely by the age of 7 years so that the skull is then a rigid box. If a suture fuses prematurely, growth cannot take place at right angles to that suture and the skull shape becomes deformed. Premature fusion of the coronal sutures between the frontal and parietal bones causes acrocephaly with deformity of the face and orbits including hypertelorism. Depression of the roof of the orbit results in exophthalmos with compression of the optic nerve giving papilloedema, optic atrophy and visual impairment. Nystagmus and strabismus are common and colobomas, cataracts and dislocation of the lens may occur. Several syndromes include this pathological process of craniostenosis. Crouzon's disease includes coronal craniostenosis with the resulting eye and facial abnormalities together with a beaked nose and a protruding lower lip. Apert's syndrome, inherited as an autosomal dominant, consists of coronal craniostenosis with fusion of the fingers, syndactyly.

VI. Craniofacial defects

These defects may present with eye abnormalities. Waardenburg's syndrome is classically diagnosed by the finding of a white forelock with nerve deafness, inherited as an autosomal dominant. The pigment defect may be localized to the eye, however, with heterochromic irides or defects in fundus pigment. The two irides may be of different colours or one segment of an iris may be different. The expression of the gene varies widely, so that iris heterochromia in one family member may point to the cause of deafness in another.

VII. Central nervous system anomalies

The eye develops as an integral part of the primitive brain and it is not surprising, therefore that major anomalies of the brain are often accompanied by structural eye defects. Septo-optic dysplasia is a sporadic condition in which the septum pellucidum of the brain is absent. Hypoplastic discs and sparse retinal vessels occur as part of optic nerve hypoplasia and there is often significant impairment of visual acuity. Structural abnormalities of the hypothalamus may lead to endocrine disorders such as growth hormone deficiency.

VIII. Dysmorphic syndromes

Many syndromes of multiple abnormalities which include eye problems are of unknown aetiology. The Rubinstein–Taybi syndrome with growth retardation and intellectual impairment, broad thumbs and great toes, characteristic face and heart abnormalities, occurs about once in every ten thousand live births. Eye abnormalities include hypertelorism, antimongoloid slant of the palpebral fissures, ptosis, cataract, colobomas and strabismus. Aicardi's syndrome is an occasional cause of the serious form of epilepsy, infantile spasms. The corpus callosum is absent and eye abnormalities are usual. One eye may be small or have a fixed irregular pupil. The fundi show punched-out areas which are in fact developmental defects of the choroid.

IX. Congenital infections

A number of maternal infections cross the placenta but only a handful have been shown to damage the fetus. Rubella is a common viral infection of children in the early school years. The symptoms are minor and non-specific. The diagnosis cannot be made clinically with any certainty because other viruses, particularly ECHO 9, produce a similar picture. If the mother develops rubella within the first 10 weeks of pregnancy, 90% of fetuses are damaged. From 10 to 20 weeks, at least 20% are involved. Affected fetuses grow poorly and have major abnormalities of the heart and brain, with cerebral palsy and mental retardation being common. Deafness and serious visual impairment contribute to the handicap. Hepatitis and osteitis are part of the generalized infection and involvement of the bone marrow leads to thrombocytopenia, a low platelet count which causes a bleeding tendency. The eyes are often involved and indeed congenital rubella was first recognized in 1941 by Gregg who described an epidemic of congenital cataracts. Glaucoma and microphthalmia may also occur and there is a characteristic 'salt and pepper' retinitis which is found in about 40% of affected individuals.

The number of cases of congenital rubella syndrome has fallen over the years due to the practice of immunization, but there are still about 20 cases a year in England and Wales with ten times as many terminations of pregnancy for proven maternal rubella. When rubella vaccine was introduced in Britain, the policy chosen was that of immunizing girls between 10 and 14 years. By 1987, 97% of pregnant women were immune to rubella but because of the large pool of natural rubella in young children, the few non-immune women were at substantial risk, hence the continuing level of rubella in pregnancy. This has forced a change in policy. Late in 1988, MMR (measles, mumps and rubella) vaccine was introduced. It is recommended that all 1 year olds and 5 year olds be given this vaccine. Hopefully this will dramatically reduce the level of natural rubella in the community so that even non-immunized women will be unlikely to catch the disease. The administration of MMR vaccine to 15 month olds has been standard practice in the USA for several years, with the result that all three diseases are relatively uncommon there.

Cytomegalovirus is the commonest infection to affect the fetus. The adult infection is asymptomatic or flu-like. When the primary infection occurs in pregnancy, at least 90% of infected babies are asymptomatic at birth but probably 20% will eventually have detectable damage, particularly hearing loss and intellectual delay. It is estimated that 300 babies are born each year in England and Wales with microcephaly and mental retardation due to congenital cytomegalovirus infection. About 25% of severely affected infants have a chorioretinitis. Strabismus and optic atrophy occur occasionally but microphthalmia and corneal opacities are rare. The infected infants continue to excrete the virus in their bodily secretions including the urine for several months. During this time they may act as a source of infection to non-immune pregnant women.

Toxoplasma gondii is a protozoon which usually affects cats but commonly infects humans. Some 30% of blood donors have serological evidence of previous infection. The adult infection is again asymptomatic or flu like but the protozoon may occasionally cause hepatitis. The congenital infection is rare in the UK, although in the USA the incidence has been estimated at 1 or 2 per 1000 live births. The affected infants are small with a large liver and spleen, intracranial calcification and hydrocephalus. Chorioretinitis is common but long-term visual problems are rare.

Rheumatoid arthritis

Juvenile rheumatoid arthritis is an uncommon but important chronic disease of childhood. It differs from the adult variety, not least in that the joint manifestations are frequently associated with inflammatory problems elsewhere, including the eyes. This condition is distinct from rheumatic fever which is a disease which follows streptococcal infection. Juvenile rheumatoid arthritis is of unknown cause but two current theories are that it may be due to an infection with an organism as yet undiscovered or alternatively that it is a form of autoimmune disease. Occasionally there is a family history of joint disease.

The condition is usefully classified into four different types and the incidence of eye problems varies from one to the other:

(1) Systematic onset or Still's disease occurs equally in the sexes and at any age through childhood. The child develops a high fever with rash and an enlarged spleen and lymph nodes. The lining of the heart or pericardium may be inflamed but severe arthritis occurs in only 25%. Iridocyclitis is not a problem in this group.
(2) Polyarticular disease also occurs at any age but the ratio of girls to boys is 8 : 1. Severe arthritis occurs in a minority but inflammation of any joint is

accompanied by low fever, anaemia and growth retardation. Eye involvement is rare.

(3) Pauciarticular disease begins in early childhood with inflammation of a few large joints, more commonly in girls. Severe arthritis is rare and there are few other manifestations, but *chronic iridocyclitis* occurs in 50% of this group.

(4) Juvenile rheumatoid arthritis is again more common in girls, with a sex ratio of 6 : 1. It is very similar to the adult form of the disease and usually begins in late childhood. Any joints may be involved but the small joints of the hands and feet are especially vulnerable. Fifty per cent have severe arthritis but fever, anaemia, vasculitis and subcutaneous nodules also occur, with bony erosions visible on X-ray. Between 10% and 20% of these children have *acute iridocyclitis*. This is often symptomatic but the condition is self-limiting and long-term sequelae are unusual.

Chronic iridocyclitis is a particularly important complication of rheumatoid arthritis in children, particularly the pauciarticular type. It is occasionally the presenting symptom of the condition but usually begins with the onset of joint problems and is itself active when the arthritis is active. The condition, which may be unilateral or bilateral, is often asymptomatic but occasionally redness, pain, photophobia and loss of visual acuity are present at the outset.

Treatment of iridocyclitis involves the use of topical steroids and dilating agents. Subconjunctival injections or even systemic steroids may be necessary and surgery may be required for the correction of sequelae. Early detection improves the outlook and it is suggested that children with rheumatoid arthritis should have a slit-lamp examination each year but that children with the pauciarticular type should be examined every 3 months.

The course of rhematoid arthritis in childhood is often prolonged but the long-term outlook is good and management is directed towards relieving symptoms and avoiding joint deformity. Medications such as aspirin and the non-steroidal anti-inflammatory drugs (e.g. naproxen) are used but physiotherapy and occupational therapy have a vital role.

Diabetes mellitus

Diabetes mellitus is a clinical syndrome, common in adults but relatively uncommon in children, characterized by a deficiency of insulin resulting in disturbed metabolism of carbohydrate, protein and fat.

Two types of diabetes are recognized. Insulin-dependent diabetes mellitus (IDDM), which in the past was known as type I, is due to a failure of the pancreas to produce insulin. In non-insulin dependent diabetes (NIDDM), or type II, the peripheral tissues are resistant to the action of insulin. NIDDM, which is the commonest type in the population as a whole, may be treated with drugs which stimulate the pancreas to produce more insulin or make the tissues more responsive to its action, or indeed with diet alone. Children with diabetes are invariably insulin dependent.

The currently fashionable theory of causation is that environmental factors trigger the diabetogenic process in genetically predisposed individuals. NIDDM has a strong genetic basis with sufferers commonly having a close relative with the disease. The pattern of inheritance in IDDM is much less clear, but diabetic children do have a higher than expected number of first degree relatives with the condition. It is known that certain HLA tissue types, namely DR3 and/or DR4, predispose the individual to IDDM, especially in Caucasians, but it is clear that other factors in the genome must also play a part.

It is thought that the usual triggering factor in children is a viral infection. One study showed that the incidence of diabetes in children paralleled the incidence of mumps in the community, with a time lag of about 4 years. Breast feeding has been shown to have some protective effect, presumably by protecting against viral infection. Other toxins may be important. In Iceland, for instance, smoked mutton eaten by pregnant women has been shown to damage the cells of the islets of Langerhans in the fetal pancreas and to trigger diabetes in some offspring. This rather curious fact serves only to illustrate the probably complex aetiology of the condition.

Once the pancreatic islet cells have been damaged by infection or toxin, the individual begins to produce antibodies to his own islet cells. These antibodies then continue to destroy the islets, causing a gradual fall in insulin production until eventually the clinical syndrome of IDDM supervenes. IDDM may therefore be thought of as end-stage islet failure due to autoimmune destruction triggered by viral infection in a genetically susceptible individual. Islet cell antibodies have been detected in children who eventually become diabetic, many months before the onset of symptoms. There have been several successful attempts to suppress the autoimmune process before the stage of complete islet failure is reached, but unfortunately the immunosuppressive drugs currently available are too toxic to make this a useful approach to the problem.

IDDM affects about 1 in 1000 children under the age of 15 years. It may occur even in the first year of life but the two peak times are between 5 and 7 years and at puberty. Although the process of islet destruction probably takes many months, the clinical condition presents fairly acutely in children. At the time of diagnosis the child has usually had symptoms for a few days or weeks. The high levels of glucose in the blood spill over into the urine, taking water with them and causing the excessive urine production and thirst which are the hallmarks of the disease. Night-time wetting in a child who has previously been dry may be the first symptom before the metabolic abnormalities lead to tiredness, weight loss and a susceptibility to staphylococcal skin infections. The presence of glucose in the urine may produce genital thrush, especially in girls. Disturbances of vision are common around the time of diagnosis. Changes in the glucose content of the lens tend to lag behind those of the blood. When the lens glucose is higher than that of the blood, water is drawn in, producing changes in the shape of the lens and hence blurring of vision.

In the absence of insulin, peripheral tissues are unable to take up glucose and instead obtain energy for their metabolic needs by burning fat. This leads to the release of various 'ketone bodies' into the blood and urine. Ketones are themselves toxic, producing abdominal pain and vomiting and, therefore, dehydration and eventually coma. In children the metabolic upset may have reached this stage of keto-acidosis at the time of diagnosis or episodes may occur later in the course of the disease when inadequate monitoring or infection lead to poor control.

The other type of 'coma' seen only in treated diabetes is that due to a low blood glucose, hypoglycaemia or so-called 'hypo'. In a 'hypo', brought on by excess insulin, inadequate food or unusual physical activity, tiredness, dizziness and sweating may sometimes give way to collapse and even convulsion. Early recognition and treatment with oral glucose should prevent the more severe symptoms of hypoglycaemia, but many patients are tempted to keep their blood glucose at an unsatisfactorily high level to avoid the risk of 'hypos'.

The management of diabetes is designed to correct the symptoms, to prevent keto-acidosis and hypoglycaemia, and to promote normal growth and development of the child. Paediatricians teach children to understand and look after their own condition so that their quality of life may be high. Children are encouraged to seek optimal control of blood glucose concentration, particularly as chronically high levels are thought to increase the risk of the various long-term complications such as eye disease. The risk of these complications increases with the length of time since diagnosis and is, therefore, particularly important in children who are likely to survive for many years. The precise relationship between blood glucose levels and the risk of complications is not understood. Some individuals with chronically high levels may remain free of problems, whereas others who seem well controlled may develop eye or kidney disease. In general, however, the risks are lowered if blood glucose concentrations are maintained at or near normal levels.

In the physiological state, insulin is secreted by the pancreas into the portal vein which carries blood from the gut to the liver, in response to an increase in the glucose concentration in that blood. The secretion of insulin is carefully regulated and blood glucose is maintained within fairly narrow limits. The intake of calories is controlled to promote normal height growth and appropriate body weight. Treatment would ideally simulate the physiological situation but in practice falls short of this.

The principle of treatment is to replace the absent insulin and to match the amount to the carbohydrate in the diet. This is achieved by giving a diet in which 50–60% of total calories are obtained from carbohydrate. Refined sugars such as sucrose are avoided as they are rapidly absorbed and cause high peaks in the blood glucose concentration. Instead sweeteners such as aspartame are used and sorbitol and fructose are allowed in moderate amounts. Carbohydrate intake is spread over the course of the day to match the absorption and action of the injected insulin and is taken as three or four main meals with snacks between them. Less than 30% of calories should come from fat and saturated fats should be especially avoided. Food which is high in fibre slows the absorption of sugars from the gut and smooths out the peaks of blood glucose.

Insulin is usually injected as a mixture of soluble and isophane insulins which are short and medium in action respectively. The current trend is towards more frequent injections with a daily dose of a long-acting insulin to provide continuous background activity and injections of short-acting insulin before each meal. These are conveniently given via a so-called pen which contains a cartridge of insulin. Another way of mimicking the physiological state involves the continuous subcutaneous infusion of insulin from a pump, again with bursts of infusion before meals.

The correct balance of carbohydrate and insulin can only be obtained if careful monitoring of blood glucose levels is carried out. Some idea of 'control' can be gained by testing the urine for glucose, in that glucose spills over into the urine only when abnormally high blood levels are reached. Regular measurement of blood glucose using the various proprietary testing strips gives more useful information. At clinic visits, blood may be taken for glycosylated haemoglobin (HbA1c) estimation. This substance is formed by the non-enzymatic attachment of glucose to haemoglobin and since the haemoglobin in red cells has a life of about 120 days, the percentage of haemoglobin which has glucose attached to it is a reflection of the mean glucose levels over the previous 2 months. Fructosamine assays have also been used to reflect control over the previous 2–3 weeks.

The long-term complications of diabetes fall into two groups, the macrovascular such as coronary artery disease and gangrene, and the microvascular such as retinopathy and kidney failure. Their importance may be judged by the statement of Knowles (1971) who, describing diabetics diagnosed in the 1940s, said, 'in any group of five diabetics followed for 25 years, one will die, two will have severe retinal, renal or arterial disease, one will have background retinopathy and only one will be free of complications.' The outlook for young people diagnosed in the 1990s is almost certainly better than this, but complications remain a major cause of handicap and death in diabetes.

Several studies have shown that adult diabetics have a two- to three-fold greater than average mortality and morbidity from coronary artery disease, stroke and peripheral vascular problems such as gangrene. It is not clear whether good control reduces the risk but other factors such as cigarette smoking, obesity and inactivity can usually be controlled.

About 25% of diabetics diagnosed before the age of 30 will die of kidney failure and many others have impaired renal function due to diabetic nephropathy. This complication progresses slowly and may be first diagnosed by the finding of small amounts of protein in the urine, usually after 5 or more years of diabetes. After 10 or more years the loss of protein is sufficient to be detected by the usual stick tests and after a further 7–10 years renal failure is evident. By this stage, proliferative retinopathy almost always accompanies the kidney disease.

Neuropathy or disease of the peripheral nerves is common in longstanding diabetes. Twenty-five years after diagnosis, about 50% have involvement of the sensory nerves. Fifty per cent of these will have no symptoms but the others will have loss of sensation, often leading to damage to the feet, pain and tingling. Abnormalities of the autonomic nervous system lead to various symptoms including impotence.

In developed countries diabetic retinopathy is the commonest cause of blindness in adults between the ages of 30 and 65 years. Retinal changes are found in 20% of individuals after 10 years of diabetes and 50% after 20. Children developing diabetes at or before the peak age of 5–7 years are, therefore, at substantial risk of eye problems. Patients with eye involvement may be asymptomatic, have some blurring of vision or even complete blindness.

Diabetic retinopathy may be classified as non-proliferative which occurs early or proliferative which occurs late. Non-proliferative retinopathy is characterized by venous dilatation and microaneurysms, with retinal haemorrhages and exudates. Venous dilatation is difficult to assess on ophthalmoscopy, but any variation from the normal arterial : venous ratio of 2 : 3 may be significant. Microaneurysms occur on the retinal capillaries, especially at the posterior pole, and vary in size from 10 μm, hardly bigger than a red cell, to 50 μm. Haemorrhages occurring deep in the retina are associated with capillary closure and take the form of 'dots and blots'. Superficial bleeds into the nerve fibre layer of the retina are splinter or flame shaped. Exudates occur deep in the retina and appear waxy in texture. 'Cotton wool spots' are due to the occlusion of arterioles with subsequent accumulation of axoplasmic debris. 'White vessels' due to opacification of the vessel walls indicate non-perfusion of the capillaries. Retinal oedema may affect the macula and threaten central vision but is difficult to diagnose on ophthalmoscopy. All of the above signs occur commonly in the posterior pole, around the disc and at the macula.

Proliferative retinopathy is far more serious in that it continues to progress until vision is threatened or lost. New vessels proliferate from the larger retinal vesels in a typical fine hairpin configuration. These vessels are irregular and tortuous and lie in front of the veins from which they arise. Connective tissue proliferates at the same time and extends across the retina and into the vitreous. Haemorrhages and scarring, with subsequent shrinkage of the scar tissue, may lead to retinal detachment. All of these changes threaten vision but haemorrhages into the vitreous are particularly serious and demand urgent treatment.

Treatment of retinopathy will vary with severity. 'Background' retinopathy with venous dilatation and microaneurysms may well stabilize with improved diabetic control and, in older patients, treatment of high blood pressure. Older girls should be aware that the oral contraceptive pill, and indeed pregnancy, may exacerbate this form of retinopathy. The next stage of maculopathy in which retinal oedema or exudates threaten central vision is treated with laser therapy to the vascular abnormalities. The best results are obtained when visual acuity at the onset of treatment is between 6/6 and 6/18, hence the need for early detection.

Proliferative retinopathy is treated by the argon laser, which burns the areas in and around the new vessel formation. These new vessels can be eliminated and useful vision maintained in 90% of patients. Some patients, however, experience field defects, night blindness or abnormal colour perception after treatment. Many patients are now free of recurrence 10 years after initial laser treatment.

The emphasis on early detection has prompted the introduction of screening programmes, many involving the use of the non-mydriatic retinal camera. This is still controversial, its critics arguing that it may miss lesions, especially in the postequatorial fundus or in front of the retina, but its use is gaining widespread acceptance.

Future developments promise well for the diabetic child. The identification of at-risk individuals and the viruses which may trigger their diabetes offers the prospect of immunization against those viruses. Safer immunosuppressive drugs may abort the diabetogenic process before clinical diabetes supervenes. So-called 'designer' insulins will be absorbed more readily and allow a more physiological response to ingested carbohydrate. Implanted glucose sensors have worked continuously in animals for more than a year and, if linked to an implanted microprocessor-controlled infusion pump delivering insulin into the peritoneum, could act as an 'artificial pancreas'. Pancreas transplants have been tried, mostly at the same time as a kidney transplant, but the graft survival is less than 50% at 4 years, the cost is high, the donors are limited and the risks substantial. More promising is islet cell transplantation in which the cells are grown in tissue culture and then injected into the portal system.

It is worth remembering that although the conditions described in this chapter may be devastating for the individual and their family, the majority of children grow up without serious problems. Even the minority with significant handicap can usually reach a satisfying and productive adult life, given early detection and proper medical and educational attention.

Further reading

ABERCROMBIE, M.L.J. (1964). Perceptual and visuomotor problems in cerebral palsy. In *Clinics in Developmental Medicine*, no. 11. Heinemann, Oxford.

BAUM, J.D. and KINMONTH, A.L. (1985). *Care of the Child with Diabetes*. Churchill Livingstone, Edinburgh.

BAX, M., HART, H. and JENKINS, S. (1981). Clinical testing of visual function of the young child. *Developmental Medicine and Child Neurology*, **23**, 92.

BEAUCHAMP, G.R. (1986). The eye and learning disabilities *Clinical Ophthalmology*, **5**, 1–12.

BEHRMAN, R.E. and VAUGHAN, V.C. (1987). *Nelson Textbook of Pediatrics*, 13th edn. W.B. Saunders, London.

BREAKEY, A.S. (1955). Ocular findings in cerebral palsy. *Archives of Opthalmology*, **53**, 852–856.

BRUSHFIELD, T. (1924). Mongolism. *British Journal of Childhood Diseases*, **21**, 241–258.

DOFT, B.H. *et al.* (1984). The association between longterm diabetic control and early retinopathy. *Ophthalmology*, **91**, 763–767.

DONALDSON, D.D. (1961). The significance of spotting of the iris in mongoloids Brushfield's spots. *Archives of Ophthalmology*, **65**, 26–31.

DRYJA, T.P. *et al.* (1984). Homozygosity of chromosome 13 in retinoblastoma. *New England Journal of Medicine*, **319**, 550–556.

FANTL, E.W. (1964). The eye in cerebral palsy. *Pediatrics*, **48**, 1964.

FORFAR, J.O. and ARNEIL, G.C. (1984). *Textbook of Paediatrics*, 3rd edn. Churchill Livingstone, Edinburgh.

GALLIE, B.L. and PHILLIPS, R.A. (1984). Retinoblastoma: a model of oncogenesis. *Ophthalmology*, 1984, **91**, 666–670.

GILBERT, F. (1983). Retinoblastoma and recessive allelles in tumorigenesis. *Nature*, **305**, 761–762.

HALL, D.M.B. (1984). *The Child with a Handicap*. Blackwell Scientific, Oxford.

HUSON, S.M., JONES, D. and BECK, L. (1987). Ophthalmic manifestations of neurofibromatosis. *British Journal of Ophthalmology*, **71**, 235–238.

JACOBS, C. (1982). *Pediatric Rheumatology for the Practitioners*. Springer Verlag, Berlin.

JONES, K.L. (1988). *Smith's Recognisable Patterns of Human Malformation*. Saunders, London.

KEITH, C.G. (1966). The ocular manifestations of trisomy 13–15. *Transactions of the Ophthalmological Society of the UK*, **86**, 435–439.

KLEIN, R., KLEIN, B.E.K., MOSS, S.E. (1984). The Wisconsin epidemiologic study of diabetic retinopathy: II. Prevalence and risk of diabetic retinopathy when age at diagnosis is less than 30 years. *Archives of Ophthalmology*, **102**, 520–526.

LANGLEY, B. and DUBOSE, R.B. (1976). Functional vision screening for severely handicapped children. *New Outlook for the Blind*, **70**, 346–350.

PEARSON, L. and LINDSAY, G. (1986). *Special Needs in the Primary School*. NFER–Nelson.

STANBURY, J.B. (1988). *The Metabolic Basis of Inherited Disease*. McGraw-Hill, Maidenhead.

SUTTON, A. (1988). Conductive education. *Archives of Disease in Childhood*, **63**, 214–217.

Swann Report (1989). *Education for All*. HMSO, London.

Warnock Report (1978). *Special Educational Needs*. HMSO, London.

4

Ocular pathology

A. Jane Dickinson, Alistair R. Fielder and Derek R. Sherwood

Introduction

An ophthalmic finding may have consequences not only for sight but also for the health of the infant or child. This presents an exciting clinical challenge, but one which may also be intimidating, as the range of conditions involving the developing visual system is vast, and many are rarely encountered in everyday practice.

It is obviously not possible to cover all paediatric ophthalmic abnormalities in a single chapter and the purpose of this chapter, therefore, is to provide an overview of certain selected topics and a bibliography which the interested reader can consult if further details are required. The chapter is arranged on an anatomical basis commencing at the front and working backwards. The following topics are covered elsewhere in this book and will not be duplicated here: measurement of vision, ophthalmic examination, amblyopia and strabismus.

The child with abnormal eyelids

It is probably unusual for eyelid problems to present to the optometrist, but both congenital and acquired disorders are fairly frequent and may be associated with other ocular changes including refractive errors. These include abnormalities of shape, position and swellings of the eyelids.

Abnormalities of shape and position

Epicanthus

This is the commonest eyelid anomaly of childhood. Arising from the upper eyelid, epicanthus consists of a fold of skin covering the medial canthus and is often seen in infancy. With growth of the facial bones epicanthus tends to, but does not invariably, regress spontaneously. When prominent, it may mislead observers to diagnose an esotropia, however, epicanthus and strabismus are both common and are not mutually exclusive! In Down's syndrome and the blepharophimosis syndrome, the fold arises from the lower eyelid (epicanthus inversus).

Coloboma

A relatively common congenital defect of the lid margin. This is usually isolated, but may be associated with other anomalies such as a dermoid (see later). Colobomas can be single or multiple, and require surgical closure, which should be undertaken promptly if there is a risk of corneal exposure.

Ptosis

The upper eyelid normally rests 1–2 mm below the upper limbus and a lower level constitutes ptosis. Surprisingly, diagnosis may not be as easy as it may seem, as hypotropia or ipsilateral enophthalmos may mimic true ptosis. Similarly proptosis, unilateral axial myopia or lid retraction of the contralateral eye, may be mistaken for ptosis of the *normal* eyelid. Thus it is important to first determine which of these possibilities is present and, as mentioned, this is not always quite as straightforward as it may appear.

Ptosis may be congenital or acquired. In general, acquired ptosis requires urgent investigation to search for any underlying cause which may be neurological. Congenital ptosis has fewer systemic connotations but will still require urgent assessment as the visual axis may be obscured and there may be an associated refractive error, clearly both are powerfully amblyogenic. Features of different types are outlined below, by far the most common being *congenital dystrophic ptosis*. A compensatory chin-up head posture may develop.

Always consider two possibilities: that ptosis may pose a risk to vision and may be the first sign of a condition which poses a risk to health. The former is obviously amblyopia, the second, fortunately rare, includes myasthenia gravis and other rare conditions. The following list is not exhaustive.

Type	**Features**
Congenital	
(1) Dystrophic	± Superior rectus weakness. A feature of many congenital syndromes such as the fetal alcohol and blepharophimosis syndromes
(2) III nerve palsy	± Medial, superior or inferior recti, or inferior oblique weakness, or mydriasis
(3) Horner's syndrome	Mild ptosis, meiosis and iris hypochromia
(4) Marcus Gunn jaw winking	Intermittent eyelid elevation, synkynetic with jaw movement
Acquired	
(1) Myogenic	Levator weakness seen in myasthenia gravis or progressive external ophthalmoplegia
(2) III nerve palsy	Similar signs to congenital form, but urgent neurological investigation required
(3) Horner's syndrome	Mild ptosis and meiosis, but iris hypochromia rare. Requires urgent neurological investigation
(4) Mechanical	Eyelid tumours, e.g. haemangioma or neurofibroma

Epiblepharon

Easily confused with entropion, but in this condition the medial portion of the eyelid is turned in by an extra fold of skin. Although the eyelashes may touch the cornea, only rarely is there the need for surgical intervention as the lashes are soft and do not usually abrade the cornea. Epiblepharon usually resolves with facial growth.

Entropion

Denotes inversion of the eyelid margin and is rare in children. Although occasionally congenital, most cases are cicatricial, arising secondary to conjunctival scarring from Stevens–Johnson syndrome, alkali burns or recurrent infection with *Chlamydia trachomatis*. Cicatricial entropion always requires surgery, to prevent potentially blinding corneal damage.

Ectropion

Eversion of the eyelid margin is very rarely congenital, but may follow traumatic scarring of the outer eyelid.

Distichiasis

Included here for completeness, this describes the eyelid with an extra row of lashes.

Swelling

Diffuse swelling

Enquiry about trauma, topical medication, or atopy may help when faced with a child who has swollen eyelids. Acute swelling, with itching and chemosis, particularly in an asthmatic or eczematous child is a common allergic phenomenon and settles quickly without treatment if the offending allergen is quickly removed. Contact dermatitis, on the other hand, is more chronic and may be due to topical substances including eyedrops. Again, avoidance is the best treatment.

These relatively minor problems should be distinguished from the potentially life-threatening condition of orbital cellulitis. Usually arising from the sinuses, this bacterial infection causes tense red painful swelling of the lids which is usually unilateral. If the infection has spread deep to the orbital septum, then conjunctival chemosis, proptosis and visual loss can occur, and eye movements will be limited and painful. These children need hospital admission for parenteral antibiotics. Other causes of diffuse eyelid swelling include neurofibromatosis and *most important* the malignant tumour – rhabdomyosarcoma. These few examples exemplify the need for the meticulous assessment of any eyelid swelling.

Localized swelling

Although most eyelid lumps are of no visual significance, large masses particularly in the upper lid can cause mechanical ptosis or astigmatism.

INFLAMMATORY

Lumps caused by *molluscum contagiosum* (*Figure 4.1*) are infectious, with umbilicated, often multiple nodules, particularly on the lid margin. They shed virus into the conjunctival fornix inducing a chronic follicular conjunctivitis. Cautery or excision of the nodules cures the conjunctivitis. *Styes* are acute infections of the eyelash follicle and usually resolve rapidly and spontaneously with warm compresses. *Chalazia*, on the other hand, are due to sterile inflammation of the meibomian glands, and often persist for months. If they fail to resolve spontaneously then incision and curettage are required, although in childhood conservative measures such as topical antibiotics are continued for longer than in the adult as surgical correction often requires a general anaesthetic.

DEVELOPMENTAL

Dermoid
As with corneal dermoids, this congenital lesion is not uncommon, and arises when ectodermal tissues become trapped in an abnormal position. They usually occur either nasally or temporally in the upper eyelid, but may extend into deeper tissues and even extend intracranially. Surgical excision is thus approached somewhat cautiously.

TUMOURS

Papillomas
These grow out from the skin with an irregular surface and are benign. They are easily excised.

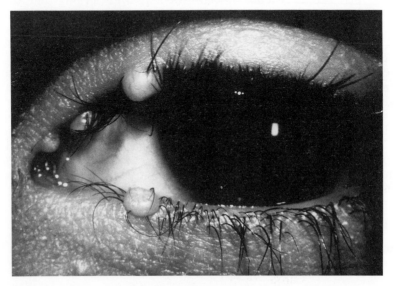

Figure 4.1. Molluscum contagiosum, infectious nodules on the eyelid margins

HAEMANGIOMAS

These are of two types. Strawberry (capillary) haemangiomas are raised, bright red lesions with an irregular surface, which appear at or near birth, but enlarge during the first year. They then involute, often to regress totally by the age of seven. Commonly associated with amblyogenic features, such as ptosis or astigmatism, treatment (intralesional steroid injections) is often used; otherwise parental reassurance is all that is required. 'Port wine' stains (naevus flammeus) are quite different. Dark and flat as the name suggests, they may be associated with developmental glaucoma, and also with choroidal and meningeal haemangiomas (Sturge–Weber syndrome).

As mentioned in children with neurofibromatosis, the *neurofibroma* may involve the eyelids and present as localized or diffuse swellings. Remember, this finding may also be associated with raised intraocular pressure.

Proptosis

The causes of proptosis in childhood fall mainly into four groups: developmental, inflammatory, neoplastic and vascular. All merit prompt investigation, the history and examination will often provide enough information to enable differentiation between these four, but tissue biopsy may be required to permit a specific diagnosis to be made. For example, rapid onset of proptosis with pyrexia suggests an inflammatory or infectious cause, whereas slow onset without pain is consistent with a benign tumour. Further investigations may include ultrasound or CT scanning to define tumours and identify swollen structures, and orbital biopsy may be required for histological confirmation prior to treatment, for example, rhabdomyosarcoma.

Important causes:

Developmental	Craniosynostoses (e.g. Crouzon's, Apert's syndromes – typical skull and face morphology
	Neurofibromatosis – orbital wall defects
	Cysts (e.g. dermoids)
Inflammatory	Pseudotumour – pain is prominent and differentiation from infection may not be easy
	Orbital cellulitis – as discussed under lid swelling
	Mucocele
Metabolic	Dysthyroid eye disease – older age group
Neoplastic	
Benign	Neurofibroma
	Optic nerve glioma
	Lacrimal gland pleomorphic adenoma
Malignant	*Primary* rhabdomyosarcoma
	Secondary neuroblastoma
	leukaemia
	lymphoma
Vascular	Cavernous haemangioma
	Arteriovenous malformation
	Carotid-cavernous fistula
	Retro-orbital haemorrhage (often traumatic)

The watering eye – epiphora

Although reflex tear production begins at birth, infants do not 'cry' tears until they are several weeks old. Clearly, excess tears can result from reflex *overproduction* induced by ocular surface irritation (corneal abrasion, foreign body, conjunctivitis), or from *obstruction* to nasolacrimal outflow, usually where the nasolacrimal duct enters the nose. The latter is the much more likely cause of tearing in children less than 1 year old. About 5% of babies have such an obstruction, but as 95% resolve spontaneously within a year, probing under anaesthetic is not generally performed unless recurrent infections develop. Simple measures usually consist of massage to the skin overlying the lacrimal sac, and topical antibiotics where conjunctivitis supervenes. Occasionally, blockage occurs at a more proximal site, as in congenital and acquired stenosis of the canaliculi and puncti, and presents a difficult therapeutic dilemma.

The red eye

Although an important and common problem, only a few of those aspects of the red eye pertinent to paediatric practice will be considered here, as this topic is well covered in many ophthalmic texts.

It is often possible even without a slit-lamp to distinguish the pattern of redness found in conjunctivitis from that induced by keratitis or uveitis. Knowledge of the visual acuity also helps, as conjunctivitis should not impair vision unless there is an associated keratitis.

Conjunctivitis

Infections – bacterial, viral or chlamydial – and allergies are all common causes of conjunctivitis, but certain features may help distinguish them. The pattern of redness in all is diffuse, and may be more pronounced in the fornices. This latter sign is important as conjunctival infection which increases towards the limbus signifies a corneal or intraocular problem.

Bacterial conjunctivitis

Bacterial conjunctivitis is almost always bilateral (although it may commence in one eye), with gritty discomfort and mucopurulent discharge. Treatment with topical antibiotics hastens recovery, particularly in the newborn, when *Neisseria gonococcus* acquired from the birth canal may cause a sight-threatening infection within the first few days. Systemic antibiotics are required in this condition.

Viral conjunctivitis

Viral conjunctivitis may be unilateral or bilateral and tends to produce a watery discharge. Slit-lamp examination reveals subconjunctival follicles. *Adenovirus* is highly contagious, and not surprisingly the most common type. Scrupulous hygiene will reduce transmission to relatives (and the examiner!), but as it is associated with an upper respiratory tract infection, droplet transmission can also occur. Although the conjunctivitis usually resolves spontaneously over a week or two, it is often accompanied by a characteristic keratitis which may cause blurring, photophobia or glare for many months. *Herpes simplex* virus type 1 (HSV) is often acquired for the first time during childhood, and this primary infection may cause eyelid vesicles and conjunctivitis (± keratitis). By contrast, *herpes zoster* infection (shingles) is rare in children, and would make one suspect immune compromise, for example, malignancy or HIV infection.

Chlamydial disease

Chlamydial disease is of two principal types. In endemic areas (hot, with very poor sanitation), recurrent infection with specific serotypes results in *trachoma*, a disease of conjunctival scarring leading to cicatricial entropion, corneal scarring and vascularization. Unfortunately most of these children never receive the treatment they need, and many go needlessly blind. Other serotypes are found in non-endemic areas such as Western Europe and USA, and these are acquired either from the birth canal in neonates, or from sexual contact later on. In neonates, this is a much less severe infection than gonococcal conjunctivitis. Antibiotics are used in all cases.

Allergic

As 10% of the population are atopic (prone to develop hay fever, asthma and eczema) and thus genetically predisposed to react to normally innocuous substances, for example, pollen, allergic conjunctivitis is extremely common. *Acute hay fever* is the commonest type with conjunctival chemosis watering and sneezing on exposure to grass pollens. When avoidance of the allergen is impossible, topical treatment to reduce the reaction can provide great relief. A more severe allergic reaction is *vernal keratoconjunctivitis* which affects especially boys, around the age of 5 years. Those with an atopic tendency are particularly prone. This condition is characterized by seasonal exacerbations and remissions which are not always confined to the spring and autumn. During the acute episode, the tarsal conjunctiva becomes swollen with giant papillae (palpebral type, *Figure 4.2*), and corneal plaques or ulcers (limbal type) may develop. In many cases the course of vernal keratoconjunctivitis lasts about 5 years, but it can persist into adult life. Topical treatment to reduce the inflammatory reaction, with steroids for exacerbations, can dramatically help an otherwise miserable condition. Sodium cromoglycate eyedrops can also be used and, as they do not have the side-effects of steroids, are preferable for prophylaxis and the control of mild episodes. The most serious hypersensitivity reaction, *Stevens–Johnson syndrome*, is fortunately rare. This is a systemic reaction provoked by certain infections and drugs and the child may be gravely ill. Conjunctival ulcers develop acutely, but the later cicatricial changes, as with trachoma, are much more visually devastating, and difficult to both prevent and treat.

Keratitis

In contrast to conjunctivitis, keratitis and uveitis cause redness which is maximal around the limbus. The appearance of a *bacterial* keratitis is of an intensely painful red eye with localized corneal clouding and, if severe, a hypopyon. Emergency hospital treatment with antibiotics is required, if corneal perforation ± endophthalmitis and possible loss of the eye are to be avoided.

The appearance of herpes simplex virus (HSV) epithelial keratitis with a dendritic

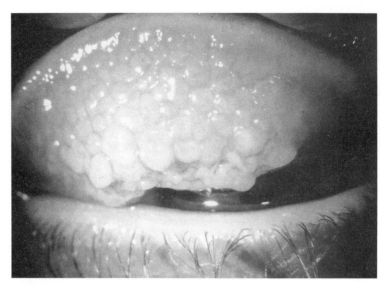

Figure 4.2. Tarsal conjunctival papillae in vernal conjunctivitis

ulcer is characteristic. Such lesions should heal without scarring, but if the stroma becomes involved then permanent damage may ensue. Steroids alone can dramatically worsen the situation and must be avoided, although they do have a place when used in conjunction with antiviral agents.

Uveitis

This is discussed under 'Disorders of the anterior visual pathway' below. Redness is often *not* a feature of uveitis in children.

Endophthalmitis

This is included here for the sake of completeness, but in routine clinical practice is rare, and even more so in children. Causes are bacterial, fungal and parasitic. The inflammatory signs are obvious and dramatic and urgent referral is mandatory if the eye is to be saved. Certain neoplastic conditions of childhood may present as a severely inflamed eye, including retinoblastoma and leukaemia.

Disorders of the anterior visual pathway

Cornea

Corneal abnormalities may be localized or diffuse. Whilst it might be expected that only lesions on or near the visual axis will affect vision, this is not always the case as the more peripherally placed lesion, such as a limbal dermoid, may also induce high degrees of astigmatism which in the paediatric age groups is strongly amblyogenic.

Corneal enlargement

The normal corneal diameter is 9.0–10.5 mm at birth, and reaches the adult value of 11.5 ± 0.5 mm within a few months.

MEGALOCORNEA

This condition is a non-progressive enlargement of the cornea which can be dominantly inherited and is not associated with raised intraocular pressure.

INFANTILE GLAUCOMA

Within the first 2 to 3 years of life, but not later, raised intraocular pressure can cause enlargement of the cornea and the globe known as buphthalmos or infantile/ congenital glaucoma (*Figure 4.3*). This is bilateral in 75% of cases, affects boys more than girls, and is inherited on a multifactorial basis. Primary infantile glaucoma is due to a maldevelopment of the anterior chamber angle and occurs in about 1:20 000 births. Glaucoma in childhood can be associated with other ocular or systemic abnormalities and it is important to consider this possibility. Ocular associations include aniridia and the so-called anterior chamber cleavage syndromes. Systemic conditions which may be associated with paediatric glaucoma are many and include Down's, Sturge–Weber (*Figure 4.4*), Marfan's and Lowe's syndromes, neuro-fibromatosis, homocystinuria and rubella embryopathy. It is important to remember that, as in the adult, secondary glaucoma can occur in trauma and retinoblastoma.

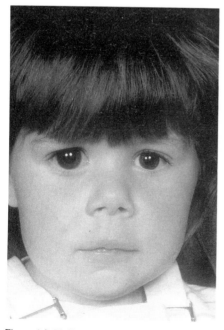

Figure 4.3. Unilateral infantile glaucoma

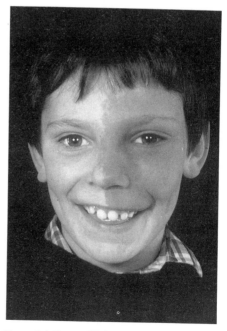

Figure 4.4. Sturge–Weber syndrome

By definition infantile glaucoma presents before the age of 1 year with photophobia, watery eyes, and blepharospasm. Surprisingly signs are often subtle and easily missed, but include unilateral or bilateral corneal enlargement, mild conjunctival injection, and corneal haze due to oedema. It is important to look for fine, slightly curved lines close to the visual axis of the cornea, and orientated just off the horizontal axis. Known as Haab's striae, these are breaks in Descemet's membrane. They also develop after traumatic forceps injury at birth, but in this latter instance they are vertically, and not horizontally directed. Vision may be reduced due to corneal oedema, but in infancy other symptoms and signs predominate and generally this passes unnoticed.

Immediate referral is essential if infantile glaucoma is suspected, for it is a potentially blinding condition. It is also pertinent to remember that many of the symptoms and signs of this uncommon condition are subtle and a high index of suspicion is needed.

Treatment is surgical. The infant is examined under anaesthesia and the following parameters are assessed: intraocular pressure, corneal diameter, gonioscopic evaluation of the anterior chamber angle, and optic disc. A variety of surgical procedures can be employed including goniotomy, trabeculotomy, and trabeculectomy. In infancy and early childhood before applanation slit-lamp tonometry can be performed, examinations under anaesthesia are required at few monthly intervals. Medical glaucoma therapy may also be required.

These patients require long-term follow-up and although visual acuity and field loss due to glaucoma can occur, other visually important sequelae also develop including refractive errors, particularly myopia, and amblyopia. Repeated refraction is mandatory to prevent unnecessary visual deficit.

Here we have only briefly considered primary infantile glaucoma. It is important to appreciate that the mode and time of presentation, and the management of the other glaucomas in childhood such as those associated with an ocular or systemic abnormality can be quite different, but cannot be dealt with here.

The photophobic child

Undue sensitivity to light is a symptom of inflammatory conditions of the anterior segment such as keratitis or corneal foreign body. One of the most important conditions is the corneal oedema of infantile glaucoma. Other causes include aniridia, albinism, cone disorders (achromatopsia and progressive cone dystrophy), and less frequently cataract.

From this wide range of conditions which are associated with photophobia it is obvious that the clinician must first, and speedily, identify that condition which requires urgent treatment such as glaucoma. Other causes also require full assessment, but the degree of urgency is less.

Small cornea/eye

Microcornea denotes a small cornea in an otherwise normally sized eye, whereas in microphthalmos the whole eye is reduced in size.

MICROPHTHALMOS

Relatively common occurring in about 1 : 2000 births. In its mildest form it is not associated with any visual deficit, however, at its most severe it presents as clinical anophthalmia, there only being a barely visible remnant of the eyeball. Between these two extremes visual function is variably affected. Microphthalmos can occur in isolation, or in association with other ocular or systemic anomalies. All modes of inheritance have been described, but 75% are sporadic. Many systemic abnormalities can be associated with microphthalmos such as chromosomal abnormalities, single gene disorders, congenital infections, including rubella, and conditions of unknown aetiology, for example, Goldenhar's syndrome. Ocular disorders can produce microphthalmos probably by two mechanisms, either by interfering with ocular growth as in persistent hyperplastic primary vitreous, or by globe shrinkage following infection.

NANOPHTHALMOS

This is a rare type of mild microphthalmos, but of particular interest to the optometrist, as the intraocular structures are slightly small but otherwise appear to be normal. Such patients have high hypermetropia and there is a high risk of angle-closure glaucoma in adult life.

Abnormalities of shape

KERATOCONUS

Strictly speaking this condition should always be called anterior keratoconus to differentiate it from the rare posterior keratoconus. This is an acquired condition usually presenting during adolescence. Usually, but not invariably bilateral, a degree of asymmetry is common. The aetiology of this condition is unknown but a small proportion are familial and the incidence is increased in atopy, vernal conjunctivitis, Marfan's and Down's syndromes. Keratoconus is also seen in conditions associated with eye poking such as Leber's amaurosis. Most patients present first to an optometrist either with frequent changes of refraction or a visual defect which cannot be corrected by spectacles. The first sign is probably an irregular retinoscopy reflex, but later fine vertical striae in the stroma at the apex of the cone can be seen, corneal nerves are prominent, and eventually the placido disc reflex is distorted. Ruptures in Descemet's membrane cause corneal oedema (hydrops) and those in Bowman's layer result in scarring.

Treatment consists of spectacle correction, but later on this may become inadequate, when rigid contact lenses are necessary. In a proportion of cases contact lenses cease to be effective and surgical treatment, either keratoplasty or epikeratophakia, should be considered.

Corneal opacification

LOCALIZED

Dermoid

This congenital lesion is a developmental anomaly in which tissues occur in an abnormal site and contain fibrous tissue, fat, sebaceous and sweat glands and hair. Dermoids are not rare and most commonly are located at the limbus (*Figure 4.5*), but they can be situated in the centre of the cornea and rarely extend into the deeper structures. Dermoids induce astigmatism (and consequently amblyopia) and

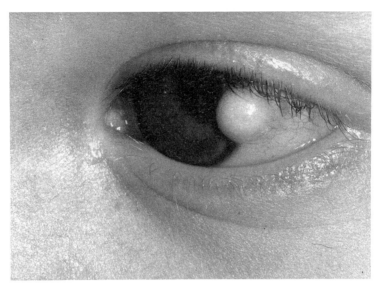

Figure 4.5. Limbal dermoid

although partial surgical removal is possible, this may not significantly improve the astigmatism. Most occur in isolation, but there can be ocular and systemic associations, such as aniridia and Goldenhar's syndrome.

Anterior chamber cleavage syndromes
Incorrectly named, these form a group of developmental conditions involving variously the cornea, anterior chamber drainage angle, iris and lens. The spectrum consists of central (Peter's anomaly), peripheral (Rieger's anomaly and sclerocornea), or a combination of both. Localized corneal central opacities are seen in Peter's anomaly, with strands from the iris to the edge of this opacity and commonly an anterior polar lens opacity. Glaucoma can develop in many of these conditions, in childhood or in adult life.

Inflammatory and traumatic
Almost too obvious to be mentioned, localized corneal scarring commonly results from keratitis and trauma.

DIFFUSE

The cloudy cornea is an important sign, not only for ophthalmic reasons but also as a guide to possible systemic disease. The first priority is to exclude the treatable infantile glaucoma, and to this end the distinguishing signs of this condition such as corneal enlargement must be sought.

Causes of diffuse corneal clouding are numerous and include the following:

Infantile glaucoma
See above.

Anterior chamber cleavage syndromes
As mentioned above these may cause localized or diffuse corneal opacification. The latter is a feature of sclerocornea.

Corneal dystrophies
Dystrophies are non-inflammatory, bilateral and symmetrical corneal lesions, and are inherited. Most do not cause symptoms until adolescence or later, but the following may be visible and cause symptoms (recurrent corneal erosions) from early childhood onwards: *Meesman's* and *Reis–Buckler dystrophies* and *recurrent corneal erosion*. Other dystrophies are often visible during childhood but do not adversely affect vision at this time. *Congenital corneal dystrophy* presents as diffuse clouding in infancy. Surprisingly, in view of the degree of cloudiness, vision is remarkably little affected.

Infections
These may be intrauterine such as rubella and syphilis, or acquired after birth as in herpes simplex, mumps keratitis and varicella.

Metabolic
Cystinosis, certain of the mucopolysaccharidoses, and the mucolipidoses can all cause corneal cloudiness. Although ocular examination of these children may aid in the diagnosis of such conditions, their systemic problems make it unlikely that they would present first to the community eye services.

Uvea

Developmental abnormalities

In this section only a few of the structural anomalies will be considered. The clinical assessment of the pupillary reactions will not be discussed.

PERSISTENT PUPILLARY MEMBRANE

Common, but rarely of significance to vision.

COLOBOMA

Failure of the fetal fissure to close in early embryonic life results in a defect along all or part of its length. Thus a coloboma may involve the iris alone (*Figure 4.6*) or spread back to involve the choroid, overlying retina and optic nerve (*Figure 4.7*). The iris coloboma has a characteristic 'keyhole' defect usually in the inferior nasal portion of the iris and *per se* has no effect on vision. A choroidal coloboma can vary in extent from a small isolated defect in the inferior fundus with no adverse effect on vision, to one involving the optic disc and macula, in which case vision is obviously severely reduced. The retina overlying the coloboma may be either thin or absent, and retinal detachment can occur. It is important to be aware of the many possible ocular and systemic associations of colobomas. They may be dominantly inherited.

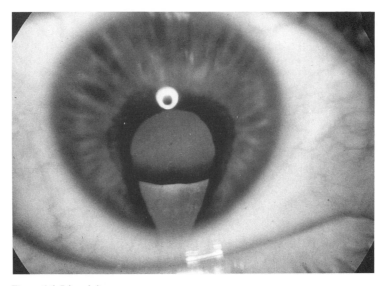

Figure 4.6. Iris coloboma

ANIRIDIA

A rare congenital disorder, either dominantly inherited or sporadic, in which the iris fails to develop. Other associated ocular anomalies are common: corneal vascularization, cataract, foveal hypoplasia and glaucoma. Vision is subnormal and patients have nystagmus. Sporadic cases can be associated with a renal tumour (Wilm's tumour) and regular abdominal ultrasound screening is required throughout early childhood to exclude this. Isolated cases may also have chromosomal abnormalities and mental retardation.

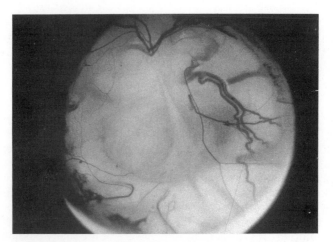

Figure 4.7. Coloboma of the optic disc

RIEGER'S ANOMALY

One of the so-called anterior chamber cleavage syndromes and characterized by iris hypoplasia, correctopia, polycoria and posterior embryotoxon. Peripheral corneal and minor lens opacities are common. Sometimes, in addition to these ocular changes, there are systemic features which include facial and dental abnormalities. The combination of Rieger's ocular anomaly and systemic abnormalities is known as Rieger's syndrome. Both the ocular anomaly and the syndrome are dominantly inherited. Glaucoma is frequent and can develop at any time of life, consequently these patients require long-term surveillance.

Uveitis

Anterior uveitis

This term describes an inflammatory response primarily of the iris (iritis) or iris and ciliary body (iridocyclitis). In these conditions compromised uveal blood vessels permit inflammatory products to enter the aqueous and to a lesser extent the posterior chamber and vitreous cavity. Although in adults uveitis is often characterized by pain, photophobia and redness, these symptoms are less frequent, or even absent, in children. Vision may be reduced by a number of mechanisms, either related directly to the inflammation or due to its long-term consequences, such as cataract or glaucoma.

JUVENILE CHRONIC ARTHRITIS

This form of arthritis affects children only and has three main subtypes. Whilst uveitis can occur in all three, it is most common in the pauciarticular group.

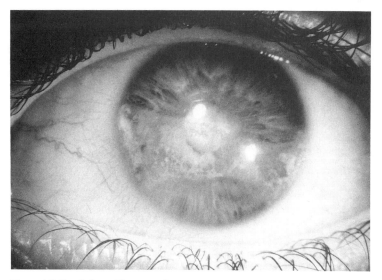

Figure 4.8. Band-shaped keratopathy in a case of chronic anterior uveitis. Note also posterior synechiae and cataract

Pauciarticular juvenile chronic arthritis affects up to four joints and about 20% of this group develop uveitis. Those most at risk of developing these ocular complications are girls with antinuclear antibody in their blood. The uveitis characteristically does not induce inflammatory symptoms, thus the eye is not red or painful and the uveitis may have existed for some time before presentation, by which time there can be reduced vision due to cataract formation. The uveitis is usually bilateral and whilst it can be mild and short lived it may be more severe with the formation of posterior synechiae, cataract and secondary glaucoma. Band-shaped keratopathy (*Figure 4.8*) is common if the uveitis is chronic and is almost diagnostic of this condition in childhood. Due to the absence of symptoms regular hospital screening is advised for all cases of juvenile chronic arthritis.

IDIOPATHIC ANTERIOR UVEITIS

Two-thirds of patients with anterior uveitis will have no identifiable underlying abnormality, although viral (varicella and herpes simplex) and bacterial infections may have an aetiological role particularly in early childhood. More important, the clinician needs to appreciate that there are several conditions which can masquerade as endogenous uveitis including *retinoblastoma*, *intraocular foreign bodies* and *acute leukaemia*.

KERATOUVEITIS

Hardly necessary as a separate heading as any acute keratitis usually induces a secondary uveitis. The most common cause is herpes simplex infection and the diagnosis is made from the typical corneal appearance. Treatment is directed to the underlying cause, and mydriatics and sometimes topical steroids are also required.

Intermediate uveitis

Formerly known as pars planitis or chronic cyclitis, this type of uveitis is not uncommon in childhood. As with many other forms in this age group, the eye is white. Posterior synechiae are characteristically absent and slit-lamp examination of the anterior chamber reveals little activity. Cells are present in the vitreous (sometimes causing floaters) and inflammatory cellular 'snowbanking' can be seen in the far periphery of the fundus if the pupil is sufficiently well dilated. Macular oedema and disc swelling may occur, and if associated with visual impairment, are an indication for treatment with either periocular or systemic steroids. In the absence of these sight-threatening features, no treatment is indicated, and the outlook is generally favourable.

Posterior uveitis

Presenting symptoms are similar to those of intermediate uveitis. Posterior uveitis (*Figure 4.9*) may be present at birth or more rarely develop during childhood.

TOXOPLASMOSIS

The protozoa *Toxoplasma gondii* may cross to the fetus if the mother is infected during pregnancy. The congenital infection thus produced may affect many systems of the body including the CNS (microcephaly, mental retardation) and eye

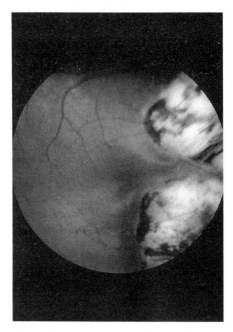

Figure 4.9. Inactive chorioretinal scars due to
congenital infection

(chorioretinitis). *Recurrent retinochoroiditis* may occur from reactivation of a
congenital lesion (never acquired) in the second, third and fourth decades of life.
This generally affects only one eye and the activity is adjacent to an old scar. Treatment with systemic steroids and sometimes antimicrobials is controversial and only
employed if the fovea is threatened.

TOXOCARIASIS

Due to an infestation by the roundworm *Toxocara catis* or *canis* and acquired by
ingestion, in early childhood, of contaminated soil or food. Ocular toxocariasis
presents as either a focal retinochoroidal lesion around the posterior pole, retinal
periphery, or as an endophthalmitis. It is clearly important that retinoblastoma is
excluded.

OTHER TYPES

Posterior uveitis may result from a number of viruses including herpes simplex,
herpes zoster, cytomegalovirus and as an opportunistic infection by any of these in
acquired immune deficiency syndrome (AIDS). Fungal infections may develop in
severely debilitated children.

Lens

The lens may become cataractous or displaced from its normal position. It is
important to appreciate that the underlying cause may have significant or even life-

threatening consequences. Cataract and lens subluxation are potent amblyogenic factors, which need to be dealt with speedily if this is to be prevented or ameliorated, and good vision achieved.

Cataract

Cataract is opacification of the lens and may result from a large variety of causes. In the paediatric age group cataract may be congenital or acquired, depending on the aetiology.

AETIOLOGY

Cataract as isolated anomaly
About 50% of cases, either sporadic or inherited, of which the dominant mode is the most common.

Cataract with ocular conditions
These are multitudinous and include: developmental anomalies (e.g. persistent hyperplastic primary vitreous, microphthalmos, aniridia, anterior cleavage syndromes, coloboma), intraocular tumours, ocular inflammations (e.g. juvenile chronic arthritis, retinopathy of prematurity), trauma and the retinal dystrophies (e.g. retinitis pigmentosa).

Cataract with systemic conditions
Too numerous, eponymous and bewildering to memorize, the most simple approach is to consider the various systems associated with cataract formation. These include: *intrauterine infection* (e.g. rubella, cytomegalovirus), *metabolic disorders* (e.g. disorders of galactose metabolism, hypocalcaemia, diabetes mellitus, Wilson's disease), *chromosomal disorders* (Down's and Turner's syndromes), *Craniofacial syndromes* (e.g. Hallerman–Streiff, Crouzon's and Rubinstein–Taybi syndromes), *skeletal disorders* (e.g. Conradi–Hunermann syndrome), *muscle disease* (myotonic dystrophy), *central nervous system disorders* (e.g. Sjögren–Larsson and Zellweger's syndromes), *renal disease* (e.g. Lowe's syndrome) and *dermatological conditions* (e.g. atopic dermatitis, Cockayne's syndrome).

MORPHOLOGY

Polar cataract
(1) *Anterior*. These are quite common (*Figure 4.10*) and rarely affect vision although they can induce a refractive error, and should therefore be followed for this reason.
(2) *Posterior*. Usually associated with a persistent hyaloid remnant, depending on size, this opacity may affect vision.

Zonular cataract
Any opacity confined to one region of the lens:

(1) *Lamellar*. White dots around the nucleus and surrounded by riders (*Figure 4.11*). Vision variably affected.
(2) *Nuclear*. Involve embryonic nucleus, vision variably affected.

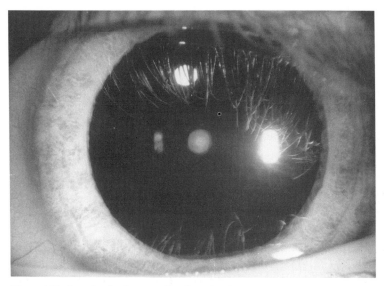

Figure 4.10. Anterior dot lens opacity of no visual consequence

(3) *Sutural.* Upright and inverted Ys. Do not affect vision.
(4) *Other types.* Coralliform, blue dot, snowflake, etc.

Total cataract
Indicating that the cataract involves the whole of the lens substance.

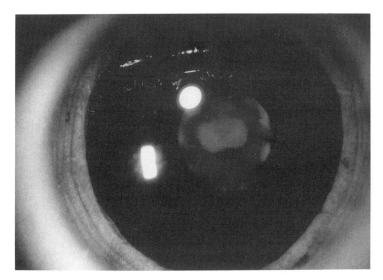

Figure 4.11. Lamellar cataract

MANAGEMENT

This is one of the most challenging aspects of paediatric ophthalmology, but space does not permit this to be discussed in detail here. Suffice it to say that even determining which cataract requires removal is not straightforward.

Investigation
(1) Exclude serious underlying ocular (e.g. retinoblastoma) or systemic pathology. Every child needs a full ophthalmic and, many, a paediatric assessment.
(2) Measure vision. Most important, but not simple.

Treatment
(1) *Surgery*. Not all cataracts need to be removed (a topic which cannot be considered here), but once it has been decided that surgery is indicated, in childhood because of the danger of amblyopia, this should be undertaken as soon as possible (for a neonate this would mean within a few days of life).
(2) *Aphakic correction*. Generally, *intraocular lens implants* are not used in children and consequently currently aphakic correction consists of *contact lenses* (usually < 18 months, or for the older child, or for the unilateral aphake), *spectacles* (for the toddler who has worn contact lenses and then become 'intolerant' around 18 months – a common occurrence), and *epikeratophakia* (this may be used in the future for the 18 month old 'intolerant' of contact lenses).
(3) *Amblyopia therapy*. Undoubtedly the major issue in the treatment of cataracts in the paediatric age group. Ensuring that the aphakic correction is *correct* and is *worn* by the infant is by far the greatest challenge for parent and surgeon/optometrist. It is important that the lens power suited to the needs of the infant or child is prescribed – remember the sphere of interest of the young infant is not 6 m, but relatively close to. Occlusion therapy is imperative for the unilateral case, but however enthusiastically performed a degree of amblyopia is the rule. Even if bilateral surgery is undertaken early on, a degree of amblyopia often results. Of course none of these issues negate the need for surgery, as even a degree of amblyopia is preferable to the untreated alternative.

Leucocoria

One of the most important ocular findings of infancy and childhood and one requiring urgent differential diagnosis is leucocoria – the white pupil. Many of these conditions are serious to sight and a few are life threatening.

All cases of leucocoria must be referred promptly for detailed investigation. The following is an incomplete list of conditions:

Tumours
Retinoblastoma

Malformations
Astrocytoma of the retina
Persistent hyperplastic primary vitreous (PHPV)
Coloboma
Myelinated nerve fibres
Retinal folds

Inherited
Familial exudative vitreoretinopathy
Incontinentia pigmenti
Retinal dysplasia – Norrie's disease, lissencephaly

Inflammations
Toxocara
Toxoplasmosis
Cytomegalovirus
Endophthalmitis

Miscellaneous
Cataract
Coat's disease
Retinopathy of prematurity (ROP)
Vitreous haemorrhage

Cataract and postinflammatory membranes must necessarily be included but are obviously straightforward to identify by routine ophthalmic examination, whilst others may present a diagnostic dilemma requiring further investigation.

Ectopia lentis

The ectopic lens may be either subluxated (*Figure 4.12*) or fully dislocated. Not common in everyday practice, it is simple to diagnose if the lens edge is visible in the pupillary aperture, or if iridodonesis is observed. However, partial ectopia can be easily missed and the clinician should be alerted to this possibility when the refractive state changes seemingly inappropriately, particularly the cylindrical component, and also anterior chamber depth varies in its different regions.

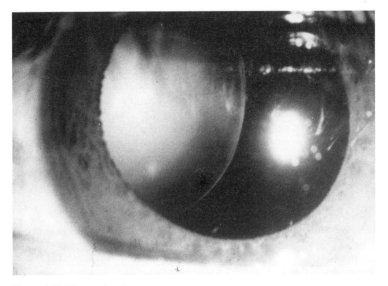

Figure 4.12. Ectopia lentis

As with so many conditions of childhood, early and correct diagnosis is important not only for ocular reasons but for the general well-being of the child. Perhaps the most obvious example is the homocystinuria in which the correct diagnosis may prevent both the progressive dislocation of the lens and certain of the serious CNS complications of this condition. Furthermore, correct diagnosis is mandatory before undertaking any surgical procedure, for without the appropriate prophylactic measures serious complications – even death – can occur.

On a practical point, although in certain conditions the lens tends to subluxate in a particular direction, this must not be used as confirmation of a definitive diagnosis as there is considerable individual variation.

AETIOLOGY

Ectopia lentis as an isolated anomaly
(1) *Simple congenital ectopia lentis.* A relatively common cause of congenital ectopia and inherited as a dominant trait.
(2) *Ectopia lentis with other ocular abnormalities.* These include spherophakia, ectopia lentis et pupillae, cataract, aniridia, infantile glaucoma, coloboma, microphthalmos, etc.

Ectopia lentis with systemic conditions
(1) *Marfan's syndrome.* A condition affecting the connective tissue of many parts of the body including the eye, cardiovascular and skeletal systems. Affected individuals are characteristically tall, with long digits, and cardiac problems. There is no diagnostic test and under certain circumstances the diagnosis of Marfan's is difficult. The lens tends to be dislocated congenitally and moves upwards. Myopia, glaucoma and retinal detachment may all occur.
(2) *Homocystinuria.* Superficially this condition may resemble Marfan's syndrome, but the joints are less mobile. Inherited as an autosomal recessive condition and due to a deficiency of the enzyme cystathione β-synthetase, these individuals excrete abnormal amounts of homocystine in the urine – the diagnostic test. These patients have a tendency to develop thromboses, especially prone to develop after surgery unless the appropriate precautions are taken. Other features include mental retardation, joint stiffness, and fair hair. Many of the effects of this condition can be prevented, or reduced by the administration of pyridoxine. The lens in homocystinuria subluxates progressively, usually inferonasally, but this is less frequent with pyridoxine treatment.
(3) *Weill–Marchesani syndrome.* Inherited as an autosomal recessive condition these patients are of short stature with short stubby fingers and toes. The lens is spherophakic and narrow angle glaucoma is common.
(4) *Other conditions.* These include Ehlers–Danlos syndrome, skeletal disorders (e.g. Crouzon's and Apert's syndromes) and sulphite oxidase deficiency.

MANAGEMENT OF ECTOPIA LENTIS

This cannot be considered here in detail. Whilst the ectopic lens can be removed surgically, this is a procedure not without difficulty and conservative measures are usually employed first. Regarding optical correction, both phakic and aphakic portions of the visual axis should be used if relevant, and in children, particular attention paid to optimizing near vision.

Vitreoretinal disorders

As there is so much clinical overlap, where relevant, disorders of the vitreous and retina will be considered together.

Vitreous

Developmental anomalies of the vitreous

PERSISTENT HYPERPLASTIC PRIMARY VITREOUS (PHPV)

In early embryonic life the first vitreous to be formed, the primary vitreous, is a vascularized structure which is normally replaced by the secondary, avascular vitreous before birth. Occasionally, parts of this primary vitreous fail to regress, leading to a spectrum of anomalies under the term persistent hyperplastic primary vitreous (PHPV).

Anterior PHPV
In its most severe form the eye is microphthalmic and the vitreous cavity is filled by a vascularized retrolental mass. Recurrent vitreous haemorrhage, cataract and secondary glaucoma may all occur. Early surgical treatment by vitrectomy improves the visual outlook and may prevent some of these complications. PHPV is one of the conditions presenting as *leucocoria* in infancy.

Posterior PHPV
In this form the white vitreous remnant is posteriorly located and may present as a lesion on the retinal surface in the macular region or as a retinal fold. It needs to be differentiated from retinoblastoma, toxocariasis and retinopathy of prematurity.

Vitreous haemorrhage

INFANCY

Retinal haemorrhages are a frequent association of normal birth and sometimes these extend into the vitreous. Usually these have resolved by about 6–8 weeks of age and if found after this time the possibility of non-accidental injury must be considered. Clearly, if the latter is suspected the situation must be handled most diplomatically.

CHILDHOOD

In the absence of trauma, vitreous haemorrhage is rare in children. It is probably never the sole diagnosis but always a feature of underlying pathology, such as retinal detachment, tumour, retinopathy of prematurity or PHPV. If the fundus cannot be examined, ultrasound examination is mandatory to enable pathology of the posterior portion of the eye to be excluded.

Vitreous inflammation

A feature of intermediate and other forms of posterior uveitis, and has already been considered.

Retina

Developmental anomalies

MYELINATED NERVE FIBRES

Perhaps the most commonly seen congenital retinal anomaly. Normally, myelination of the retinal nerves ceases at the optic disc, but on occasion patches of myelinated fibres within the fundus are seen (*Figure 4.13*). Sometimes connected to the disc, the appearance is characteristic – a spray of white, with a fibrillated margin, which obscures vessels.

RETINAL PIGMENT EPITHELIAL CHANGES

Hypertrophy, clumping and hyperplasia of the retinal pigment epithelium are all congenital anomalies which are not infrequently seen in practice, appearing either as a single pigmented lesion or as the well-known multiple areas of pigmentation: 'bear track'. Of no visual consequence, they need to be differentiated, particularly in adult life, from choroidal naevi and melanoma.

ASTROCYTIC HAMARTOMA

These are white lesions, often multiple, overlying retinal vessels. Almost flat in early childhood, they become more bulky with time (*Figure 4.14*) and can be confused with retinoblastoma. Astrocytic hamartoma or retinal phakoma can occur as an isolated

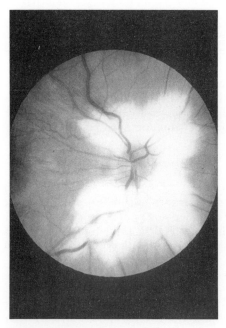

Figure 4.13. Myelinated nerve fibres

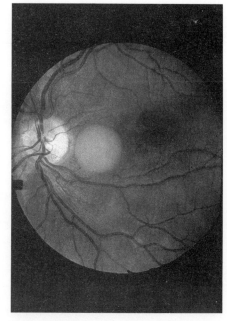

Figure 4.14. Astrocytic hamartoma

anomaly, but is more likely to be associated with tuberose sclerosis or neurofibromatosis. As both conditions have important and widespread consequences the identification of such a lesion requires referral.

Ocular tumours

Benign tumours or malformations in the retina are all extremely rare, but one of the most frequently observed is the astrocytic hamartoma of tuberose sclerosis, indeed this may be observed as an incidental finding during routine clinical examination.

RETINOBLASTOMA

Although rare, retinoblastoma is the commonest intraocular tumour of childhood, with an incidence of around 1 : 20 000 births. There is no sexual predilection, and it may be sporadic, inherited as an autosomal dominant trait, or as part of the chromosomal 13 deletion. About 40% are inherited, and this includes all bilateral cases. Thus even in the absence of a positive family history bilateral disease heralds the onset of a new mutation. Inherited tumours are often bilateral and multifocal. Most children present before the age of 3 years with strabismus, visual loss, pain or hyphaema, though the best known form of presentation is the white pupil (*leucocoria*). Investigation involves excluding other conditions presenting with leucocoria, and usually includes ocular ultrasound, full paediatric assessment and CT scanning. Treatment, depending on the features of the individual case, is by radiotherapy, photocoagulation, chemotherapy, and/or enucleation of the eye. The success rate is around 80%, but a proportion develop tumours remote from the eye in early adult life.

OTHER OCULAR TUMOURS

Primary
These are exceptionally rare but include uveal melanoma and medulloepithelioma.

Secondary
This may occur in leukaemia, neuroblastoma, histiocytosis, lymphoma and in others even less frequently.

Retinopathy of prematurity

Formerly known as retrolental fibroplasia (RLF), retinopathy of prematurity (ROP) is a potentially blinding condition affecting, almost exclusively, infants born prematurely.

As ROP only affects immature retinal blood vessels it cannot develop after this structure is fully vascularized, soon after term. In the early 1950s it was discovered that oxygen therapy was an important factor in the development of this condition, but it is now known that there is more to its pathogenesis as, despite meticulous care and oxygen monitoring, ROP still occurs and at present is not entirely preventable. Other important risk factors are the degree of immaturity (low birth weight or gestational age), and factors related to neonatal illness, particularly adverse neurological events.

Its clinical course is divided into acute and cicatricial phases, both staged according to a new internationally agreed classification system:

Acute ROP
This develops in the neonatal period at the junction of the vascularized and peripheral non-vascularized retina. Characteristically, but not exclusively, acute retinopathy involves the temporal periphery of the retina. There are five stages:

Stage 1 – demarcation line, the accumulation of mesenchymal cellular precursors of retinal vessels.
Stage 2 – ridge, the demarcation line now extends out of the plane of the retina.
Stage 3 – ridge with frank neovascularization. New vessels are now visible.
Stage 4 – retinal detachment, subtotal.
Stage 5 – retinal detachment, total.

All acute stages 1 and 2 undergo spontaneous resolution, but some infants with stage 3 and all with stages 4 and 5 are less fortunate and proceed to develop cicatricial ROP.

Cicatricial ROP
Grade 1 – small mass of opaque tissue in the periphery of the fundus, without retinal detachment.
Grade 2 – larger peripheral mass, with localized detachment; some retinal traction may be present.
Grade 3 – large mass incorporating a traction retinal fold to the optic disc.
Grade 4 – retrolental tissue covering part of the pupil.
Grade 5 – retrolental tissue covering the entire pupil.

The correlation of ophthalmoscopic findings and visual function can be difficult, but in general grade 1 cicatricial ROP does not significantly affect vision whereas the functional consequences of the more advanced grades become increasingly severe.

This classification has recently been modified and cicatricial disease is also now known as regressed ROP, however within the context of this chapter this offers no advantage over the scheme quoted above and has not been quoted here.

Although acute ROP does not fall into the domain of the optometrist in everyday practice, cicatricial disease does, for the patient, of any age, may present with myopia (a common sequel of severe acute ROP), a retinal fold, retinal detachment, or at its most severe, as leucocoria. Probably the most commonly encountered mode of presentation in routine practice is the myopic patient with so-called 'dragging' of the optic disc (*Figure 4.15*). The term 'dragging' is used to denote vessels which are drawn towards the periphery (usually temporal), so that the angle between the major vascular arcade is narrowed, or even drawn into a fold. The central retina can be displaced by this process causing macular ectopia and a pseudodivergent strabismus. It is also important to recall that this is a possible cause of retinal detachment. To conclude, although most infants with acute ROP undergo complete resolution, if more severe it can lead to sequelae, ranging in severity from the visually insignificant to total blindness.

OPHTHALMIC SEQUELAE OF PREMATURITY

Infants born prematurely can suffer other visual pathway defects besides ROP.

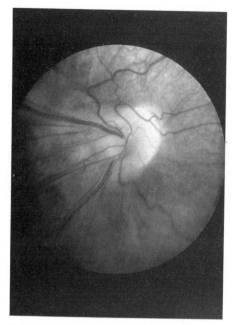

Figure 4.15. Dragged optic disc due to cicatricial retinopathy of prematurity

These are the result of both ocular and neurological insults suffered in the perinatal period. These include mildly reduced acuity, refractive errors (particularly myopia), optic atrophy and ocular movement disorders. The latter include strabismus (11–20%) for those with birthweights under 1500 g, gaze and saccadic palsies, and nystagmus.

Retinal detachment

Separation of the retina from the retinal pigment epithelium is far less common in childhood than in adulthood. A traumatic break in the retina accounts for most cases (rhegmatogenous), but vitreoretinal traction (e.g. ROP) or exudation of fluid (e.g. Coat's disease) may be responsible. Half of all traumatic cases occur at the ora serrata (dialysis), but are surgically repaired similar to breaks elsewhere. Treatment of non-rhegmatogenous detachment, or the giant tears associated with the very high myopia of Stickler's syndrome, is more complex.

Hereditary retinal disorders

Albinism

In this condition there is a congenital defect of the pigment epithelium of the eye with hypopigmentation of the iris and retina. There are various clinical types. The *oculocutaneous* types in which skin and eye are involved and are either tyrosinase positive or negative, depending on the presence of this enzyme in the skin and hair bulb. These two forms are inherited as autosomal recessive traits and can be distinguished clinically as without the enzyme tyrosinase, the hair remains white throughout life and vision is poor. In contrast, the hair of tyrosinase-positive patients darkens with age and the vision is less severely affected. The *ocular* type is confined to the eye and being X linked affects only males. Other rare types will not be considered here.

In albinism the fundus and iris are hypopigmented, the fovea hypoplastic with absence of the foveal reflex, and there is almost total decussation of optic nerve fibres at the chiasm (normal about 60%) which can be detected by visual evoked potential. Clinically patients with albinism are photosensitive, have reduced acuity, nystagmus, ametropia often with astigmatism, and commonly strabismus. It must be emphasized that, although clinical intuition would have most of us believe otherwise, albinism can be a difficult diagnosis to make. It is essential that every patient with nystagmus is examined carefully by slit-lamp biomicroscopy for iris transillumination and the fundus is scrutinized for the foveal reflex. Albinism has a non-progressive clinical course.

Refractive correction may help, but be warned, even the child with a large astigmatic error may not find the correction of sufficient benefit to warrant the wearing of spectacles. Despite reduced distance acuity, near vision is usually excellent. Tints are often a great help.

Cone disorders

ROD MONOCHROMATISM

In this rare condition, also known as achromatopsia, cones are either totally or partially absent, consequently acuity is reduced (around 3–6/60), colour vision defective and visual function is particularly poor under photopic conditions. Inheritance is via an autosomal recessive trait except for a rare incomplete form which is X linked. The classic mode of presentation is a photosensitive infant with poor vision and nystagmus who prefers scotopic to photopic conditions. At this stage the differential diagnosis includes: infantile glaucoma, inflammation of the anterior segment, such as keratitis, and albinism. Later in childhood the reduced acuity and defective colour vision become even more obvious.

Abnormal ocular findings are often absent early on, although later in life subtle pigmentary macular stippling may be observed. Not surprisingly, before colour vision can be tested, the diagnosis of achromatopsia is difficult and although it may be suspected on clinical grounds, it can only be confirmed by electroretinography (ERG). The ERG is present at 2 Hz (a test of rod and cone function), but absent at 30 Hz (cone function only). Except for the X linked form in which myopia is the rule, children with achromatopsia are often hypermetropic (as in Leber's amaurosis) and, whilst this can diminish with age, astigmatic errors often subsequently develop.

Visual functions in achromatopsia are stationary. These patients can be helped considerably by correction of any refractive error, particularly the prescription of tints (even side shields may be required in early childhood, when the photosensitivity is particularly troublesome), and low vision aids for close work (N5 can often be achieved with help).

PROGRESSIVE CONE DYSTROPHY

This rare disorder is either sporadic, dominantly or recessively inherited and causes reduced acuity commencing in childhood. Unlike achromatopsia the clinical course of this conditions is, as the name implies, progressive. Changes at the macula become increasingly obvious. As with all retinal dystrophies, electrophysiological investigations are helpful, and in many instances, mandatory in establishing the diagnosis.

Pigmentary retinopathies

A group of progressive hereditary disorders which primarily affect both retinal photoreceptor and pigment epithelial function. As the alternative term rod-cone dystrophy implies, both types of receptors are involved, though rod dysfunction predominates. The ophthalmic variants and systemic associations are a multitude and most confusing to the clinician in general ophthalmic or optometric practice who only rarely encounters such a patient. Here it is neither possible nor appropriate to discuss all pigmentary retinopathies, for this the reader is directed to larger texts.

The first symptom of all rod disorders is nightblindness and whilst this symptom is easily elicited in the adult it is not reported by an affected child who is not at all surprised that vision is severely reduced at night.

INVESTIGATION OF THE PIGMENTARY RETINOPATHIES

The associations listed below offer important guides to which systemic investigations are appropriate in an individual child. However it is important to remember that in childhood, despite a severe visual deficit, ophthalmic signs are commonly either absent or minimal, and easily missed. Bearing in mind the difficulty of ophthalmic examination in some infants and children, particularly if mentally retarded, the clinician must have a high index of suspicion. Examination techniques are covered elsewhere in this book, but it must be emphasized that for most of these conditions a precise diagnosis can only be made following electrophysiological investigations. In childhood these consist of an electroretinogram (ERG) (ensuring that rod and cone functions are tested individually), visually evoked potential (VEP), and for the older child (about 7–8 years) an electro-oculogram (EOG). Details of many of these tests are contained in Chapter 17.

RETINITIS PIGMENTOSA

This is the best known pigmentary retinopathy, and should be reserved for cases of unknown aetiology, with no non-ocular associations (except Usher's syndrome). Several inheritance patterns exist of these progressive disorders of which the autosomal recessive and X linked forms can present in childhood and progress rapidly to blindness in early adult life. Autosomal dominant retinitis pigmentosa (RP) presents later in life and visual function sometimes can be retained for many years, even into the sixth decade.

Nightblindness is the first symptom. The visual field gradually becomes severely constricted. Acuity may be preserved even in the presence of a tubular field, but is eventually affected by cataract, macular changes, or the RP process. Ophthalmoscopic signs include the classical bone-spicule pigmentation (a relatively late feature), vessel attenuation and later disc pallor. Complications include cataract and macular oedema. Electrodiagnostic tests are employed in establishing the diagnosis, both EOG and ERG are reduced. These tests are also often, but unfortunately not always, helpful in the screening of female carriers of X linked disease, who can also exhibit minimal or no clinical signs.

Although retinitis pigmentosa is basically untreatable, refraction is essential, as many of these patients are myopic. The other remediable aspects of the disease, namely cataract and macular oedema, are late complications and thus not necessary before adulthood.

PIGMENTARY RETINOPATHY WITH SYSTEMIC INVOLVEMENT

An important aspect of management is the exclusion or diagnosis of the multitude of other conditions which may present with pigmentary retinopathy. Often loosely called RP, the term pigmentary retinopathy is preferred as they often bear little resemblance to classical retinitis pigmentosa. Their recognition often requires a high index of suspicion, but in view of the serious problems which may arise if untreated, full ophthalmic and paediatric assessment is mandatory. The list of conditions is vast and only a few of the most important are mentioned in order to give the reader a feel for the range of possible associations:

Deafness
These associations are many of which the best known is Usher's syndrome, an autosomal recessive condition with the classical RP retinal appearance. Others include: Alstrom's, Refsum's and Alport's syndromes, Leber's amaurosis, mitochondrial cytopathy, etc.

Endocrine dysfunction
Diabetes mellitus occurs in Alstrom's syndrome or mitochondrial cytopathy.

Mental retardation
In the Laurence–Moon–Bardet–Biedl syndrome a retinal dystrophy is associated with mental retardation, obesity, renal failure, genital hypoplasia and extra digits. Mental retardation is also a feature of a number of childhood retinal disorders including Batten's disease and Cockayne's syndrome.

Metabolic
Refsum's disease – rare, with severe neurological complications including ataxia and deafness. Its recognition is essential, as a phytanic acid free high-calorie diet can prevent both neurological and visual deterioration.
Abetalipoproteinaemia – a disorder of lipoprotein metabolism, and like Refsum's an autosomal recessive condition, in which the progressive retinal dystrophy and neurological complications can be prevented by treatment, in this case with vitamins E and A.
Mucopolysaccharidoses – a group of conditions in which mucopolysaccharides accumulate in many tissues of the body. Corneal clouding develops in some of these and a pigmentary retinopathy in most.

Heart block
One of the most important aspects of mitochondrial cytopathy, a condition in which ptosis, progressive external ophthalmoplegia, heart block, short stature, renal problems, etc. are associated. The pigmentary retinopathy is quite subtle and unlike retinitis pigmentosa in its early stages.

Ataxia
Already mentioned in association with abetalipoproteinaemia and Refsum's sydrome, ataxia is also a feature of other neurological disorders such as olivopontocerebellar atrophy.

Juvenile Batten's disease
A most serious association, children present between 4 and 8 years with progressive visual failure and behavioural problems. The course is one of neurological regression and eventual death. The earliest ophthalmic signs are a subtle bull's eye maculopathy and later optic atrophy and retinal pigmentation.

LEBER'S CONGENITAL AMAUROSIS

A well-known cause of congenital blindness and not to be confused with Leber's optic atrophy. Affected infants present with very poor vision (often blind) and nystagmus within the first few months of life. Inheritance is via an autosomal recessive trait. Fundal findings are frequently absent initially, but retinal pigmentary stippling, vessel attenuation and optic atrophy develop later. High hyperopia is common. The diagnosis rests on finding an unrecordable or severely reduced ERG, and this can be performed in even the youngest of children. Eye poking is common but not pathognomonic for this condition as it is seen in many causes of blindness where the cause lies in the anterior visual pathway itself (i.e. it is not a feature of cortical visual impairment). Although many infants with Leber's amaurosis have no systemic abnormalities, the range of possible associations is wide and includes mental retardation, renal, cardiac abnormalities and eye movement disorders.

OTHER PIGMENTARY RETINOPATHIES

Retinal pigmentation can also develop in many other conditions such as: following trauma, congenital infections (rubella, herpes simplex and varicella), previous retinal problems (retinopathy of prematurity or retinal detachment) and certain medications.

Macular disorders

In routine clinical practice these are extremely rare, and whilst it is virtually impossible to remember the names of all individual conditions, think of a macular disorder when confronted with a child with poor vision and what appears to be a normal ophthalmoscopic appearance. As with so many paediatric ophthalmic conditions, signs are either absent or subtle and a high index of suspicion is required.

STARGARDT'S DISEASE

Characterized by progressive and symmetrical atrophy of the macula, this autosomal recessive disease may start in adolescence. Despite loss of central vision and colour defects, the fundus is often initially normal and these patients are often thought to be hysterical. With time the so-called 'bull's eye' develops at both maculae, often accompanied by retinal flecks around the posterior pole. Progression of visual deterioration tends to be similar for individuals of the same pedigree, but ultimately

6/60 vision results. Electrodiagnostic tests are not always abnormal early on, but fluorescein angiographic changes, which predate fundal changes, may be diagnostic.

BEST'S DISEASE

Another rare familial disorder (autosomal dominant), Best's disease or *vitelliform dystrophy* begins in childhood and passes through a number of aptly named clinical stages. The initial lesion has the appearance of an egg yolk at the macula, and may remain stationary for many years, with surprisingly little visual impairment (e.g. 6/9). During adolescence, the cyst takes on a 'scrambled egg' appearance with further visual loss, and sometimes appears like a 'pseudohypopyon'. Eventually, rupture of the lesion leads to atrophy and further loss of vision. A grossly abnormal EOG with a normal ERG is virtually diagnostic even in the preclinical stage, and is also valuable in screening family members.

X-LINKED RETINOSCHISIS

Although rare, this condition, which affects only boys, is mentioned because it should be considered in a young male with reduced vision for no apparent cause. When examined critically the macula contains microcysts and many also have peripheral retinoschisis.

OTHER MACULAR DISORDERS

These include the already mentioned cone abnormalities, dystrophies of the pigment epithelium and inner retina and will not be discussed here.

Vascular disorders of the retina

CAPILLARY HAEMANGIOMA

Retinal capillary haemangiomas may occur in isolation, or be part of a systemic disorder – *von Hippel–Lindau* – in which angiomatous tumours can develop in the brain and abdomen. Although very rare, it is autosomal dominantly inherited, and regular screening for not only patient, but also family members is thus important. Cryotherapy or laser can be employed to ablate the retinal lesions although large lesions have a poor prognosis.

COAT'S DISEASE

In this condition the retinal vessels are telangiectatic (dilated and tortuous). Affected children present in the first few years of life with large areas of subretinal exudation associated with dilated and tortuous retinal blood vessels in the affected region. Coat's disease is one of the causes of leucocoria and can present as a painful blind eye. The abnormal blood vessels can be treated by laser photocoagulation or cryotherapy, but some cases still progress to phthisis bulbi. The condition affects boys more than girls and is usually uniocular.

Acquired retinal disorders

DIABETES MELLITUS

In contrast to the elderly, all young patients with diabetes mellitus are insulin dependent, and rarely develop visible retinal changes until the disease has been present for 10–15 years. Annual retinal screening through dilated pupils can probably be left until after puberty, as retinopathy requiring treatment is rare before that time. Laser photocoagulation can largely prevent the blinding complications of this disease. Throughout the world, much of this screening is performed by optometrists, though to a lesser extent in the paediatric age group.

At a retinal level, the disease principally damages the microvascular circulation (retinal capillaries); the earliest visible changes being microaneurysms and intraretinal haemorrhages which both appear as small red dots. As the damaged vessels leak, hard whitish exudates appear – often in a circle around a microaneurysm – and these changes anywhere outside the macula constitute *background retinopathy*. By definition the visual acuity is normal, and no treatment is required. If there is leakage within the macular area, however, then acuity may be reduced, and this is termed *exudative maculopathy*. This responds readily to photocoagulation, though if diffuse leakage and ischaemia of the macula develop, the outlook for acuity becomes very poor. The other main complication is *proliferative retinopathy*, where retinal ischaemia induces neovascular tufts to sprout forwards from retinal veins including those on the disc. Before the new vessels are visible there may be fluffy-edged 'cotton wool spots' (these are not exudates) indicative of nerve ischaemia. Untreated, new vessels have a high risk of causing vitreous haemorrhage, tractional detachment and rubeotic glaucoma leading to total blindness, but with panretinal photocoagulation this should be avoidable.

Other retinal disorders

LEUKAEMIA

Ocular involvement can be detected in 10% of children with leukaemia, and in addition to anterior uveitis, there may be changes in the choroid, retina, optic nerve and orbit. The most common retinal picture is of dilated sheathed veins, white-centred haemorrhages and cotton wool spots.

CHERRY RED SPOT

A rare but classic sign, the cherry red spot at the macula indicates an accumulation of pale material in the surrounding ganglion cells around the foveal pit. The importance of recognition cannot be overemphasized, as it is a diagnostic feature of several serious systemic metabolic disorders including Tay–Sach's, Sandhoff's and Niemann–Pick diseases.

Optic disc

Developmental anomalies

Optic nerve hypoplasia

A relatively common congenital anomaly in which the number of optic nerve axons is reduced. Subtle degrees are difficult to diagnose, but have little effect on the visual acuity or field, whereas the most severe cases are associated with profound visual impairment (even blindness) and an abnormally small optic nerve head, showing the characteristic double ring sign. No treatment is available, but the frequent association with ocular anomalies and most important endocrine or neurological abnormalities make full ophthalmic and paediatric assessment essential.

Optic nerve drusen

Buried hyaline bodies within the nerve head, must not be confused with the same term used to describe white flecks in the retina. Optic disc drusen are commonly bilateral and can be inherited (autosomal dominant). Over the years they gradually increase in size, calcify, and become visible as discrete refractile masses on the surface of the disc (*Figure 4.16*). Although they can give rise to haemorrhages, field defects or visual loss, in early childhood their main significance lies in the fact that discs containing buried drusen appear swollen (*Figure 4.17*). In order to distinguish this so-called *pseudo* papilloedema from true papilloedema look for spontaneous venous pulsation, anomalous vessel branching and an absent disc cup, all found with drusen. Photographs to show autofluorescence are diagnostic.

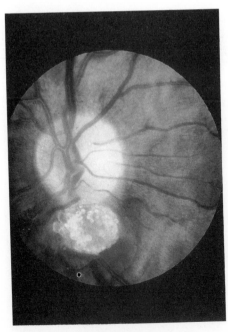

Figure 4.16. Large drusen of the optic disc

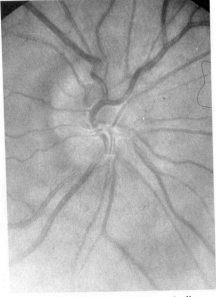

Figure 4.17. Buried drusen of the optic disc, causing a 'swollen' appearance

Coloboma

Disc coloboma may occur in isolation or be part of a chorioretinal coloboma (*Figure 4.6*). The effect on visual function depends upon the extent of the defect.

The tilted disc

Relatively common and often associated with astigmatic refractive errors and slightly reduced corrected acuity (around 6/9–6/12). Field defects occur frequently and may cause confusion with a lesion compressing the chiasm. In clinical practice of course this presents a dilemma as such a patient may also harbour an intracranial tumour.

Acquired disc anomalies

Optic atrophy

The causes of optic atrophy are a multitude, but fall into several main groups. A variety of familial forms have been described, but optic atrophy can be the first sign of serious, even life-threatening, underlying pathology. Optic atrophy is not a diagnosis, merely a sign (*Figure 4.18*) and its identification is not always easy, particularly in highly pigmented fundi or myopes. Furthermore the clinician must be aware that correlating disc appearance and acuity is fraught with difficulty, as applies to many ophthalmoscopic findings of the optic disc and macula.

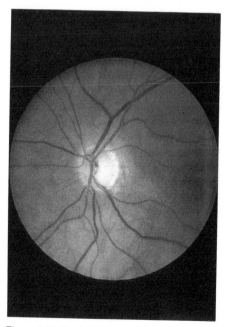

Figure 4.18. Optic atrophy – the degree of pallor cannot be equated with acuity

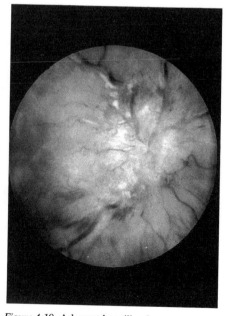

Figure 4.19. Advanced papilloedema

The following is an incomplete list of causes:

Prenatal   Infection, drugs, alcohol, or developmental brain disorders.
Perinatal   Birth asphyxia, postnatal brain ischaemia.
Familial   Various forms, ± neurological abnormalities.
                Dominant optic atrophy – commonest form, relatively mild and rarely identified before school age.
                Recessive optic atrophy – severe, rare, present in infancy.
                Leber's optic atrophy – onset in teenage years, with the sudden loss of the vision of one eye, followed within a few months by the other. Usually affects males.
Ocular   Secondary to longstanding retinal disease such as the retinal dystrophies, pigmentary retinopathies, glaucoma, etc.
Compressive   Tumours of the optic nerve (glioma), or chiasm (e.g. cranio-pharyngioma), or secondary to raised intracranial pressure.
Miscellaneous Intrinsic brain disease, meningoencephalitis, toxins, trauma, etc.

Papilloedema

This term refers to disc swelling secondary to raised intracranial pressure. The optic disc is pink, spontaneous venous pulsation is lost, and if severe there may be haemorrhages adjacent to the disc (*Figure 4.19*). Although careful visual field assessment may reveal an enlarged blind spot, it is unusual for the visual acuity to fall significantly unless the papilloedema is very severe or has been present for some time. Clearly, urgent referral for full ophthalmological and neurological investigation, probably including CT scanning, is mandatory.

Nystagmus

Nystagmus is defined as a rhythmic oscillation of the eye(s). Few signs instil such a feeling of inadequacy in the clinician as it is difficult to describe and has a wide range of associations ranging from the trivial to the potentially lethal. It is important to emphasize that nystagmus is simply a sign and not a diagnosis, and whilst certain patterns are suggestive, rarely are they pathognomonic of a particular diagnosis. Furthermore its presence provides little or no clue to the level of vision which can range from normal, or near normal, to blindness. Here only certain clinical aspects will be mentioned.

Nystagmus is characterized by the following features:

Direction This may be horizontal, vertical or rotational and refers to the direction of the fast phase.
Waveform The terms 'jerk' and 'pendular' indicate, very crudely, the nature of the waveform, but do not help classify the nystagmus and are of little if any clinical help.
Frequency The rate of the oscillation (velocity) is of little diagnostic help, although certain forms tend to be more rapid (voluntary) than others (the slow nystagmoid movement of the blind).
Amplitude Linked with frequency.

Classification

Physiological

Under this heading the following are included: end-point, rotational, caloric, optokinetic (OKN) and voluntary nystagmus. Not of clinical concern, however certain aspects of physiological nystagmus such as rotational nystagmus and OKN are useful supplementary diagnostic aids in paediatric ophthalmic practice. Both can be used as qualitative tests of vision and eye movements in infancy.

Pathological

Acquired central nervous system disease

Nystagmus can occur in many CNS disorders including those involving the cerebellum, brainstem and vestibular regions. In children the patterns of nystagmus are often quite variable and therefore have limited localizing and diagnostic value. Although uncommon, because of their serious implications, these causes must be considered first and without delay. Sometimes, but not invariably, the child's general health and behaviour may indicate a neurological basis. Remember nystagmus may be the first clue to a serious neurological disorder.

GAZE-EVOKED NYSTAGMUS

This type occurs on eccentric gaze and is seen as part of a supranuclear gaze paresis. Its direction depends on the site of the lesion and may be anywhere in the brainstem or cerebellum. Apart from structural brainstem abnormalities such as internuclear ophthalmoplegia, gaze-evoked nystagmus is often caused (in the adult) by drugs affecting the CNS – tranquillizers, anticonvulsants, etc.

VESTIBULAR NYSTAGMUS

Disorders of any part of the vestibular mechanism (ear to brainstem) can give rise to nystagmus which characteristically exhibits a torsional element. Causes range from infection to intracranial tumour.

DOWN- AND UP-BEAT NYSTAGMUS

Both may be forms of vestibular nystagmus and indicate pathology of the brainstem, or its connections: the former is caused by lesions low down in the brainstem (near the craniocervical junction) and the latter by disorders of cerebellum or medulla.

SPASMUS NUTANS

An intriguing and variable triad consisting of nystagmus, abnormal head posture and head nodding. Commences in the first year of life and usually spontaneously remits within 2–3 years. Spasmus nutans has a particular propensity to be uniocular. Although benign it is important to recognize that as this condition can be associated with intracranial tumours all affected children must be appropriately investigated.

SEE-SAW NYSTAGMUS

One eye elevates and intorts whilst the other depresses and extorts. Characteristically, but not invariably, caused by tumours in the region of the optic chiasm.

CONVERGENCE-RETRACTION NYSTAGMUS

Due to lesions of the midbrain such as a tumour. On attempted up-gaze the eyes rhythmically converge and retract.

Sensory deprivation nystagmus

Bilaterally reduced vision in early childhood (before about 6 years of age) results in nystagmus. Interestingly this only holds true if the cause of the visual deficit lies in the anterior visual pathway: cortical blindness does not therefore produce nystagmus. This form of nystagmus does not develop until about 3 months of age and is seen in two forms:

(1) Wandering eye movements of the blind. In this situation the eye movements are slow, wandering and variable in direction.
(2) Nystagmus indistinguishable from congenital nystagmus. Probably only differing from the blind child by the severity of the visual defect and not aetiology. Here the nystagmus is uniplanar and horizontal in all positions of gaze. This is produced by any cause of reduced vision lying in the anterior visual pathway, such as albinism, achromatopsia, Leber's amaurosis, optic nerve hypoplasia, etc.

ASYMMETRIC NYSTAGMUS

Rarely nystagmus can be either uniocular or asymmetrical and occurs in monocular blindness, spasmus nutans and chiasmal tumours.

Congenital nystagmus

Intentionally, the acquired causes of nystagmus have been mentioned before congenital although in practice congenital or infantile nystagmus is probably the commonest form encountered. However, it must be a diagnosis of exclusion and can only be diagnosed when other types have been considered and excluded. The term congenital is quite confusing as the nystagmus is rarely present at birth and usually develops after about 2 months of age. An identical clinical picture can be produced by a variety of visual pathway disorders, therefore congenital nystagmus is best subdivided into two categories:

(1) *Idiopathic congenital nystagmus.* No associated ocular or neurological pathology. Sometimes inherited, by autosomal dominant, recessive and X-linked traits.
(2) *Secondary congenital nystagmus.* Associated with pathology in the CNS or visual pathway pathology (any cause of reduced vision in childhood, see above).

CLINICAL FEATURES

Congenital nystagmus is bilateral and symmetrical, with the oscillation in the horizontal meridian in all positions of gaze (there are rare exceptions to this). The intensity of the nystagmus increases on fixation but decreases in certain positions, the 'null' position, in which position acuity is improved. Abnormal head movements sometimes develop. In the idiopathic type, visual acuity is relatively good (can even be near normal) and improves slightly during life. Near vision is good.

MANAGEMENT

This is aimed at gaining an improvement of visual acuity, by altering the position of the null point, by prisms or extraocular muscle surgery. A variety of other treatment modalities have been tried such as with certain drugs, acupuncture, pleoptics, etc. Each have their advocates but have not gained general acceptance. In practice, congenital nystagmus rarely requires treatment and surgery is only contemplated when to achieve the null position an extreme compensatory head posture has to be adopted.

LATENT NYSTAGMUS

This appears when one eye is covered – the fast phase is AWAY from the occluded eye. The contradictory term *manifest latent nystagmus* applies when there is subtle nystagmus under binocular viewing conditions which increases when one eye is occluded. Latent nystagmus is quite common. In practice this condition should be remembered when the acuity of each eye individually is unexpectedly low. The finding of a normal binocular acuity will suggest this diagnosis.

Clinical examination of a child with nystagmus

Nystagmus must always be taken seriously, and the diagnosis of idiopathic congenital nystagmus should not be resorted to until the child has been fully examined and investigated. The extent of these investigations will be dictated by clinical circumstances, but must include at the very least a full ophthalmic examination. The value of electrophysiology must not be underestimated, for significant retinal pathology may be ophthalmoscopically undetectable as in Leber's amaurosis or achromatopsia. As full and urgent neurological assessment may be required, it is mandatory that if there is a possibility of a neurological basis to the nystagmus such children are referred to the general practitioner immediately.

Disorders of the posterior visual pathway

Delayed visual maturation

This is probably the commonest cause of blindness in early infancy. By definition in all infants vision improves with time. However the reader must be aware of the spectrum of delayed visual maturation (DVM).

There are three types:

(1) DVM as an isolated abnormality in which there are no significant ocular and

non-ocular abnormalities. Complete and rapid recovery is the rule, usually by 3–5 months of age.

(2) DVM associated with severe neurodevelopmental delay. In this group recovery is slower and less complete and the developmental problems persist.

(3) DVM associated with nystagmus with or without ocular abnormalities. The example most commonly seen is albinism. In this type of DVM, during the period of blindness nystagmus does not commence until around the time of visual improvement, usually between 3 and 6 months of age.

Electrophysiological tests are of value as the finding of a normal ERG precludes a retinal basis for the visual problem. As a variety of visual evoked potential (VEP) results have been reported in DVM the value of this test is limited. It is important that the reader appreciates that differentiating between the three types in infancy is not always straightforward.

Cortical visual impairment

Although the term cortical blindness is commonly used, cortical visual impairment (CVI) is preferred as a degree of improvement frequently occurs. The word degree must be emphasized, for although full recovery may occur following trauma (e.g. relatively minor closed head injuries), depending on the extent of neurological damage sustained, this is not always so and occasionally total blindness persists. Apart from the visual defect, ophthalmic examination is normal including the pupillary responses. Interestingly in contrast to childhood visual impairment from a disorder of the anterior visual pathway (eye, optic nerve and optic chiasm), nystagmus is not a feature.

Causes include, prenatal insults, malformations, intrauterine infections, perinatal asphyxia, neurodegenerative disorders and trauma.

Clearly such children require full ophthalmic and neurological assessment. Unfortunately in this condition the VEP has proved to be of relatively little value, although the preservation of the ERG excludes the retina as the site of the defect.

Poor vision and a normal ophthalmic examination

In infants apart from disorders of the posterior visual pathway, several of those affecting the anterior visual pathway may also have, apart from the reduction of vision, a normal ophthalmic examination. For instance, infants with either achromatopsia or Leber's congenital amaurosis may appear clinically normal, and older children with early retinitis pigmentosa or Stargardt's disease may develop visual symptoms long before ocular signs become apparent. In certain other instances subtle signs are not identified, nevertheless the effect is the same – the infant or child has a visual defect for which there is no visible explanation.

Causes in infancy:

Delayed visual maturation   All types
Retinal dystrophies   e.g. Leber's amaurosis, cone dysfunction
Optic nerve anomalies   Strictly, not a category, but signs can be subtle
Cortical visual impairment

In the older child other conditions cause bilaterally reduced vision of a mild to severe degree. Treatable causes must always be considered first, such as visual loss due to *optic atrophy* resulting from compression by an intracranial tumour. At this age certain of the *pigmentary retinopathies* (e.g. mitochondrial cytopathy and Laurence–Moon–Bardet–Biedl syndrome) may present, as may progressive cone dysfunction. *Macular dystrophies* present with minimal if any signs in childhood (e.g. Stargardt's disease). Certain *neurodegenerative disorders* present initially in childhood with visual failure (Batten's disease and leukodystrophy), neurological signs appearing later.

Functional (hysterical) visual loss is a not uncommon cause of visual loss in young school children and adolescents, particularly girls. Its onset cannot always be determined but sometimes follows a routine ophthalmic examination, particularly one at which some concern has been expressed (usually ill-founded) or other ophthalmic triggering factor such as a conjunctivitis. This is commonly bilateral and ophthalmic examination including pupil and optokinetic responses are normal. Careful examination usually enables functional and organic causes of visual loss to be readily differentiated but there are a number of examination techniques which will aid this process. These include, for bilateral loss of vision, optokinetic responses, visual threats of varying types, observing the child negotiate obstacles, and obtaining a fusional response to a base-out prism. For unilateral deficits base-out prisms can again be used, and also the use of two cancelling cylinders in front of each eye. If the visual fields can be tested, they are often found to constrict in a spiral fashion. Diplomatic management is important, and it goes without saying that *all other causes of visual loss must always be excluded before resorting to this diagnosis.*

Investigation of the infant or child with poor vision and a normal ophthalmic examination

Take a detailed history and perform a clinical ophthalmic examination. The presence of nystagmus excludes DVM and most cortical visual impairment, and is a clue to the presence of an anterior segment abnormality. High hypermetropia is frequent in both Leber's amaurosis and achromatopsia. Electrodiagnosis is essential in many to establish a precise diagnosis, and the test of most clinical value is the ERG, taking care to distinguish rod and cone responses. Paediatric evaluation is also often helpful in many instances.

Ocular trauma

Birth trauma

Haemorrhages from birth trauma are common, usually transient, and generally outwith the remit of the optometrist. Globe damage from forceps may split Descemet's membrane leading to transient corneal oedema, which must be distinguished from developmental glaucoma. The vertical or oblique splits (parallel lines in the cornea) persist and significant astigmatism and amblyopia occur.

Accidental and non-accidental trauma

Accidental ocular trauma is relatively common and will usually present promptly to the hospital casualty department. Occasionally, however, even penetrating trauma goes unrecognized and may present to the optometrist. Non-accidental injury may be suspected with many types of trauma, particularly subconjunctival haemorrhage, eyelid bruising or burns, hyphaema, retinal or vitreous haemorrhage. If such an injury is suspected the situation must obviously be dealt with very diplomatically and it is essential that the child is referred to the family doctor or local hospital, with the appropriately diplomatic letter (which if accompanying the child should not contain this suspicion). Ascertain *that day that the appointment has been kept.*

Blunt trauma can damage the bony orbit, soft tissue or eyeball. When a bony fracture causes entrapment of the periocular tissues, this is known as a 'blow-out'. Diplopia and numbness over the cheek are common, due possibly to both intraorbital haemorrhage and entrapment. As the former will improve as the bruising resolves, muscle restriction may require surgical intervention. X-rays are mandatory.

Penetrating trauma often involves the cornea, with collapse of the anterior chamber, and calls for urgent surgical repair. An eye shield which avoids any pressure on the eye may be helpful in the interim. As mentioned penetrating injuries, such as by a small metallic foreign body, may cause little discomfort, do not always reduce vision, and produce subtle signs visible only on slit-lamp examination. The short- and long-term consequences of a retained intraocular foreign body are too well known to be reiterated here. A careful history is helpful in alerting to this possibility and referral for the appropriate assessment and X-ray is mandatory.

Conclusion

In this chapter we have briefly considered some of the pathological conditions affecting the developing visual pathway. Inevitably this list is incomplete. As many of these disorders are rare and may never be encountered in a lifetime of general clinical practice, full and immediate recall cannot be expected. Hopefully, this section will enable the clinician to appreciate that more pertinent than knowledge of a rare syndrome is the understanding of the importance and urgency of certain potentially sight-threatening or lethal situations. Often without detailed knowledge of the underlying pathology a degree of urgency can be ascribed (e.g. sudden onset of nystagmus, 6th nerve palsy and unsteadiness of gait) and acted upon, to enable the appropriate investigations (in the case quoted for an intracranial tumour) to be undertaken without delay. As mentioned time and again, certain signs are subtle and easily missed; listen carefully to the history provided by the child or parent. Observations by parents are rarely without basis, although the interpretation by either parent or clinician can be difficult. Finally, remember – certain ophthalmic signs are the first clue to a systemic diagnosis.

Further reading

CRAWFORD, J.S. and MORIN, J.D. (eds) (1983). *The Eye in Childhood.* Grune and Stratton, New York.
HARLEY, R.D. (ed.) (1983) *Pediatric Ophthalmology*, 2nd edn. W.B. Saunders, Philadelphia.
ISENBERG, S.I. (ed.) (1989). *The Eye in Infancy.* Year Book Publishers, Chicago.
TAYLOR, D. (1990) *Pediatric Ophthalmology.* Blackwell Scientific Publications, Oxford.

5

Perceptual development in early infancy

Alan Slater

Introduction

The past thirty years have seen a rapid increase in our understanding of perceptual development in infancy. The main focus of the research has been visual perception, with less on auditory perception, and little on the senses of taste and smell. Other senses of course, particularly audition, provide important information, but it is clear that humans have evolved to rely heavily on vision at all ages.

The young infant is a fairly helpless creature, and to the casual observer their manual and motor behaviours often appear random, uncoordinated, and unrelated to what is going on around them. Clearly, therefore, in order to answer questions such as 'How much can a baby see and hear?', 'How do perceptual abilities develop?' 'What sense can the baby make of his or her perceived world?', we need ways of measuring infants' abilities that do not rely upon immature motor systems. Not surprisingly, therefore, advances in our understanding of infants' vision and hearing have depended upon the development of techniques for communicating with infants. As we shall see, it turns out that infants display considerable perceptual competence at a surprisingly early age: while vision at birth is fairly poor, even the newborn perceives an organized and structured world. Vision develops rapidly in the early months, and visual experience has a criticial facilitating effect on its development.

The first part of this chapter concentrates on visual development, the obvious starting point being the newborn baby's visual world.

The visual world of the newborn

Unlike the other senses (the possible exception is the sense of smell), there is no opportunity for visual experience prior to birth. It is therefore not surprising that the visual world of the newborn is quite different from that of the adult. *Figure 5.1* shows schematic horizontal sections through the (left) eyes of the adult and the neonate to illustrate differences in overall size, in the shape of the lens, and in the depth of the anterior chamber. At birth, the eye, like the brain, is relatively well developed, and both increase in volume about three to four times compared with the rest of the body which increases about 21 times to reach adult size: this differential growth accounts for the relatively large head size of the infant and small child. At the time of normal birth (i.e. at term) the peripheral retina of the eye is quite well developed, but the central retina (the macular region and the fovea) are poorly developed and undergo

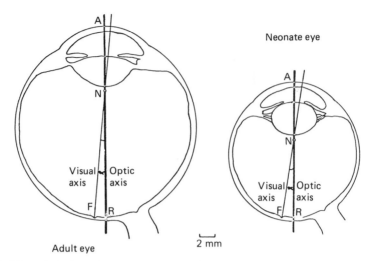

Figure 5.1. Schematic horizontal sections through the (left) eyes of the adult and neonate (to scale), to illustrate differences in gross size, in the shape of the lens, and in the depth of the anterior chamber. F, fovea; R, retina

considerable post-term changes: the fovea is quite well developed by 6 months of age, by which age visual acuity has developed to near-adult levels (see below) but even at 45 months of age there are morphological differences from the adult (Abramov *et al.*, 1982; Yuodelis and Hendrickson, 1986; Fielder, Moseley and Ng, 1988).

Despite its immaturity, which is further discussed below, it is clear that the visual system is functional at birth. One behavioural state that can be distinguished is known as 'alert inactivity' and is the state (often too rare from the parents' point of view!) where the baby is wide awake and alert, but not fussing or crying. In this state the casual observer can see that the eyes move together in a coordinated or conjugate fashion, and the baby gives every indication of actively exploring its visual world. Detailed studies of newborns' eye movements, both in the presence and absence of patterned visual stimulation, have confirmed this view. Haith (1980) has described a number of dispositions or 'rules' that guide visual activity in newborns and which help infants begin the task of learning about their newly experienced visual world. The first four of these 'rules' are the following:

Rule 1: If awake and alert and light not too bright, open eyes.
Rule 2: If in darkness, maintain a controlled, detailed search.
Rule 3: If in light with no form, search for edges by relatively broad, jerky sweeps of the (visual) field.
Rule 4: If an edge is found, terminate the broad scan and stay in the general vicinity of that edge.

While many researchers would disagree with the precise form of these rules, there is general agreement that the newborn is biologically prepared to explore the visual environment, and is able actively to seek out and attend to some forms of stimulation in preference to others. More detailed consideration of this is given later: in the next section we consider the visual information detected by the newborn.

Basic visual capacities and their development

It is not surprising to find that the visual information detected by the newborn is very impoverished when compared with that detected by the adult. Sensitivity to contrast differences is poor. A black and white pattern gives a contrast approaching 100%, and under good viewing conditions adults can discriminate between shades of grey giving contrast values of less than 1%; a contrast value of 30–40% is close to the newborn's threshold of detectability. Visual acuity, the ability to detect fine detail, is also poor. The most commonly used procedure to measure visual acuity is the visual preference method, often called preferential looking, or PL. In this procedure black and white stripes or gratings of the sort shown in *Figure 5.2* are shown to the infant, each stripe pattern paired with a grey patch of equal overall luminance: the width of the stripes is progressively reduced and when the infant no longer looks at the stripes in preference to the grey patch it is assumed that the acuity threshold has been reached. A second method uses visual evoked potentials: electrical activity of the visual area of the brain to the repeated presentation of a grating is recorded, and the smallest stripe width that reliably gives a different evoked potential from that to a grey patch gives an estimate of the threshold. The third procedure uses following movements of the eyes (optokinetic nystagmus) to a moving grating, and the angular size of the smallest stripe width that elicits the response is used as the measure of visual acuity.

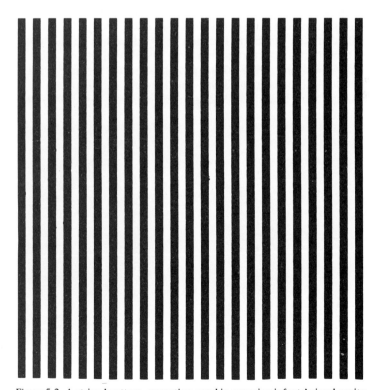

Figure 5.2. A striped pattern, or grating, used in assessing infants' visual acuity

Most methods and investigators find acuity of ≈ 6/240 soon after birth (Fulton, Hansen and Manning, 1981; Banks and Dannemiller, 1987; Brown, Dobson and Maier, 1987; von Noorden, 1988). As a rough guide *Figure 5.3* gives an indication of how the mother's face might look to a newborn infant, and how she might look to us: while the image is degraded and unfocused for the newborn, enough information is potentially available for the infant to learn to recognize the mother's face.

As measured by the visually evoked potential, acuity increases rapidly to approach adult levels within the first year (e.g. Marg *et al.*, 1976; Hamer *et al.*, 1989) whereas preferential looking indicates a slower development, taking at least 2 years to reach adult levels (Mayer and Dobson, 1982). These techniques reflect the activity of different levels of the visual system and employ different stimulus parameters and scoring criteria (Dobson and Teller, 1978). The evoked potential is always the more sensitive (Sokol and Moskowski, 1985) but with identical stimuli the two methods can give highly correlated results (Cannon, 1983). Optokinetic nystagmus findings are similar to those of preferential looking but are heavily influenced by field size (Schor and Narayan, 1981). The monocular asymmetry of optokinetic nystagmus in infants (Naegle and Held, 1982b) and amblyopes (Westall, Woodhouse and Brown, 1989) and the extent to which the technique assesses midbrain as opposed to cortical function (Naegle and Held, 1982a), make it a rather unsatisfactory measure of developing acuity.

Visual acuity improves because of the increasing specificity and resolution of the cortical neurones (Hickey and Peduzzi, 1987; Brown, Dobson and Maier, 1987) promoted by the combined effects of the increased density of the foveal cones, (≈ 4×, Yuodelis and Hendrickson, 1986) and the enlargement of the retinal image that follows from growth of the eye (≈ 1½×, Streeten, 1969).

The spatially complex function of vernier acuity develops quickly over the first 6 months, but then improves more slowly and is still well below adult levels at 14 months (Manny and Klein, 1985). By 3 months contrast sensitivity for low spatial frequencies is adult-like (Norcia, Tyler and Hamer, 1988), phase discrimination becomes demonstrable (Braddick, Atkinson and Wattam-Bell, 1986), though this is

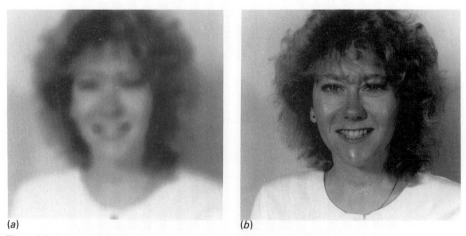

(a)   (b)

Figure 5.3. A face as it might appear to a newborn (a) and to us (b)

limited by the normal phase variation across the pupil (Charman and Walsh, 1985), and the critical fusion frequency is normal (Regal, 1981).

Accommodation is initially poor, but since acuity is poor at birth it is likely that the 'fine tuning' afforded by accommodation changes makes little difference to the clarity of the perceived image: as Banks put it, 'instead of stating that young infants see relatively clearly at one distance and not others, it is more accurate to say that they see equally unclearly across a wide range of distances' (Banks, 1980, p. 663). Accommodation responses improve along with changes in acuity, so that from 2 months, or earlier, all normal infants alter their accommodation in the appropriate direction as the distance of a visual target changes (Howland, Dobson and Sayles, 1987). The typical refractive errors of infancy do not impede the development of acuity because the depth of focus of the eye, $\simeq 1$ D at 1 month reducing to $\simeq 0.5$ D by 3 months (Green, Powers and Banks, 1980; Boltz, Manny and Katz, 1983), gives adequate tolerance until the accommodation becomes more accurate after 4–5 months (Braddick *et al.*, 1979; Banks, 1980; Brookman, 1983; Dobson *et al.*, 1983).

It is worth noting that some common myths about early vision can be dispelled. It is certainly not the case that babies are born blind, neither is it true that their vision is 'locked on' at a particular distance from the eyes. The immediate input to the visual system is the image that falls on the two-dimensional retinae of the eyes. Although in no sense do we (or infants) ever 'see' this retinal image, a commonly expressed view is that, since this image is upside down and reversed from right to left, at birth infants see the world similarly distorted. The simplest experiment convinces us that babies see the world 'the right way round': if a light is shone to the left, or right (or up or down) of the baby's looking positions the baby will turn its eyes in the correct direction to localize, or look at, the light. Of course, if the visual world were inverted or reversed the babies would look in the opposite direction, which they don't! This type of procedure can be used to measure infants' effective field of view. Schwartz *et al.* (1987) measured visual field size in newborn, 1-month-old and 2-month-old infants. Each of the trials began when the infant was fixating a centre target, a white sphere, and a second white sphere was then moved at a rate of approximately 2–3° per second from a peripheral position toward the centre. An observer reported the direction of any eye movement that the infant made away from the centre target, and the infant's field of view was defined as the angular deviation of the peripheral target towards which directionally appropriate eye movements were made. Curiously, the older infants appeared to be more 'captured' by the central target than the younger ones, which gave them somewhat smaller visual field sizes than newborns: newborns were able to detect targets that were 40° from their looking position, a field of view that is appreciably smaller than that of adults who can detect targets over 80° to left or right of where they are looking.

Newborn infants display some degree of colour vision. Adams, Maurer and Davis (1986) reported that newborns differentiated grey from green, from yellow and from red. For each of these colours they preferred to look at colour and grey checker-boards compared to grey squares, matched for overall luminance. However, the newborns showed no evidence of discriminating between grey and blue. At 1 month the absolute spectral sensitivity threshold is $\simeq 50 \times$ that of the adult; improving to $\simeq 10 \times$ by 3 months. At this age spectral sensitivity matches the CIE scotopic curve (Powers, Schneck and Teller, 1981) and infants display broadly trichromatic colour perception (Varner *et al.*, 1985; Teller and Bornstein, 1987).

By being physically separated in space the two eyes provide slightly different images of the perceived world. Detection of these differences, or disparities, provides the basis for an important binocular cue to stereopsis, and several studies suggest that stereoscopic depth perception emerges around 3 months of age (see Braddick and Atkinson, 1983). Stereoscopic disparities of $\simeq 45$ minutes of arc are detectable at $\simeq 4$ months by evoked potential (Petrig *et al.*, 1981), preferential looking (Birch, Shimojo and Held, 1985) or by the eye movements produced by a moving random dot stimulus (Fox *et al.*, 1980; Archer *et al.*, 1986). For the first several months, the development of acuity and binocularity proceeds in parallel with considerable independence and mutual tolerance (Birch, Gwiazda and Held, 1983), so much so that stereopsis is immediately present when the deviation of congenital esotropes is corrected with prisms or surgery (Birch and Stager, 1985; Mohindra *et al.*, 1985; Archer *et al.*, 1986; Rogers *et al.*, 1986; Stager and Birch, 1986).

Early visual perception

Newborn and older infants, when shown pairs of stimuli, will display consistent preferences between them, in the sense of looking more at one member of the pair. The preference for patterned over unpatterned stimuli has been used on innumerable occasions, as we have already seen, to provide estimates of visual acuity and its development. Newborn infants will also prefer moving to stationary, large to small, three-dimensional to two-dimensional, high-contrast to low-contrast stimuli (Slater, 1989). However, preferential looking is not very helpful in answering other questions we may want to ask about infants' visual abilities: for example, if we want to find out if infants can discriminate, say, between a square and a circle, it is unlikely that they will 'prefer' one to the other if both are shown side by side. In order to investigate infants' discriminative abilities one procedure that has proven to be particularly useful is *habituation*: if one stimulus is presented repeatedly over a period of time infants will spend progressively less time looking at it (i.e. they habituate), and they will often subsequently *dishabituate* (show recovery of attention) when a different, novel stimulus is shown. If the novel stimulus is shown paired side by side with the familiar (habituated) stimulus, infants will typically spend more time looking at the novel one. Habituation procedures work with infants from birth. For example, after newborns had been habituated to one of four simple geometric shapes (a square, cross, circle or triangle) they gave novelty preferences when the familiar shape was paired with one they hadn't seen before (Slater, Morison and Rose, 1983): *Figure 5.4* shows a newborn infant being tested for this sort of discrimination. While this provides evidence of early shape discrimination, the basis of the discrimination is unclear since any two shapes will differ in features such as orientation of lines and angles, overall size, density of contour, enclosed versus open, and so on. These sorts of 'low order' variables are discriminated by newborns and they may be discriminating between configurations on the basis of these features rather than on the basis of 'true' form perception. An experiment by Cohen and Younger (1984) illustrates this. Six- and 14-week-old infants were habituated to a simple stimulus consisting of two connected lines which made either an acute (45°) or obtuse (135°) angle. On subsequent test trials the 6 week olds dishabituated to a change in the orientation of the lines (where the angle remained unchanged), but *not* to a change in angle alone, while the 14 week olds did the opposite in that they recovered attention to a change in angle, but not to a change in orientation. This suggests that shape perception in infants 6 weeks and younger may be dominated by attention to lower-order variables such as orientation. However, in a recent experiment (Slater,

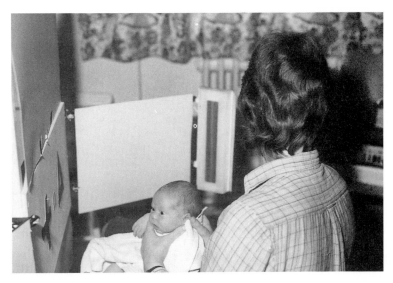

Figure 5.4. A newborn baby being tested

Mattock and Brown, 1989) newborns were shown either an acute angle or an obtuse angle which changed its orientation on each of six habituation or familiarization trials. On subsequent test trials all the infants looked more at the novel angle: thus, those familiarized to the acute angle spent longer looking at an obtuse angle when the two angles were shown side by side, and vice versa for those familiarized to the obtuse angle – the stimuli presented on the familiarization and test trials are shown in *Figure 5.5.* This finding demonstrates that, from birth, infants are able to perceive angular relationships, which may be the basic elements or building blocks of form perception.

Beyond about 2 months of age infants give clear evidence of perceiving wholes, rather than parts of visual stimuli (Aslin and Smith, 1988), and can classify and categorize stimuli on the basis of perceiving similarities and differences between different examples. For example, recognizing that several different rectangles are members of a class separate from a square or a circle.

Depth perception

We have seen earlier that sensitivity to binocular disparity, stereopsis, as a cue to depth, appears around 3 months of age. Motion-carried, or *kinetic* depth cues are responded to even earlier. Newborn infants will selectively fixate a three-dimensional stimulus in preference to a photograph of the same stimulus, even when they are restricted to monocular viewing and the major depth cue is *motion parallax* (Slater, Rose and Morison, 1984). Appreciation of *pictorial* depth cues – those cues to depth that are found in static scenes such as might be found in photographs – has been found from about 5 months. One such cue is relative size, the larger of two otherwise identical figures usually being perceived as the closer. Yonas, Cleaves and Pettersen (1978) used the 'Ames window', a trapezoidal window rotated around its vertical axis. When adults view the two-dimensional Ames window monocularly a

Familiarization

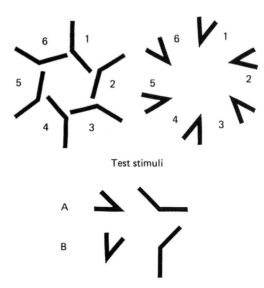

Test stimuli

Figure 5.5. Familiarization and test stimuli used in an experiment on form perception. Half the infants were familiarized to the six variations of the obtuse angle (upper left), half to the six variations of the acute angle (upper right)

powerful illusion is perceived of a slanted window with one side (the larger) closer than the other. Yonas *et al.* reported that 6-month-old infants wearing an eye patch (to remove binocular information) are twice as likely to reach for the larger side of the distorted window than for the smaller side, suggesting that this depth cue is detected by this age.

Organization in visual perception

One of the most important characteristics of visual perception is that it is organized: we perceive a world of objects, people and events, which move and change in a unified, coherent fashion. Important organizational features of visual perception are the visual constancies, such as brightness, shape and size constancy, and these are probably present at birth. Shape constancy is where we see an object as its true shape even when it is seen at an angle relative to our line of sight: we see a plate as round, even if we see it tilted. Evidence of shape constancy at birth was reported by Slater and Morison (1985). They familiarized newborns (mean age 1 day, 23 hours) to a shape, either a square or a trapezium, which changed in slant during the familiarization trials. On subsequent test trials the newborns gave a strong novelty preference for a different shape when this was paired with the familiarized shape, the latter in a different orientation from any seen earlier.

Size constancy refers to the fact that we see objects as their real sizes despite the changes that occur to the size of their retinal images as their viewing distance from an observer changes: thus, a 6-foot man 20 feet from us gives half the retinal image size as the same man 10 feet away, but we see him as the same size. Newborn infants also display size constancy. Slater, Mattock and Brown (1990) familiarized newborns to a single object (a cube) which was shown at different distances, hence regularly changing its retinal image size while its real size was constant. On subsequent test trials these newborns looked longer at a *different-sized* object when this was shown paired with the familiar one, even though these two objects were at different distances calculated to give them the same retinal image size.

These experiments are a convincing demonstration that infants at all ages perceive real objects, and their true shapes and sizes, and do not perceive a fleeting world of changing retinal images.

Perception of faces

The human face is a highly attractive and salient stimulus to the human infant. The face is three dimensional and contains regions of high contrast and, when seen by the infant faces are usually animated or moving. These aspects of stimulation by themselves are highly salient to newborn and older infants, which ensures that the face will be attention-getting and holding, but the interesting question is whether there is a predisposition to respond to the face other than as a collection of stimuli. The question becomes, 'do infants have an innate perceptual knowledge of the face?' There is no easy answer to this question, but certain lines of evidence suggest that we can offer a tentative 'yes'. Newborns quickly learn some of the characteristics of faces and, 49 hours from birth, they showed a reliable preference for their mother's face when paired with that of an adult female stranger (Bushnell, Sai and Mullin, 1989). Such evidence of early learning may be only a specific example of a more general learning ability, but there is other evidence of a special response to the face. Newborn infants will follow with their eyes a head shape bearing normal facial features more intently than one with the features scrambled, and they will do this within 5 minutes from birth – that is, before they have seen a real face (Goren, Sarty and Wu, 1975; Dziurawiec and Ellis, 1986). Further compelling evidence for early face perception is the suggestion that newborns will imitate adult facial gestures. An early report of neonatal imitation of mouth opening, tongue protrusion, and lip pursing was by Meltzoff and Moore (1977). Similar reports of newborn facial imitation have also appeared (i.e. Reissland, 1988), which implies that infants have an inborn representation of the face on to which they can map their own facial movements. Finer facial discriminations, i.e. between male and female, young and old faces, and between facial expressions, are learned in later months, but the newborn's predisposition to attend to faces, and what seems to be an innate knowledge of faces, makes an excellent starting point.

Overview

The newborn is amazingly competent at structuring the visual world, but their world is not the same as ours. As one authority speculates: 'Perhaps their experience is like ours during those first few moments when we awaken in a strange room: we see everything, but nothing makes sense' (Gordon, 1989, p. 70). Their visual world will lack meaning, familiarity and associations, and as acuity and other basic visual functions improve infants' experiences will quickly add this meaning and order. Some of the ways in which this may manifest itself are considered in the next section.

Objects, events and encounters

From the 1970s there has been a growing increase in the number of studies which have shown moving and changing 'dynamic' stimuli to their infant subjects. Much of this research is inspired by J.J. Gibson's (1979) theory of 'direct perception'. According to Gibson, perception of basic stimulus invariants is direct in that it does not need enhancing as a result of particular experiences. In line with this approach many researchers have argued that visual perception is most meaningful, and is most meaningfully studied, under conditions of change. A few illustrative experiments are described here.

Kellman and Spelke (1983) and Kellman, Spelke and Short (1986) described a series of experiments investigating young infants' perception of partly occluded objects. Four-month-old infants were habituated to a stimulus, usually a rod, which moved back and forth behind a block which occluded its centre portion (as in the upper part of *Figure 5.6*). Following habituation, the babies were shown two test displays without the occluder, one being the complete rod, the other being the top and bottom parts of the rod, with a central gap where the occluder had been (the test trials, *Figure 5.6*). Either of these test stimuli could have been the familiarized stimulus, and the question of interest was, what were the babies seeing during the habituation trials? If they saw the rod as connected or complete behind the block, then the discontinuous rod pieces would be the novel of the two test stimuli. If they saw the rod as being in two separate parts, then the complete object would be novel. Their results clearly supported the first of these possibilities: the babies spent more time looking at the discontinuous object on the test trials. However, when newborn babies were tested with the same arrangement they looked at the *continuous* rod, suggesting that an understanding of object coherence and unity is learned in the early months of life (Slater *et al.*, 1990). Nevertheless, infants' understanding of the world of objects improves rapidly, and an experiment by Baillargeon, Spelke and

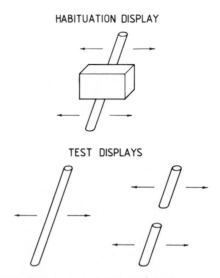

HABITUATION DISPLAY

TEST DISPLAYS

Figure 5.6. Habituation and test displays: during habituation the rod moved back and forth behind the occluder

Wasserman (1985) suggest that 5-month-old infants can appreciate the continuous existence of a *completely invisible* object. Their babies were shown a solid block, which was then hidden by a screen, but which should have prevented or blocked a moving drawbridge from travelling through a full 180° rotation. They spent more time looking at the 'impossible' complete 180° rotation than at a 'possible' 120° rotation, suggesting that they were aware not only of the block's continuous existence behind the screen, but that they 'knew' that its presence constituted an obstacle to the drawbridge's movement.

These experiments investigated infants' understanding of occluded objects by using what have been called *events*, defined as dynamic changes to the optic array which do not require activities of the infant observers. An *encounter* is where the observer is actively involved (Butterworth, 1989), and an example of infants' responses to encounters is in the 'moving room' procedure, in which the whole of the visual environment moves relative to the infant. Lee and Aronson (1974) and Butterworth and Cicchetti (1978) tested infants who were seated or held inside a small room in which the floor (and the baby) was stationary, but the three walls and the ceiling were made to move towards and away from the baby. In these studies the babies (like adults) lose balance, and the loss of balance is always appropriate to the direction of movement (i.e. if the room moves towards them they sway, or lurch forwards). Under normal circumstances the flow patterns of visual information that occur in the 'moving room' correspond to those that occur when the baby moves, or sways backwards and forwards: their presence in the absence of the baby's movement disrupts the infant's normal, visually guided, postural control.

In summary, babies enter the world with an immature visual system, but the basic visual capacities develop quickly in early infancy. The immediate visual input is that which impinges upon the flat, two-dimensional retinae, but at no age do infants perceive a two-dimensional world, and from birth infants perceive *distal* cues in the sense of perceiving the world 'out there' rather than responding only to proximal retinal cues. Visual perception is active and organized at birth, and babies soon learn to perceive shapes as wholes, and to classify and categorize visual stimuli. Studies of 'dynamic' perception tell us that from birth infants use visual information to guide their own movements in the world, and that by 4 or 5 months they perceive a world of coherent, spatially connected, unified, whole and permanent objects.

A sensitive period in visual development

In the 1960s and 1970s many experiments were carried out on animals, particularly kittens and monkeys, which have led to the conclusion that the developing visual system and the visual cortex can be changed by abnormal visual experiences, and that these changes are most readily produced if the abnormal experiences occur early in the animal's life. Reviews of this work are given by Barlow (1980) and Bornstein (1989). We shall see later that this work has important implications for human visual development.

To illustrate this research I will describe two types of unusual environments and their consequences for the kitten visual system. Kittens are born with their eyes closed, and normal eye opening occurs after about 1 week. From that point, and for another 4 months, imagine that we rear the kittens as follows:

(1) *A stripy world*. Kittens are kept in complete darkness for 23 hours of the day. For the other 1 hour they have a ruff placed around their necks (so that they cannot

see their own bodies) and are shown either: (a) only horizontal stripes, or (b) only vertical stripes.

(2) *No binocular experience.* This can occur in one of three ways:

(a) *Alternating monocular vision.* On alternating days kittens are allowed the use of the left then the right eye, but never both eyes at once.

(b) *Monocular vision.* One eye (say the left) is kept permanently closed, either by patching or by suture, while vision is allowed to the other (the right) eye.

(c) *Strabismus.* Kittens are reared with a permanent squint, usually induced by surgical means. This can be either a divergent squint (exotropia or 'wall-eyed'), or convergent squint (esotropia or 'cross-eyed').

These abnormal visual experiences have predictable consequences for the visual system, which can be described with reference to the normal cat's visual system. All visual perception depends on brain processes, which are responsible for interpreting and making sense of the images that fall on the retinae. Many parts of the brain, both subcortical and cortical, are involved in visual processing, and the part we shall consider here is the visual, or striate, cortex, located in the back of the head. Neurophysiologists have investigated the functioning of the visual cortex using, among other procedures, single-cell recording. With the use of very fine electrodes it is possible to record the responses of individual cells of the cortex to patterns of light (usually simple stimuli such as edges, bars, stripes, or slits of light) that fall on the retina. In the cat's visual cortex, cells can be found which respond specifically to orientation: each cell gives a response to a stimulus in a highly specific orientation (horizontal, vertical, or diagonal) and cells are found which detect all possible orientations. Normally, too, the majority of cells in the visual cortex (perhaps 70–80%) receive connections from both eyes, in the sense that they give their strongest response when corresponding areas of the retinae of both eyes are stimulated with the same stimulus. Almost certainly these 'binocular cells', and cells that are attuned to detect stimulation falling on slightly disparate areas of the retinae, are implicated in normal binocular vision.

The consequences for our abnormally reared kittens are the following. Those reared in the 'stripy world' will have many visual cortical cells that are attuned and respond to the perceived orientation, but very few that respond to retinal stimulation in the opposite orientation. There are also behavioural consequences. Kittens who have experienced a 'horizontal world' will happily jump onto chair seats, but will bump into vertical chair legs: they simply don't see them. Conversely, kittens reared in a 'vertical world' will avoid chair legs and other vertical objects, but will not see horizontally orientated stimuli. For the binocularly deprived kitten the numbers of binocularly driven cortical cells are much reduced, from the normal level of 70–90% to as little as 7% or lower. Behaviourally, these kittens do not have binocular vision, or stereopsis. Other effects will depend upon the precise nature of the deprivation. Those (group (2a)) who experienced alternating monocular vision will have two eyes, each with normal acuity. This may not seem too unusual, but from a physiological point of view it is puzzling: as Barlow (1980, p. 84) expressed it, 'to me, that is almost as surprising as to find that you can chop a car in half to produce two motorcycles'. The kittens in group (2b) reared with monocular vision, will have good vision in the seeing (in our example, the right) eye, but the occluded left eye will be amblyopic. Indeed, the defect may be so bad that the amblyopic, sometimes called 'lazy' eye is barely functional, and if vision becomes restricted to that eye the kitten may not be able to manoeuvre around its visual world. The deficit associated with early strabismus is likely to vary with the type of squint: exotropic kittens will probably have two functional, but monocular eyes, while esotropic kittens will probably have one good (monocular) eye, while the other is amblyopic.

What is important to note about these cases is that the effects of early deprivation are confined to a critical or sensitive period early in development. For the kitten this sensitive period begins at normal eye-opening and ends about 3–4 months later: a kitten that is reared normally for this period, and then subjected to deprivation, will show no long-term effects of the deprivation. However, deprivation for the duration of the sensitive period will have long-lasting permanent effects: the horizontally reared kitten will *never* see vertical parts of the world. We do know, however, that if the deprivation is reversed within the sensitive period the changes that would otherwise result are reversed, or at least reduced in intensity. This alerts us to the likelihood that if we wish to prevent many visual problems we need to be able to detect and treat them at an early period of development.

The human parallel

The types of deprivation experiment that have been carried out with animals cannot, for obvious ethical reasons, be repeated with humans, but there is convincing evidence that human visual development goes through a similar sensitive period during which abnormal visual experiences can leave permanent damage. We have known for many years that if an infant is born with a squint and this is not surgically corrected then normal stereoscopic vision will not develop, and amblyopia in one eye may well set in. These are not uncommon problems: somewhere between 2% and 8% of children develop strabismus and/or amblyopia. However, if an infant's squint is corrected immediately then normal vision is likely to result. This knowledge was used by Banks, Aslin and Letson (1975) and by Hohmann and Creutzfeldt (1975) who investigated the sensitive period for human visual development. Both groups of researchers tested adults who had a history of strabismus in childhood. Their subjects varied in the age at which their squints were first diagnosed (at birth or later in infancy), and also in the age at which the squint was surgically corrected. All subjects were given a test of binocularity and both groups of researchers concluded that the sensitive period for human visual development ended at about 2½–3 years.

This is an inevitable simplification of a complex story, and two caveats may be added to demonstrate the complexity of the problem. First, all individuals are different, and for some the sensitive period may extend as long as 5 years from birth. Second, there seem to be some infants who, despite correction, seem inevitably destined for squint and/or amblyopia: Wattam-Bell *et al.* (1987) describe infants who initially displayed binocular vision but subsequently developed strabismus, and there are other infants who become amblyopic for no apparent reason.

Nevertheless, we can be sure that if we are to prevent many visual problems from developing, detection and treatment in infancy and early childhood is essential.

Detection of infants 'at risk'

In recent years a number of techniques have been developed to test infants' vision and to detect problems at the time when treatment is most likely to be efficacious, namely during the sensitive period. Before describing two of the most useful testing procedures it is first worth asking what sorts of infants are particularly 'at risk' for developing visual problems? For convenience we can divide these into three groups:

(1) Prematures.
(2) Parents with visual problems.
(3) Infants with visual problems.

(1) Premature infants

Infants born prematurely are at risk for visual handicap. The very worst disorder, known as retrolental fibroplasia, which is a consequence of being given too much oxygen while in the incubator, can result in total blindness: fortunately such cases are becoming rarer as an awareness of the problem has resulted in careful monitoring of oxygen therapy given to prematures. However, retinal problems (often called retinopathy of prematurity, or ROP) are still a common consequence of an early birth. Unfortunately, the premature infant can spend the first few weeks or even months of its life in a special care baby unit, which is usually constantly (for 24 hours of the day) and brightly illuminated, experiencing light levels which can cause permanent retinal damage in laboratory animals. Despite the deleterious effects that premature birth may have on the visual system we still have very little knowledge of these effects. Problems can result from neurological damage (which are often associated with early labour), high light levels, phototherapy, and the fact that the infant is born at a time when visual development is rapid, and hence vulnerable to assault: from 28 to 40 weeks from conception, the time of most premature births, is one of the most active periods of ocular growth.

Premature infants are much more at risk than full term infants for visual problems of strabismus, deficits in colour vision, myopia, and reduced visual acuity: children who were born prematurely are likely to have visual acuities at the lower end of the normal range. These and other visual problems associated with premature birth are discussed by Fielder, Moseley and Ng (1988), from whose excellent review this brief summary is derived. It is important to emphasize that the majority of premature infants develop with no visual problems of any kind, but premature birth is a potential indicator of risk.

(2) Parents with visual problems

Parents who have (or have had) visual problems are more likely than 'visually normal' adults to have children who have, or develop, visual problems. This indicates the congenital (rather than environmentally caused) origin of many visual problems and typical adult histories include cataracts, early strabismus, myopia, hyperopia, astigmatism and amblyopia.

(3) Infants with visual problems

These are infants with cataracts, an obvious squint, or with latent squint, or with apparent difficulties in fixating. Infant visual problems are often associated with birth complications and with indications of neurological impairment, such as cerebral palsy, or oxygen starvation at birth. Some otherwise completely normal infants develop visual problems, for example if the two eyes have differential refractive indices (perhaps if one eye is short-sighted, the other long-sighted) there is a risk of amblyopia developing in one eye.

Coordination between the senses

There is evidence that the senses are coordinated from birth. We can distinguish at least two types of sensory coordination. One is where information from one modality specifies or has consequences for information from another. Examples are visually guided reaching, or turning in the direction of a sound source. With respect to the latter, Butterworth (1983) has argued that when newborn babies turn their eyes in the direction of a sound stimulus they *expect* the sound to have a visual consequence – they expect to see the thing that produced the sound. This suggests that, from birth, infants can differentiate the sensory information given by the different modalities. A second type of sensory coordination is where different modalities provide equivalent information. Meltzoff and Borton (1979) gave evidence for the detection of intersensory equivalence in an habituation experiment. One month olds were familiarized to one of two dummies (pacifiers) which was placed in the babies' mouths. One dummy had a smooth nipple while the other, nubby nipple had protuberances on it. Following familiarization the babies were shown visual replicas of the two dummies and they showed a reliable visual preference for the one they had previously perceived orally. This experiment gives evidence of early intermodal matching, supporting the view that there is an innate unity of the senses.

Taste, olfaction and audition

Research on taste and olfaction has concentrated on newborn infants, with a paucity of research in the later months of infancy. The newborn infant is as well equipped with taste buds as at any later time in life, and distinguishes between the four basic taste sensations – sweet, salty, sour and bitter – as shown by differential sucking and ingestion of solutions, and by facial gestures (Crook, 1987; Rosenstein and Oster, 1988). While taste has a number of 'primary' sensations this does not appear to be the case for olfaction, and perhaps because of this infants' responses to a great variety of chemical olfactory stimuli have been studied. Space does not permit a detailed description of these studies: suffice it to say that the sense of smell is clearly active from birth. There is also evidence that newborns will learn about and orient towards preferred odours: Macfarlane (1975) found that 6-day-old infants would orient towards their mother's breast pad in preference to one from another lactating mother. The chemical senses are probably important in the early control of feeding and serve to enhance the intake of nutritious foods and to inhibit ingestion of non-nutritive, harmful or toxic substances (Crook, 1987).

After vision, hearing is the modality which has received the greatest attention, and much of the research has focused on speech perception. While the fetus experiences an auditory environment that is quite different from the adult's, there is good evidence both for auditory perception, and for learning about auditory stimuli, before birth. De Casper and Spence (1986) had pregnant women recite a passage of speech aloud, in a quiet room, every day during the last 6 weeks of pregnancy. Shortly after birth (an average of 2 days 8 hours) the infants preferred the mother's previously recited passage to one spoken by a female stranger: in this experiment 'preference' was indexed by the baby being more prepared to change sucking patterns to hear the mother's voice. While auditory thresholds at birth are much higher than for adults it is known that thresholds reduce during infancy, and that infants display good discrimination between stimuli that differ in intensity and/or pitch during the first year (Bremner, 1988).

Infants also make discriminations between speech sounds which may suggest that they are innately attuned to the phonetic characteristics of human speech. For example, there is an auditory continuum known as voice onset time (VOT) which separates pairs of phonetic units – /ba/ and /pa/, /ga/ and /ka/, /ta/ and /da/ – and infants as young as 1 month discriminate these sounds across the boundaries of the continuum, but not within categories (i.e. Eimas *et al.*, 1971). More recently it has been discovered that other species, including chinchillas, rhesus monkeys and Japanese monkeys (macaques), give the same discrimination performance, perhaps suggesting that as language evolved it capitalized on general auditory perceptual mechanisms for sound discrimination, rather than developing specific mechanisms for processing speech (Kuhl and Miller, 1975; Kuhl and Padden, 1982).

The fine distinctions between general auditory and speech-specific mechanisms will exercise researchers in the years to come. It cannot be doubted, however, that human infants are uniquely predisposed to acquire speech. Since research on young infants has focused on their discrimination between isolated speech sounds we do not know when they discriminate words as separate auditory segments. However, comprehension of speech sounds is clearly present in the second half of the first year, and the baby's first words are uttered towards the end of the first year, indicating responsivity to word meanings from an early age.

Conclusion

As we have seen, there is evidence that all of the senses are functioning from birth and the newborn infant is perceptually surprisingly competent. With respect at least to the sense of vision, this early competence is accompanied by considerable vulnerability. Any sustained disruption to normal development, for example, unilateral cataract, ptosis, strabismus, anisometropia, etc., results in subnormal acuity of the eye, loss of stereo and in severe cases failure of the fixation reflexes and nystagmus (Parks, 1986). If early visual problems are not detected and treated early in life, the danger, if not the certainty, is that it will lead to permanent damage to the developing child.

References

ABRAMOV, I., GORDON., J., HENDRICKSON, A. *et al.* (1982). The retina of the newborn infant. *Science*, **217**, 265–267.

ADAMS, R.J., MAURER, D. and DAVIS, M. (1986). Newborns' discrimination of chromatic from achromatic stimuli. *Journal of Experimental Child Psychology*, **41**, 267–281.

ARCHER, S.M., HELVESTON., E.M., MILLER, K.K. and ELLIS, F.D. (1986). Stereopsis in normal infants and infants with congenital esotropia. *American Journal of Ophthalmology*, **101**, 591–596.

ASLIN, R.N. and SMITH, L.B. (1988). Perceptual development. *Annual Review of Psychology*, **39**, 435–473.

BAILLARGEON, R., SPELKE, E.S. and WASSERMAN, S. (1985). Object permanence in five-month-old infants. *Cognition*, **20**, 191–208.

BANKS, M. (1980). The development of visual accommodation during early infancy. *Child Development*, **51**, 646–666.

BANKS, M. S. and DANNEMILLER, J.L. (1987). Infant visual psychophysics. In *Handbook of Infant Perception*, vol. I. edited by P. Salapatek and L. Cohen. Academic Press, New York.

BANKS, M.S., ASLIN, R.N. and LETSON, R.D. (1975). Sensitive period for the development of human binocular vision. *Science,* **190**, 675–677.

BARLOW, H.B. (1980). Theories of cortical function and measurement of its performance. In *Neurobiological Basis of Learning and Memory,* edited by Y. Tsukuda and B.W. Agroroff, John Wiley, New York.

BIRCH, E.E., GWIAZDA, J. and HELD. (1983). The development of vergence does not account for the onset of stereopsis. *Perception,* **12**, 331–336.

BIRCH, E.E., SHIMOJO, S. and HELD, R. (1985). Preferential-looking assessment of fusion and stereopsis in infants aged 1–6 months. *Investigative Ophthalmology and Visual Science,* **26**, 366–370.

BIRCH, E.E. and STAGER, D.R. (1985). Monocular acuities and stereopsis in infantile esotropia. *Investigative Ophthalmology and Visual Science,* **26**, 1624–1630.

BOLTZ, R.L., MANNY, R.E. and KATZ, B.J. (1983). Effects of induced optical blur on infant visual acuity. *American Journal of Optometry and Physiological Optics,* **60**, 100–105.

BORNSTEIN, M.H. (1989). Sensitive periods in development: structural characteristics and causal interpretations. *Psychological Bulletin,* **105**, 179–197.

BRADDICK, O.J. and ATKINSON. J. (1983). Some recent findings on the development of human binocularity: a review. *Behavioural Brain Research,* **10**, 71–80.

BRADDICK, O.J., ATKINSON, J., FRENCH, J. and HOWLAND, H.C. (1979). A photorefractive study of infant accommodation. *Vision Research,* **19**, 1319–1330.

BRADDICK, O.J., ATKINSON, J. and WATTAM-BELL, J.R. (1986). Development of the discrimination of spatial phase in infancy. *Vision Research,* **26**, 1223–1239.

BREMNER, J.G. (1988). *Infancy.* Blackwell, Oxford.

BROOKMAN, K.E. (1983). Ocular accommodation in human infants. *American Journal of Optometry and Physiological Optics,* **60**, 91–99.

BROWN, A.M., DOBSON, V. and MAIER. J. (1987). Visual acuity of human infants at scotopic, mesopic and photopic luminances. *Vision Research,* **27**, 1845–1858.

BUSHNELL, I.W.R., SAI, F. and MULLIN, T. (1989). Neonatal recognition of the mother's face. *British Journal of Developmental Psychology,* **7**, 3–15.

BUTTERWORTH, G.E. (1983). Structure of the mind in human infancy. In *Advances in Infancy Research,* vol. 2, edited by L.P. Lipsitt and C.K. Rovee-Collier, Ablex Publishing Corpn., Norwood, New Jersey.

BUTTERWORTH, G.E. (1989). Events and encounters in infancy. In *Infant Development,* edited by A. Slater and G. Bremer. Erlbaum, Sussex.

BUTTERWORTH, G.E. and CICCHETTI, D. (1978). Visual calibration of posture in normal and motor retarded Down's Syndrome infants. *Perception,* **7**, 513–525.

CANNON, M.W. (1983). Contrast sensitivity: psychophysical and evoked potential methods compared. *Vision Research,* **23**, 87–95.

CHARMAN, W.N. and WALSH, G. (1985). The optical phase transfer function of the eye and the perception of spatial phase. *Vision Research,* **25**, 619–623.

COHEN, L.B. and YOUNGER, B.A. (1984). Infant perception of angular relations. *Infant Behavior and Development,* **7**, 37–47.

CROOK, C.K. (1987). Taste and olfaction. In *Handbook of Infant Perception,* vol. 1, edited by P. Salapatek and L.B. Cohen, Academic Press, New York.

DE CASPER, A.J. and SPENCE, M.J. (1986). Prenatal maternal speech influences newborns' perception of speech sounds. *Infant Behavior and Development,* **9**, 133–150.

DOBSON, V., HOWLAND, H.C., MOSS. C. and BANKS, M.S. (1983). Photorefraction of normal and astigmatic infants during viewing of patterned stimuli. *Vision Research,* **23**, 1043–1052.

DOBSON, V. and TELLER, D.Y. (1978). Visual acuity in human infants: a review and comparison of behavioural and electrophysiological studies. *Vision Research,* **18**, 1469–1483.

DZIURAWIEC, S. and ELLIS, H.D. (1986). Neonates' attention to face-like stimuli: Goren, Sarty and Wu (1975) revisited. Paper presented at the Annual Conference of the Developmental Section of the British Psychological Society, University of Exeter, September 1986.

EIMAS, P.D., SIQUELAND, E.R. JUSCZYK, P. and VIGORITO, J. (1971). Speech perception in infants. *Science,* **171**, 303–306.

FIELDER, A.R., MOSELEY, M.J. and NG, Y.K. (1988). The immature visual system and premature birth. *British Medical Bulletin,* **44**, 1093–1118.

FOX, R., ASLIN, R.N., SHEA, S.L. and DUMAIS, S.T. (1980). Stereopsis in human infants. *Science,* **207**, 323–324.

FULTON, A.B., HANSEN, R.M. and MANNING, K.A. (1981). Measuring visual acuity in infants. *Survey Ophthalmology,* **25**, 325–332.

GIBSON, J.J. (1979). *The Ecological Approach to Visual Perception.* Houghton Mifflin, Boston.

GORDON, I.E. (1989). *Theories of Visual Perception.* John Wiley, Chichester.

GOREN, C.C., SARTY, M. and WU, P.Y.K. (1975). Visual following and pattern discrimination of face-like stimuli by newborn infants. *Pediatrics,* **59**, 544–549.

GREEN, D.G., POWERS, M.K. and BANKS, M.S. (1980). Depth of focus eye size and visual acuity. *Vision Research,* **20**, 827–835.

HAITH, M.M. (1980). *Rules that Babies Look By.* Ablex Publishing Corp., Hillsdale, NJ.

HAMER, R.D., NORCIA, A.M., TYLER, C.W. and HSU-WINGES, C. (1989). The development of monocular and binocular VEP acuity. *Vision Research,* **29**, 397–408.

HICKEY, T.L. and PEDUZZI. J.D. (1987). Structure and development of the visual system. In *Handbook of Infant Perception,* vol. I, edited by P. Salapatek and L. Cohen. Academic, New York, pp. 1–42.

HOHMANN, A. and CREUTZFELDT, O.D. (1975). Squint and the development of binocularity in humans. *Nature,* **254**, 613–614.

HOWLAND, H.C., DOBSON, V. and SAYLES, N. (1987). Accommodation in infants as measured by photo-refraction. *Vision Research,* **27**, 2141–2152.

KELLMAN, P.J. and SPELKE, E.S. (1983). Perception of partly occluded objects in infancy. *Cognitive Psychology,* **15**, 483–524.

KELLMAN, P.J., SPELKE, E.S. and SHORT, K.R. (1986). Infant perception of object unity from translatory motion in depth and vertical translation. *Child Development,* **57**, 72–86.

KUHL, P.K and MILLER, J.D. (1975). Speech perception by the chinchilla: voiced–voiceless distinction in alveolar plosive consonants. *Science,* **190**, 69–72.

KUHL, P.K. and PADDEN, D.M. (1982). Enhanced discriminability at the phonetic boundaries for the voicing feature in macaques. *Perception and Psychophysics,* **32**, 542–550.

LEE, D.N. and ARONSON, E. (1974). Visual proprioceptive control of standing in human infants. *Perception and Psychophysics,* **15**, 529–532.

MACFARLANE, A. (1975). Olfaction in the development of social preferences in the human neonate. In *Parent–infant interaction* (CIBA Foundation Symposium 33). Elsevier, Amsterdam.

MANNY, R.E. and KLEIN, S.A. (1985). A three alternative tracking paradigm to measure vernier acuity of older infants. *Vision Research,* **25**, 1245–1252.

MARG, E., FREEMAN, D.N., PELTZMAN, P. and GOLDSTEIN, P.J. (1976). Visual acuity development in human infants: evoked potential measurements. *Investigative Ophthmalology and Visual Science,* **15**, 150–153.

MAYER, D.L. and DOBSON, V. (1982). Visual acuity development in infants and young children, as assessed by operant preferential looking. *Vision Research,* **22**, 1141–1151.

MELTZOFF, A.N. and BORTON, R.W. (1979). Intermodal matching by human neonates. *Nature,* **282**, 403–404.

MELTZOFF, A, N. and MOORE, M.K. (1977). Imitation of facial and manual gestures by human neonates. *Science,* **198**, 75–78.

MOHINDRA, I, ZWAAN, J., HELD, R. *et al.* (1985). Development of acuity and stereopsis in infants with esotropia. *Ophthalmology,* **92**, 691–697.

NAEGLE, J.R. and HELD, R. (1982a). Development of optokinetic nystagmus and effects of abnormal visual experience during infancy. In *Spatially Orientated Behavior,* edited by M. Jeannerod and A. Hein, Springer, New York, pp. 155–174.

NAEGLE, J.R. and HELD, R. (1982b). The postnatal development of monocular optokinetic nystagmus in infants. *Vision Research,* **22**, 341–346.

NORCIA, A.M., TYLER, C.W. and HAMER, R.D. (1988). High contrast sensitivity in the young human infant. *Investigative Ophthalmology and Visual Science,* **29**, 44–49.

PARKS, M.M. (1986). Pediatric ophthalmology and strabismus. In *Transactions of the New Orleans Academy of Ophthalmology, 34th Annual Session.* Raven, New York.

PETRIG, B., JULESZ, B., KROPFL, W. *et al.* (1981). Development of stereopsis and cortical binocularity in human infants: electrophysiological evidence. *Science,* **213**, 1402–1405.

POWERS, M.K., SCHNECK, M. and TELLER, D.Y. (1981). Spectral sensitivity of human infants at absolute visual threshold. *Vision Research,* **21**, 1005–1016.

REGAL, D.M. (1981). Development of critical flicker frequency in human infants. *Vision Research,* **21**, 549–555.

REISSLAND, N. (1988). Neonatal imitation in the first hour of life: observations in rural Nepal. *Developmental Psychology,* **24**, 464–469.

ROGERS, G.L., BREMER, D.L., LEGUIRE, L.E. and FELLOWS, R. (1986). Clinical assessment of visual function in the young child: a prospective study of binocular vision. *Journal of Pediatric Ophthalmology and Strabismus,* **23**, 233–235.

ROSENSTEIN, D. and OSTER, H. (1988). Differential facial responses to four basic tastes in newborns. *Child Development,* **59**, 1555–1568.

SCHOR, C. and NARAYAN, V. (1981). The influence of field size upon the spatial frequency response of optokinetic nystagmus. *Vision Research,* **21**, 986–984.

SCHWARTZ, T.L., DOBSON, V., SANDSTROM, D.J. and HOF-VAN DUIN, J. (1987). Kinetic perimetry assessment of binocular field shape and size in young infants. *Vision Research,* **27**, 2163–2175.

SLATER, A.M. (1989). Visual memory and perception in early infancy. In *Infant Development,* edited by A. Slater and G. Bremner, Erlbaum, Sussex.

SLATER, A.M., MATTOCK, A. and BROWN, E. (1989). Development of Shape and Object Perception from Birth. Paper presented at the Child Vision Research Society, University of Cambridge, July 1989.

SLATER, A.M., MATTOCK, A. and BROWN, E. (1990). Size constancy at birth: newborn infants' responses to retinal and real size. *Journal of Experimental Child Psychology,* **49**, 314–322.

SLATER, A.M. and MORISON, V. (1985). Shape constancy and slant perception at birth. *Perception,* **14**, 337–344.

SLATER, A.M., MORISON, V. and ROSE, D. (1983). Perception of shape by the new-born baby. *British Journal of Developmental Psychology,* **1**, 135–142.

SLATER, A.M., MORISON, V., SOMERS, M. *et al.* (1990). Newborn and older infants' perception of partly occluded objects. *Infant Behavior and Development,* **13**, 33–49.

SLATER, A.M., ROSE, D. and MORISON, V. (1984). New-born infants' perception of similarities and differences between two- and three-dimensional stimuli. *British Journal of Developmental Psychology,* **2**, 287–294.

STAGER, D.R. and BIRCH, E.E. (1986). Preferential-looking acuity and stereopsis in infantile esotropia. *Journal of Pediatric Ophthalmology and Strabismus,* **23**, 160–165.

STREETEN, B.W. (1969). Development of the human retinal pigment epithelium and the posterior segment. *Archives of Ophthalmology,* **81**, 383–394.

TELLER, D.Y. and BORNSTEIN, M.H. (1987). Infant color vision and color perception. In *Handbook of Infant Perception,* vol. I, edited by P. Salapatek and L. Cohen. Academic, New York, pp. 185–236.

VARNER, D., COOK, J.E., SCHNECK, M.E. *et al.* (1985). Tritan discriminations by 1- and 2-month-old human infants. Vision Research, **25**, 821–831.

VON NOORDEN, G.K. (1988). A reassessment of infantile esotropia. XLIV Edward Jackson Memorial Lecture. *American Journal of Ophthalmology,* **105**, 1–10.

WATTAM-BELL, J., BRADDICK, O.J., ATKINSON, J. and DAY, J. (1987). Measures of infant binocularity in a group at risk for strabismus. *Clinical Vision Sciences,* **1**, 327–336.

WESTALL, C.A., WOODHOUSE, J.M. and BROWN, V.A. (1989). OKN asymmetries and binocular function in amblyopia. *Ophthalmology and Physiological Optics,* **9**, 269–276.

YONAS, A., CLEAVES, N. and PETTERSEN, L. (1978). Development of sensitivity to pictorial depth. *Science,* **200**, 77–79.

YUODELIS, C. and HENDRICKSON, A. (1986). A qualitative and quantitative analysis of the human fovea during development. *Vision Research,* **26**, 847–855.

6

Amblyopia

J.A.M. Jennings

Introduction

Amblyopia is the major cause of defective vision in the young with an incidence of a few percent (2.5%, Burian and von Noorden, 1974; 5%, Atkinson *et al.*, 1984). It is more apparent in the central visual field than the periphery (Levi, Yap and Greenlee, 1988) and the loss in sensitivity is greatest under the active inhibitory conditions of simultaneous vision (Awaya and von Noorden, 1972). The effect of this inhibition on monocular acuity is the clinical condition of amblyopia (Chavasse, 1939; Hallden, 1982). It is commonly associated with strabismus and anisometropia although it can result from visual deprivation, cataract or ptosis. The reduction in acuity persists despite correction of the refractive error and is not the result of any pathological processes within the eye. Although reduced acuity is its most obvious defect, amblyopia is a complex functional anomaly affecting many aspects of visual performance.

Site of amblyopia

Retinal image – accommodation and amblyopia

The ocular media are clear at birth (Hansen and Fulton, 1989) and although the muscles of the ciliary body are poorly differentiated (Grose, 1988) as early as the first few weeks there is some deliberate accommodation. This becomes more accurate over the next 4 or 5 months (Banks, 1980; Brookman, 1983; Dobson *et al.*, 1983).

In amblyopia the better eye controls and closely coordinates the accommodation of both eyes (Winn and Heron, 1990). Under monocular conditions the amblyopic accommodative response is abnormal (Schor and Ciuffreda, 1983). Its amplitude is reduced and the response curve is flattened like that of a normal subject who accommodates on a low spatial frequency stimulus. As the amblyopia responds to treatment the accommodative facility recovers (Hokoda and Ciuffreda, 1986), indicating that the dysfunction is secondary to rather than the cause of amblyopia.

The typical refractive errors of infancy (see below) do not impede the development of acuity because of the depth of focus of the eye ($\simeq 1\,D$ at 1 month reducing to $\simeq 0.5\,D$ by 3 months, Green, Powers and Banks, 1980; Boltz, Manny and Katz, 1983), which gives adequate tolerance until the accommodation becomes more accurate.

Receptor amblyopia

Enoch (1959) proposed that amblyopia could be due to misalignment of the outer segments of the cones whose wave guide properties make cone function critically dependent upon orientation. It has been claimed that 3–5 days occlusion flattens the Stiles-Crawford function suggesting an active role for receptor orientation in amblyopia. Subsequent work has demonstrated a phototropic factor influencing the outer segments (Applegate and Bonds, 1981), but no effect of occlusion on adult receptor alignment (Applegate et al., 1986; Enoch et al., 1987). It appears unlikely that receptor amblyopia is a significant factor in strabismic and anisometropic amblyopia.

Retinal ganglion cells

At birth the peripheral retina appears well developed but the central 5° is markedly different from its adult structure. The inner nuclear and ganglion cell layers extend across the fovea. This rod-free foveal area is very large, $\simeq 1$ mm in diameter. The foveal cone inner segments are short and thick and almost all the outer segment develops after birth. The fovea only adopts completely adult characteristics by about the age of 2 years (Yuodelis and Hendrickson, 1986). The foveal optic nerve fibres are myelinated first; all fibres are myelinated by about 5 months. At the lateral geniculate nucleus there is rapid cell growth in the first 6 months with adult characteristics being achieved by about 2 years (Hickey and Peduzzi, 1987).

The visual acuity improves in the first few months because of the increasing specificity and resolution of the cortical neurones (Brown, Dobson and Maier, 1987; Hickey and Peduzzi, 1987) promoted by the combined effects of the increasing density of the foveal cones ($\simeq 4\times$, Yuodelis and Hendrickson, 1986) and the enlargement of the retinal image that follows from growth of the eye ($\simeq 1\frac{1}{2}\times$, Streeten, 1969). This early development does not depend upon normal visual stimulation (Birch and Stager, 1985), indicating that amblyopia is not a failure of the initial stages in the development of acuity.

Ikeda proposed that amblyopia was a retinal anomaly caused by an inappropriate or defocused retinal image (Ikeda and Tremain, 1979). She was able to demonstrate loss of resolution in the central ganglion cells of cats with surgically induced strabismus. However, other investigators (Cleland et al., 1982) found the ganglion cells to have normal resolution. Crewther, Crewther and Cleland (1985) were able to induce retinal dysfunction only when the strabismus was caused by surgery so drastic as to inhibit normal eye movements and probably disrupt proprioceptive feedback (Steinbach, 1987).

Subsequent work has shown that both the retina (Hess et al., 1985) and the lateral geniculate cells have normal resolution, suggesting that cell size is more a function of the metabolic demands of its connections than a reflection of its performance (Blakemore and Vital-Durand, 1986). Even in the absence of normal visual experience, the peripheral visual system develops to be functionally normal with the retina and the lateral geniculate nucleus transmitting high resolution information from the amblyopic eye. Recent work of Blakemore (Collinge, 1989) shows that unlike visually deprived or anisometropic animals, strabismic monkeys, who are deeply amblyopic on behavioural assessment, have cortical neurones with normal responses to high spatial frequency stimuli presented to the amblyopic eye.

The exact nature of the cortical anomaly in amblyopia remains unknown but its pervasive influence results in anomalies of temporal resolution, reaction times and motion detection (Bradley and Freeman, 1985; Chelazzi *et al.*, 1988; Steinman, Levi and McKee, 1988), and subtle differences between anisometropic and strabismic amblyopia.

Strabismic and anisometropic amblyopia

Most anisometropic amblyopia is accompanied by strabismus and sometimes eccentric fixation. However, both experimental work and clinical observation show differences in the natures of strabismic and anisometropic amblyopia.

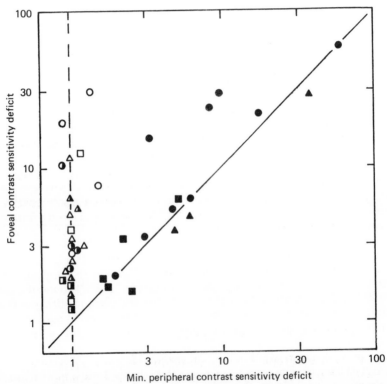

Figure 6.1. A comparison of the loss of central and peripheral contrast sensitivity in strabismic and anisometropic amblyopes. The figure shows the contrast sensitivity deficit in amblyopes with strabismus (open symbols), anisometropia (filled symbols) and both (half-filled symbols) for spatial frequencies of 0.8 cycles/degree (□), 3.2 cycles/degree (○), 6.4 cycles/degree (△), n = 17. The contrast sensitivity loss at the fovea is plotted against the minimum loss anywhere in the central 30°. Data points falling on the vertical dotted line indicate an exclusively central contrast sensitivity loss whereas points on the oblique line indicate a general depression of contrast sensitivity over the retina. Non-strabismic anisometropic amblyopia (filled symbols) tends to a general depression of sensitivity, whereas strabismic amblyopia (open symbols) and strabismic anisometropic amblyopia (half-filled symbols) have a contrast sensitivity loss restricted to the central region. (After Hess and Pointer, 1985)

In anisometropic amblyopia peripheral grating acuity and vernier acuity are equally reduced by adjacent crowding contours. In strabismic amblyopia these acuities have the normal relationship – vernier acuity deteriorates more steeply with peripheral angle than is found for grating acuity (Levi and Klein, 1985). Vernier acuity stimuli have a wide spatial frequency content and it may be that the abnormal discrimination of phase in amblyopia (Hess, Bradley and Piotrowski, 1983; MacCana, Cuthbert and Lovegrove, 1986) is related to the strabismic/anisometropic differences. The reduction in vernier acuity may indicate a more generalized anomaly as it is also defective in the good eye of strabismic, but not anisometropic, amblyopes (Levi and Klein, 1985).

Amblyopia is relatively less severe at mesopic levels (Levi, Yap and Greenlee, 1988) and if a strabismic amblyope dark adapts for several minutes through a 1% transmission grey filter (neutral density 2.0), acuity and contrast sensitivity is little affected. In anisometropic and organic amblyopia the lower light level causes a reduction in acuity and contrast sensitivity (Hess, Campbell and Zimmern, 1980; France, 1984).

With good observers, Amsler charts have been used (Lang, 1969) to detect subjectively the area of central macular inhibition in anisometropia and to distinguish this from the more eccentric area of inhibition in strabismic amblyopia (Lang, 1972).

Comparison of contrast senstivity in the central and peripheral retina of anisometropic and strabismic amblyopes (*Figure 6.1*) shows a systematic difference in the distribution of the amblyopic defect. In non-strabismic anisometropia there is a uniform depression in contrast sensitivity over at least the central 30°, whereas in strabismic amblyopia, whether accompanied or not by anisometropia, the reduced sensitivity is restricted to the foveal region. The presence of strabismus is critical in determining whether or not the peripheral contrast sensitivity is defective. This is confirmed by comparison of central and peripheral (50°) contrast sensitivity functions in a non-strabismic anisometropic amblyope and an isometropic strabismic amblyope (*Figure 6.2*). In both subjects the non-competitive monocular parts of the visual field show no amblyopia (Hess and Pointer, 1985).

The subtle differences between the amblyopias imply different causes. Strabismus dominates any coexisting anisometropia and imposes the strabismic characteristic of an exclusively central retinal defect. Anisometropic amblyopia, like visual deprivation, is more broadly distributed over the retina.

Prediction and prevention of amblyopia

For the prevention of amblyopia to be a realistic objective it is necessary not only to recognize the cause but to be able to counteract it without introducing any other problems. For example, the incidence of amblyopia could be minimized by alternately occluding the eyes from birth, with the unfortunate side-effect that all binocular vision would be lost!

Heredity and amblyopia

The hereditary nature of amblyopia and squint has been noted since Hippocrates (Cantolino and von Noorden, 1969; Jay and Elston, 1987). A very high incidence of

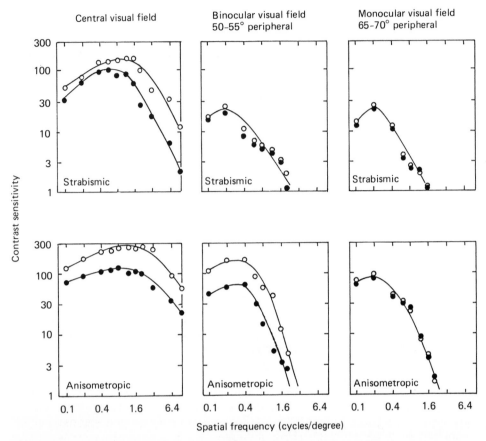

Figure 6.2. Central and peripheral contrast sensitivity in strabismic and anisometropic amblyopia. The figure shows contrast sensitivity functions of the normal (○) and the amblyopic (●) eyes of a strabismic amblyope, upper graphs, and a non-strabismic anisometropic amblyope, lower graphs. In strabismic amblyopia the anomaly is restricted to the central field. In the anisometrope amblyopia is also present in the peripheral binocular field. Neither subject has amblyopia in the peripheral monocular field. (After Hess and Pointer, 1985)

strabismus (40%) has been found in the children of treated amblyopes (Sarniguet-Badoche and Pincon, 1982). However the mode of inheritance is multifactorial, perhaps with some environmental predisposing influences, making specific prediction impossible (Dobson and Sebris, 1989). The effect of having a close relative with amblyopia or strabismus was evaluated in 105 non-strabismic infants (Wattam-Bell *et al.*, 1987) who were monitored from 10 to 26 weeks of age, eight of these developed strabismus over the course of the study, five times the normal incidence of early strabismus. However, 19% of the infants were >4 D hypermetropic, ≃4× normal incidence. A group of nine infants (Dobson and Sebris, 1989) with normal refractive errors at 8 months (<+2.75 D) but having two or more close relatives with strabismus or amblyopia, all remained non-strabismic at 3 years. The refractive error itself seems to be the critical hereditary factor.

Strabismus

Unilateral strabismus is usually accompanied by amblyopia. Obviously, alternators and persistent cross-fixators rarely have significant amblyopia. Larger strabismuses, perhaps because they are noticed and treated earlier, in fact tend to achieve better final acuities than smaller deviations (Neumann, Friedman and Abel-Peleg, 1987). Very low birth weight infants (< 1500 g) are particularly at risk of strabismus and amblyopia (Van Hof-Van Duin *et al.*, 1989), as are children with Down's syndrome or cerebral palsy.

Refractive error

In the newborn, refractive error is widely distributed (mean + 2.00 D, s.d. ± 2 D). The spread diminishes over the first year under the influence of emmetropization to produce a typical refractive error at 1 year of ≃ + 1.00 D (Banks, 1980). Amblyopic eyes emmetropize less effectively and remain more hypermetropic (Lepard, 1975; Nastri *et al.*, 1984). Large refractive errors are unusual, only ≃ 5% of 6–9 month olds have hypermetropia > + 3.50 D and only ≃ 0.5% have myopia > −3.00 D (Atkinson *et al.*, 1984).

Premature infants tend to be myopic (Banks, 1980), but normal, low birth weight infants (< 2000 g) have unremarkable refractive errors (Shapiro *et al.*, 1980). As the eye develops the temporal side of the globe grows more quickly than the nasal side. Hence, at birth the fovea–disc distance is relatively large and it remains fixed from birth to maturity (Streeten, 1969). This results in the large angle K of the newborn (≃ 9°, Slater and Findlay, 1972), which may contribute to the high incidence of against-the-rule astigmatism in the infant (Fulton *et al.*, 1980).

Astigmatism of 1–2 D is typical and regresses spontaneously over the first 12 months as the cornea becomes more spherical (Howland and Sayles, 1985) without causing any permanent meridional deficits, although vernier acuity may be reduced (Gwiazda *et al.*, 1986). Remaining astigmatism diminishes over the next year or two (Abrahamsson, Fabian and Sjöstrand, 1988) towards the typical adult incidence of only ≃ 30% of eyes having > 1 D of astigmatism (Satterfield, 1989).

The minority of children whose astigmatism persists or even increases (Abrahamsson, Fabian and Sjöstrand, 1988) are likely to get meridional amblyopia if left uncorrected (Atkinson *et al.*, 1987). This is a permanent, cortical, loss in contrast sensitivity for gratings of the habitually most defocused orientation, despite optimum refractive correction of the astigmatism (Thibos and Levick, 1982). The Snellen chart is not very sensitive at detecting meridional defects though they are usually associated with hypermetropia and general amblyopia (Atkinson *et al.*, 1987).

Anisometropia is generally associated with amblyopia except when the refractive error encourages alternation as in emmetropia in one eye and low myopia in the other.

The relationship between the refractive error at 1 year and the later incidence of amblyopia and strabismus has been extensively studied. Children with > + 3.50 D in any meridian, about 4% of the population, were found to have a 48% chance of amblyopia being present at 3½ years (Ingram *et al.*, 1986a). However, attempting to influence this outcome, by provision of spectacles to the at-risk group at the age of 1 year (Ingram, 1987) or at 6 months (Ingram *et al.*, 1990b), had no effect on the subsequent incidence of amblyopia. Two-thirds of the infants in the study who became strabismic were not abnormally hypermetropic at 1 year of age and it was noticed that in these the amblyopia responded better to treatment (Ingram *et al.*, 1985).

Ingram proposed two sorts of amblyopia (Ingram, 1987), an early-onset intractable amblyopia related to hypermetropia and strabismus, and a later-onset amblyopia which is amenable to treatment. His conclusion is that though some amblyopias can be predicted they cannot be prevented, casting doubt on the value of routine vision screening of infants (Ingram *et al.*, 1986b, 1990b).

The relationship between hypermetropia, strabismus and amblyopia was confirmed by Dobson and Sebris (1989). A group of high hypermetropic infants ($\geq +4.00$ D at 8 months) had an incidence of strabismus of 38% at 3½ years. The incidence was 24% in the $+3.00 -+4.00$ D group while those with $< +3.00$ D hypermetropia at 1 year had only a 4% (i.e. normal) incidence.

In a study using isotropic-photorefraction rather than retinoscopy (Atkinson *et al.*, 1987), an 'at-risk' criterion of $> +3.50$ D was applied to non-strabismic infants of 6–9 months. One group of high-hypermetropes had spectacles prescribed; an undercorrection of $\simeq 1$ D to minimize the disruption of emmetropization (Repka *et al.*, 1989). A matched group was left uncorrected. At 4 years of age the incidence of squint was 25% for the non-spectacle-wearing hypermetropes whereas for the spectacle wearers the incidence was similar to the normal controls. These data are more encouraging than Ingram's (Ingram *et al.*, 1986b, 1990b) findings and indicate that refractive management might prevent some strabismus and amblyopia.

Rather surprisingly, in both Atkinson's (Atkinson *et al.*, 1987) and Ingram's (Ingram *et al.*, 1990b) studies the acuities of the uncorrected, non-strabismic, hypermetropes were significantly worse than in hypermetropes who had worn a refractive correction.

Statistically refractive error is a good predictor of amblyopia but a causal relationship has not been established. A general strategy of early refractive correction would certainly not prevent the two-thirds of squints which are not associated with excessive hypermetropia and at best would require several infants to wear spectacles 'unnecessarily' for each amblyopic squint prevented.

Clinical investigation of amblyopia

Reduced vision in one eye has little effect on everyday behaviour and is rarely noticed by either the young child or the parent. Diplopia or asthenopic symptoms are unusual, indeed children with persistent headaches should always be referred for further investigation. If strabismus is present within the first year amblyopia is probable and the prognosis for recovery of acuity is poor (Dickey and Scott, 1987). A detailed history is essential to establish the mode and age of onset, the dates, nature and success of previous treatment.

Although a history is essential to determine the background of the visual anomalies, the actual diagnosis of amblyopia in the infant (Ellis *et al.*, 1988) relies heavily on careful observation of eye position and eye movements, the assessment of binocularity, the refractive error and the estimated acuities.

Eye position

Infants will intermittently fixate a pentorch and the positions of the corneal reflexes can be compared (Slater and Findlay, 1972, 1975a, b; Brodie, 1987; Quick and

Boothe, 1989). Only large deviations can be detected (Paliaga, 1989), but the fixing and following ability of the eyes can be compared. Both eyes should follow with equal facility to all extremes of gaze. Any tendency to turn the head to keep the fixation target in the field of the preferred eye suggests amblyopia (Sarniguet-Badoche and Pincon, 1982). The large angle K of the infant ($\approx 9°$; Slater and Findlay, 1972) helps to counteract the impression of convergence produced by the epicanthal folds but it complicates the estimation of the angle of any deviation (Brodie, 1987). A large K should be carefully distinguished from exotropia.

It is easier to hold the attention of infants at near rather than distance so the cover test is often better done with the thumb, while attempting to control fixation with a flashing light or a toy held in the other hand. Any difference in the infant's reaction to the covering of one eye rather than the other should be considered suspicious.

A deeply amblyopic eye may not move to take up fixation when the good eye is covered. Small lateral movements of the target encourage the patient to fixate and help to indicate whether attention is being maintained.

Motor fusion

5Δ or 10Δ base-out placed before one eye of a normal binocular child results in a fusional convergence movement indicating normal binocular function. This reflex should be established by 6 months (Aslin, 1977). Although the response is encouraging in that it objectively demonstrates binocular vision, it does not exclude the presence of some slight amblyopia.

Stereopsis

Experimentally stereopsis is detectable at 4 months (e.g. Archer *et al.*, 1986) but the attention and cooperation required for clinical measurement makes it only routinely possible after at least 2 years.

Stereopsis is a very powerful diagnostic aid since the presence of random dot stereopsis preculudes squint (Reineke and Simons, 1974; Cooper and Feldman 1978, 1981) or substantial amblyopia (Walraven, 1975). The Lang random dot stereo test (Lang, 1984) is sometimes effective with very young children (<1 year, Stidwill, 1985). The Titmus 'fly' can be expected to elicit a response in 3 or 4 year olds and any amblyopia causes a proportional reduction in stereo acuity (Levy and Glick, 1974). With the Titmus test care must be taken in the interpretation of low 'stereo' scores because the lateral displacements creating the disparity are visible as monocular cues in the coarser stimuli (Cooper and Warshowsky, 1977). Clinically measured stereoscopic acuity increases up to early teens, probably as a result of the younger children's lack of attention (Heron *et al.*, 1985). Under ideal conditions and high motivation the stereoscopic acuity of children (3–5 year olds) is similar to adults (Fox, Patterson and Francis, 1986). In infants, the smaller eye separation, $\approx 40\,mm$ in the newborn (Aslin and Jackson, 1979), means that a particular disparity is associated with more physical depth (Lang, 1984).

Refractive error

Refractive error in children can be accurately measured by cycloplegic retinoscopy. Cyclopentolate gives a satisfactory level of cycloplegia (Robb and Petersen, 1968). Departure from the typical range of refractive error or any anisometropia is cause for concern.

Alternative methods of measuring refractive error have been developed based on video or photographic recording of the coaxially illuminated pupil (Howland and Howland, 1974; Bobier, 1988; Wanger and Waern, 1988; Hsu-Winges *et al.*, 1989). Although the accuracy of these methods is typically not high and the refractive range can be limited (Howland *et al.*, 1983; Braddick and Atkinson, 1984), refractive screening of large numbers of children is greatly facilitated (Atkinson *et al.*, 1987).

All measures of refractive error based on light reflection from the fundus suffer from a systematic error caused by the difference between the perceptual layer of the retina and the reflecting surface (Glickstein and Millodot, 1970). This error varies inversely with the square of the eye's focal length. In the infant's eye of $\simeq 16$ mm axial length (Streeten, 1969; Larson, 1971) and $\simeq 85$ D power (Lotmar, 1976) this amounts to an overestimation $\simeq 0.50$ D of hypermetropia.

Visual acuity

Most methods and investigators find acuity of $\simeq$ 6/240 soon after birth (Banks and Dannemiller, 1987). As measured by the visually evoked potential, acuity increases rapidly to approach adult levels within the first year (e.g. Marg *et al.*, 1976), whereas preferential looking indicates a slower development, taking at least 2 years (Mayer and Dobson, 1982). Complete agreement would be surprising since these two techniques assess activity at different levels of the visual system and use different stimulus parameters and scoring criteria (Dobson and Teller, 1978). The evoked potential is always the more sensitive but with identical stimuli the two methods can give highly correlated results (Cannon, 1983). Optokinetic nystagmus findings are similar to those of preferential looking but are heavily influenced by field size (Schor and Narayan, 1981). The monocular asymmetry of optokinetic nystagmus in infants (Naegele and Held, 1982b) and amblyopes (Westall, Woodhouse and Brown, 1989) and the extent to which the technique assesses midbrain as opposed to cortical function (Naegele and Held, 1982a), make it an unsatisfactory measure of developing acuity.

Preferential looking is a successful technique up to about 18 months, after which the child's mobility and curiosity reduce concentration (Dobson *et al.*, 1985). From 3 years matching tests such as Sheridan–Gardner (Fern and Manny, 1986) or Kay Pictures (Kay, 1984) are usually satisfactory. The Snellen distance chart remains difficult for most children up to the age $\simeq 10$ years, particularly when used with a mirror.

The single symbols of the Sheridan–Gardner and Kay tests are very successful with young children (Fern and Manny, 1986) but there is no 'crowding' (Fern *et al.*, 1986) resulting in an overestimate of the acuity of amblyopes. Multiple character charts (Elliott, 1985; Rodier, Mayer and Fulton, 1985; Atkinson *et al.*, 1988) have the test letter surrounded by 'crowding' stimuli to minimize this defect. On all tests, any consistent difference in acuity between the eyes, however small, should be considered suspicious.

Many different picture charts have been produced but problems of standardization and child comprehension make them generally unreliable (Fern and Manny, 1986). The infant's ability to retrieve small cake decorations (hundreds and thousands) is a crude measure of visual function and is not a reliable indicator of amblyopia.

Ophthalmoscopy

It is obviously essential to exclude the possibility of an organic cause for the reduced acuity. Cycloplegia provides ideal conditions for careful ophthalmoscopy and evaluation of the quality and locus of fixation.

Mass screening

Mass screening of infants for amblyopia has frequently been suggested and pilot schemes initiated (e.g. Dholakia, 1987). There is disagreement about the practicality and cost effectiveness of screening (Ingram *et al.*, 1986b; Reineke, 1986; Ingram *et al.*, 1990a) because of its basic difficulty and the limited success of methods of prevention and cure. However, some screening projects (Atkinson *et al.*, 1987; Vital-Durand, 1989) suggest that early refractive correction may prevent some amblyopias.

Quantifying amblyopia

Visual acuity

The initial acuity needs to be carefully measured if progress is to be accurately assessed. A perfunctory measurement with unfamiliar apparatus will exaggerate the original defect and then spurious improvement occurs as familiarity and motivation increase.

The same method of acuity measurement should be used on each occasion, both line and single letter acuity being measured. The acuities are best left as the Snellen fraction so that the actual testing distance is apparent. Three metres is usually the most satisfactory testing distance for children (Fern and Manny, 1986; Atkinson *et al.*, 1988).

Although not all may be clinically practical, a broad range of measurements helps to quantify progress of treatment, for example, contrast sensitivity, accommodation, convergence eye movement records, visually evoked potentials (Thorn and Comerford, 1983).

Contrast sensitivity

The contrast sensitivity function provides a more comprehensive measure of visual disability than is apparent from visual acuity alone. It describes the amblyopic defect across the whole spatial frequency range (*Figure 6.2*) (Hess, 1977b; Bradley and Ohzawa, 1986; Ciuffreda and Fisher, 1987). With appropriate clinical apparatus (Verbaken and Johnston, 1986; Reeves and Hill, 1987; Rubin, 1988) and techniques (Brown and Woodhouse, 1986) the effect of treatment on the contrast sensitivity function can be monitored (Rogers, Bremer and Leguire, 1987; Tytla *et al.*, 1988). The contrast sensitivity function does not correlate well with Snellen acuity, probably because of the single frequency nature of the test. Vernier acuity with its more complex spatial frequency content correlates better with Snellen measures (Levi and Harwerth, 1982) but is differently affected in anisometropic and strabismic amblyopia (Levi and Klein, 1985). The discrimination of phase is suspect (Hess, Campbell and Greenhalgh, 1978; Hess, Bradley and Piotrowski, 1983; MacCana,

Cuthbert and Lovegrove, 1986) and the amblyope's characteristic description of the test chart as high contrast but distorted (Barbeito, Bedell and Flom, 1988), may reflect impaired phase analysis and poor orientation specificity (Skottun, Bradley and Freeman, 1986).

Eccentric fixation

The frequent association of eccentric fixation with amblyopia became apparent with the development of the projection ophthalmoscope. Estimates of the incidence of eccentric fixation in amblyopia vary wildly (Burian and von Noorden, 1974), 50% is a rough average. In deep amblyopia fixation can be several degrees from the fovea and it sometimes varies over a wide area (von Noorden, 1970). The maximum possible acuity at any retinal eccentricity is known from normal data (*Figure 6.3*), any

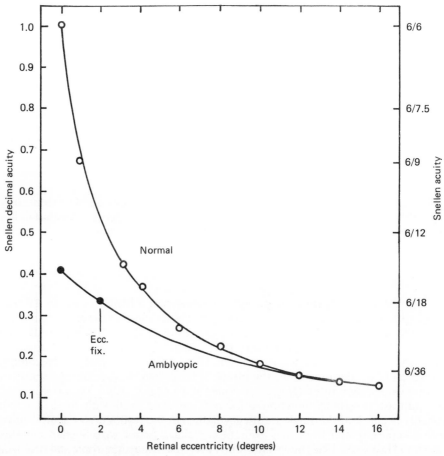

Figure 6.3. Visual acuity and retinal eccentricity. The upper curve shows the normal variation in Landolt C acuity with eccentricity (mean of five). The lower curve is that of an amblyope with 2° eccentric fixation. The foveal acuity is ≃ 6/15 and that at the eccentric fixation point acuity is ≃ 6/18. Acuity remains highest at the fovea but the relative loss is greatest centrally. (After Kirschen and Flom, 1978)

inhibitory influences will further reduce acuity below this value (Hess, 1977a; Kirschen and Flom, 1978).

Occlusion of the amblyopic eye (inverse occlusion) has been recommended as it was feared that conventional occlusion would consolidate rather than eradicate eccentric fixation (Arruga, 1962). The benefit of inverse occlusion has never been substantiated (von Noorden, 1965) and more recent theories of eccentric fixation (Schor, 1978) make it implausible.

The foveal function in amblyopia is controversial. Evidence has accumulated that the deep foveal scotoma envisaged by Worth (1905) and Chavasse (1939) is not present (Linksz, 1952; von Noorden, 1970; Kirschen and Flom, 1978; Flom, Kirschen and Bedell, 1980; Hallden, 1982; Hess and Pointer, 1985; Mehdorn, 1989). Central acuity is obviously subnormal (*Figure 6.4*), but it remains better than the acuity of any other part of the retina (Bradley *et al.*, 1985; Levi, Yap and Greenlee, 1988). The reason that eccentric fixation is adopted is not to facilitate use of best available acuity but because the habitual strabismic deviation causes an adaptive after-effect which modifies the subsequent monocular localization (Schor, 1978).

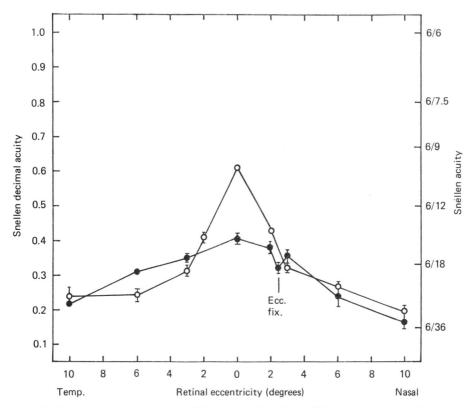

Figure 6.4. Visual acuity in the good eye (○) and the amblyopic eye (●) of an 8° esotrope with 2.4° eccentric fixation. The data are threshold values for 55% negative contrast Landolt C stimuli. The vertical bars or the symbol dimensions represent ± 1 standard error. The acuity is higher at the fovea than at the point of eccentric fixation. Clinically, acuity was 6/6 and ≃ 6/24 in the normal and amblyopic eyes. (After Flom, Kirschen and Bedell, 1980)

Objectives of amblyopia treatment

Functional amblyopia is secondary to early-onset strabismus, anisometropia, astigmatism or more gross sensory deprivation, for example, cataract, ptosis. The underlying cause must be found and treated lest it persists and reasserts its influence.

In early-onset strabismus a stable level of amblyopia is established by school age and restoration of normal binocular vision and equal acuities is rarely possible (Deller, 1988; von Noorden, 1988). Parents and children should be aware that the objectives of treatment are almost always limited to improving acuity, reducing angles of strabismus and enhancing binocularity. A 'cure' is rarely possible.

The minimum justification for treatment is that each eye should be encouraged to develop its best possible vision as an insurance against the surprisingly high incidence of accidental loss of the good eye (Tommila and Tarkkanen, 1981). More ambitiously, the improvement in acuity may be preparation for reviving simultaneous vision prior to aligning the visual axes by surgery, refraction or orthoptic exercises. In non-strabismic anisometropes substantial improvement in both the acuity and stereopsis may be possible.

Experimental occlusion

The treatment of amblyopia by covering the 'good' eye is probably the oldest orthoptic therapy. It is immediately impressive in that it restores the squinting eye to the primary position in the orbit. Its influence on visual acuity may have been an unexpected side-effect. Either Saint-Yves in 1722 (Garzia, 1987) or de Buffon (1743) is credited with the first published account of the use of occlusion for amblyopia treatment.

It is apparent that some amblyopes respond to occlusion and some do not. Ingram, Rogers and Walker, 1977; Ingram, 1987) proposed that early-onset amblyopia, left untreated for 3 months, is subsequently irredeemable, a concept similar to 'amblyopia of arrest' (Chavasse, 1939).

Short-term effects of occlusion

Over the past 25 years much has been learned about the effects of monocular occlusion at various ages on the development of the visual system of the cat and monkey. Despite interspecies differences there are obvious parallels with the amblyopic child.

Studies on young cats, $\simeq 5$ weeks (e.g. Presson and Gordon, 1979), show that alternating occlusion results in very few binocularly driven neurones in the visual cortex. The visual acuity of both eyes is maintained but most neurones are driven by either one eye or the other. Alternate occlusion a few weeks later, $\simeq 12$ weeks old, has much less effect.

Constant monocular occlusion causes most cortical cells to be driven by the fixing eye. Only those cells which would normally be monocularly driven by the occluded eye remain under its influence (Leventhal, 1984). The effects of monocular occlusion can be largely overcome by reversing the occlusion so that the previously deprived eye is used. As little as 1 hour a day of monocular experience for the initially occluded eye produces an improvement in the visually evoked potential and a shift in the cortical dominance in 6-week-old cats (Rauschecker, Schrader and von Grünau,

1987). Careful control of the periods of initial and reverse occlusion can enhance the proportion of binocularly driven cells but never restore normality (Crewther, Crewther and Mitchell, 1983).

Long-term effects of occlusion

Although reverse occlusion is undoubtedly effective, its long-term influence is complex. If after a period of reverse occlusion a cat is then allowed its first experience of simultaneous vision, the improved acuity of the originally occluded eye is quickly lost and the acuity of the originally good eye, which reduced during the period of reverse occlusion, recovers but not to its initial value (*Figure 6.5*) (Mitchell, Murphy and Kaye, 1984). Competition between the eyes makes the acuity of the better eye deteriorate even before the fellow eye has recovered causing bilateral amblyopia (Murphy and Mitchell, 1987). In the end the good eye is a little worse and the bad eye is not much better than after the initial period of deprivation.

This effect is permanent and subsequent monocular occlusion is ineffective in the adult cat (1 year). Enucleation of the better eye has been found to permit an improvement in the acuity in the remaining eye (Mitchell and Murphy, 1984). Similarly enucleation in adult monkeys (4 year olds) also promotes slow but substantial recovery from longstanding strabismic amblyopia (Harwerth *et al.*, 1986). It may be that the removal of the eye and its afferent innervation enhances cortical plasticity (Buisseret and Singer, 1983; Steinbach, 1987).

Cats and monkeys show some differences in their response to occlusion. Monkeys do not retain significant binocular connections after a single period of occlusion, so

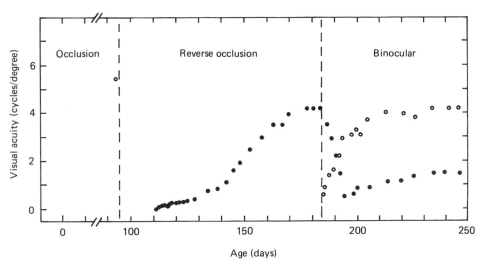

Figure 6.5. Changes in the visual acuity of the initially open eye (○) and the initially occluded eye (●) of a cat. At 94 days the unoccluded eye (○) has normal acuity of ≃ 5.5 cycles/degree. The occlusion is reversed and the acuity of the initially deprived eye (●) recovers to ≃ 4 cycles/degree. At 184 days binocular viewing is permitted for the first time. The newly developed acuity of the initially deprived eye (●) immediately deteriorates and stabilizes at ≃ 2.5 cycles/degree. The acuity of the 'good' eye (○) is found to have reduced to ≃ 0.5 cycle/degree during the period of reverse occlusion. Under binocular conditions it recovers to ≃ 4 cycles/degree, less than its acuity at 94 days. (After Mitchell *et al.*, 1984)

binocular experience does not promote a partial recovery of the amblyopic eye as happens in cats. In monkeys, reverse occlusion completely reverses the effects of the initial deprivation and the absence of binocularity prevents the competition which, in cats, leads to significant bilateral amblyopia (Crawford *et al.*, 1989; Harwerth *et al.*, 1989).

Long periods of monocular occlusion, even from birth, do not seem to cause strabismus in cats (Mitchell, Murphy and Kaye, 1984; von Noorden, 1985a) or monkeys (Harwerth *et al.*, 1989), but daily alternating occlusion from birth does result in strabismus and alternating suppression (Tumosa *et al.*, 1983). The speed of the acuity changes in young animals suggests a role for pharmacological agents affecting synaptic neurotransmission (Sillito, 1979; von Noorden, 1985a).

In strabismic infants the monocular acuities start to develop normally. An amblyopic difference in acuity can only be demonstrated after $\simeq 8$ months (Birch and Stager, 1985; Mohindra *et al.*, 1985). At this early age amblyopia responds quickly to occlusion showing a trade-off between the acuities of the eyes (Thomas, Mohindra and Held, 1979) similar to that described in cats (Mitchell, Murphy and Kaye, 1984). Von Noorden (1985b) describes 'idiopathic amblyopia' in clinical patients. Once competition between the eyes has been established the acuities 'see-saw' even if the original anisometropia or strabismus is no longer present.

A study of patients who had lost the vision of their good eye through accident or disease in middle age showed that there were substantial improvements in acuity in about a third of the 203 cases (Vereecken and Brabant, 1984). So it appears that at least in some cases partial recovery of monocular acuity is possible at almost any age.

The reverse occlusion data implies that the good eye of amblyopes may also have some restriction of function. In adult amblyopes Kandel, Grattan and Bedell (1977) found small ($\simeq 5$ minutes) nasal eccentric fixation in the good eye. Vernier acuity is reduced in the good eye of strabismic but not anisometropic amblyopes (Levi and Klein, 1985). In amblyopes who had been occluded, the good eye has a reduced response to high spatial frequencies in motion detection tasks (Bromley, Javadnia and Ruddock, 1987). Both Day, Orel-Bixter and Narcia (1988) and Dobson and Sebris (1989) report that the acuity of the good eye of esotropes is significantly subnormal, perhaps as a result of occlusion or the slight deprivational effects of uncorrected hypermetropia (Atkinson *et al.*, 1987; Ingram *et al.*, 1990b).

Occlusion is very effective at promoting large changes in acuity and cortical organization in young animals (e.g. Presson and Gordon, 1979). The period of developmental plasticity can be extended by various means, for example, dark-rearing (Blakemore and Price, 1987; Wright, Wehrle and Urrea, 1987; Mitchell, 1988), modification of the proprioceptive input to the cortex (Buisseret and Singer, 1983; Steinbach, 1987) or by pharmacological effects (Kasamatsu and Pettigrew, 1979; Singer, 1985; von Noorden, 1985a). Even in adult animals a slow recovery of acuity occurs if they are made to be critically dependent upon visual information and hence 'highly motivated' (Singer, Tetter and Yinon, 1982a, b).

Refractive error and occlusion

In neonatal chickens (Gottlieb, Fugate-Wentzek and Wallman, 1987), cats (Yinon and Koslowe, 1984) and monkeys (Smith *et al.*, 1987) monocular lid suture causes large, generally myopic, refractive errors. The growth of the eye seems to be under local influences since sectioning of the optic nerve does not prevent the refractive change (Raviola and Weisel, 1985; Wildsoet and Pettigrew, 1988). Similar myopic anisometropia occurs in human infants who are visually deprived from birth by unilateral cataract or corneal opacity (Raviola and Weisel, 1985). Clinical occlusion of amblyopes later in childhood has not been found to affect the refractive error. Paradoxically, the amblyopic eye is usually more hypermetropic than the fixing eye (Lepard, 1975; Nastri et al., 1984).

Stereopsis and occlusion

Disruption of binocular vision whether by naturally occurring strabismus or by occlusion has a detrimental effect on stereopsis (Ross-Dommasch and Morris, 1987). The experimental evidence from work with cats (Timney, 1984) suggests that a brief period of monocular vision (10 days) in early life ($\simeq$40 days old) permanently destroys stereopsis without causing amblyopia or a strabismus, despite unrestricted previous and subsequent binocular experience. Similar periods of monocular vision earlier or later than $\simeq$40 days have minimal effect on binocularity. In monkeys, Crawford et al. (1984) found that dissociation between 30 and 60 days with large oblique ophthalmic prisms resulted in no amblyopia or strabismus but permanent loss of stereopsis. Animal experiments show that abnormal visual experience early in life can cause loss of stereopsis without loss of motor fusion (Crawford et al., 1983; Harwerth et al., 1989), demonstrating the relative independence of stereoscopic disparity analysis and disparity-driven vergence control (von Noorden, 1985a; McKee and Mitchison, 1988; Rose, Blake and Halpern, 1988).

Infants, even infantile esotropes, show signs of stereopsis when their visual axes are aligned either with prism or by surgery (Birch and Stager, 1985; Mohindra et al., 1985; Archer et al., 1986), but if the visual axes are not permanently aligned by some time about the end of the first year, the opportunity for stereopsis is irretrievably lost. Although results remain disappointing, clinical data confirm that early surgery gives the best chance of some level of binocularity (e.g. Deller, 1988).

Clinical occlusion

The optimum occlusion routine is controversial. Animal work strongly favours brief periods of occlusion spread over many days (e.g. Crewther, Crewther and Mitchell, 1983; Mitchell et al., 1986). However, these studies refer largely to young non-strabismic animals which are dark-reared when not receiving their allocation of visual experience. This is quite different from the visual environment of the strabismic child.

In amblyopic children more than 5 years old, there is little danger of occlusion amblyopia (Burian and von Noorden, 1974) and clinical experience confirms that the recommendations of Worth (1905) remain valid and sensible.

> I order the fixing eye to be continuously occluded for a time. It is not a good plan to order the eye to be occluded for part of each day only; apart from the fact that this is not nearly so rapid and effective as continuous occlusion, the child usually cries every time the shade is applied, so the treatment is seldom properly carried out. When the better eye is continuously covered, the child soon becomes accustomed to the shade, so that, after a day or two, he usually ceases to object to it. ... I examine the child again at the end of two or three weeks. If the vision of the deviating eye be improved sufficiently, the shade is discontinued. If not, the fixing

eye is occluded for a another month, after which the child is again examined. If occlusion of the fixing eye is going to do much good, one usually finds a very great improvement in the vision of the squinting eye within a fortnight.

Constant total occlusion with an adhesive eye patch (Opticlude, 3M Medical Products Division) is the most effective regimen. The patch only needs replacing when it falls off or becomes unacceptably grubby. The refractive correction is worn constantly to optimize the acuity and to minimize the deviation. The acuities of both eyes are reviewed every week. Acuities for line and single letter are measured on each occasion, as is contrast sensitivity if possible. As Worth (1905) noted, 2 weeks of constant occlusion is usually sufficient to discover if progress can be made. In successful cases improvement occurs in a few days and there is a noticeable increase in the confidence the child places in the amblyopic eye. If there is no sign of any improvement after 2 weeks it is neither kind nor productive to persist.

If occlusion is successful it is continued for a few more weeks until it is apparent that no more improvement is possible. The final level of acuity is rarely perfect, for example, 6/9. Examination often reveals a microtropia (Helveston and von Noorden, 1967) which forms a satisfactory and stable conclusion to the treatment.

Animal work shows that excessive early occlusion destroys binocularity and encourages an abnormal level of interocular competition. It may be that any period of occlusion in the first year of life is hazardous, even bandaging for injuries should be carefully considered. Despite these risks, Blakemore and Vital-Durand (1986) report that correction of abnormal refractive errors and brief periods of occlusion immediately on detection of any acuity difference, shows promise as a management strategy for high-risk infants (Collinge, 1989).

The risk of provoking a strabismus by occluding an anisometropic amblyope is thought to be small, for example, 'What may be at risk after unilateral or alternate patching during infancy is not the patient's ability to fuse but his stereopsis. Loss of stereopsis is a small price to pay for the advantage of regaining normal vision in a formally amblyopic eye or preventing the development of amblyopia by patching' (von Noorden, 1985a). Despite this firm advice, prudence dictates that occlusion of children should be brief and carefully monitored.

Other forms of treatment

Penalization

As an alternative to occlusion, the near vision of one eye can be blurred by instilling atropine (Worth, 1905; Cantonnet and Filliozat, 1938). If the amblyopic eye is over-plussed by $+3.00\,D$ and atropine instilled into the other eye, then the good eye will be used for distance vision and the amblyopic eye for near vision – near-vision penalization. The advantage of the method is that binocular vision is maintained rather than disrupted, latent nystagmus remains latent and the embarrassment of wearing an occluder is avoided. It is less effective than conventional occlusion and is more appropriate for mild amblyopia and intermittent deviations (Flynn and Cassady, 1978; Deller, 1979). The daily instillation of atropine drops is a disadvantage and the legality of the extended therapeutic use of a drug by a British optometrist is doubtful.

Prism therapies

Prism equal to the angle of the squint, placed before the good eye, causes a version movement of both eyes and the amblyopic fovea is 'stimulated passively'. Combining the prism with near penalization has a claimed ≃70% cure rate for amblyopes up to mid teens (Brack, 1976; Haasse, 1976). The deviation is said to be stable over many months (Haase, 1976), and is apparently not influenced by prism adaptation (Sethi, 1986; Morley, Lindsey and Judge, 1988).

Adverse prism has been used in association with conventional occlusion in order to disrupt eccentric fixation (Mallett, 1979). The rationale is that adverse prism, base out for exo-eccentric fixation or base in for eso-eccentric fixation, forces the eye to move beyond its habitual monocular posture and helps to re-establish foveal fixation.

Pleoptics

Foveal fixation and enhanced hand-eye coordination can be encouraged by selective stimulation of the fovea and peripheral retina with after-images. A whole range of these 'pleoptic' techniques have been developed (Duke-Elder, 1973). The claims of these methods have not been sustained and intensive inpatient treatment is not thought to be justified by the results (Garzia, 1987). Despite the fading of enthusiasm for pleoptic methods (Nawratski, 1976), techniques such as after-image transfer (Caloroso, 1972), the Nutt auto disc (Lyle and Wybar, 1967) and 4 Hz flashing stimuli (Mallett, 1985) remain useful methods, although never formally substantiated, for older and less easily occluded amblyopes.

Rotating gratings

Viewing rotating gratings (Dobson, 1933; Campbell et al., 1978) has not proved any more effective than other demanding visual tasks performed while occluded (Garzia, 1987).

Antisuppression exercises

Non-strabismic amblyopia is best managed without intensive occlusion (Pickwell, 1976) and the attendant risk of precipitating a strabismus. The non-strabismic amblyope is the ideal patient for short periods of occlusion (≃1 hour/day) within a binocular regimen (Mitchell et al., 1986). The occlusion is more effective if reinforced with detailed hand–eye coordination tasks, for example 'frogspawn' (Pickwell, 1984). The full refractive correction should be worn constantly and in anisometropia, aniseikonia is best minimized with contact lenses (Winn et al., 1988). If the deviation can be eradicated by surgery or refraction, even if only at one distance, then orthoptics, for example, Holmes stereoscope cards, physiological diplopia, home computer exercises, may reduce the amblyopia as normal binocular vision is encouraged (Pickwell, 1984; Somers, Happel and Phillips, 1984).

Effectiveness of amblyopia treatment

Success of treatment

The effect of amblyopia treatment is variable with a typical success rate of ≈40%. Success can be defined as 6/9 or an improvement of several lines (e.g. Birnbaum,

Koslowe and Sanet, 1977; Jenkins and Pickwell, 1982). The recent comprehensive review by Garzia (1987) stresses the importance of a full refractive correction combined with conventional occlusion and demanding visuomotor activities, for example detailed drawing exercises.

Influence of age

Younger children tend to recover their acuity more quickly (von Noorden, 1965), leading to the suggestion that occlusion is ineffective above a certain age, for example 'After about seven years of age usually not much improvement in vision can be obtained, though I have met with many exceptions to this rule' (Worth, 1905). In early-onset strabismus best results have been achieved when treatment starts before 18 months (Neumann, Friedman and Abel-Peleg, 1987), but a further study has shown no relationship between the age of onset, the duration of the squint and the final acuity in conventionally managed, squinting, children (Ingram et al., 1990b). Up to late teens, there is little evidence that the age of starting treatment has any effect on the probability of success (Birnbaum et al., 1977; Vereecken and Brabant, 1984; Hokoda and Ciuffreda, 1986). It may be that the greater motivation of older patients balances their decreasing plasticity.

Hazards

The art of amblyopia treatment is to balance the conflicting demands of monocular and binocular vision. Occlusion, the most effective method of enhancing monocular acuity, is obviously disruptive of binocular vision. In infantile strabismus the prognosis for normal binocular vision is very poor, good monocular acuity for each eye is the most realistic objective. In later-onset strabismus a binocular infrastructure has been established and it is reasonable to try to enhance both acuity and binocularity.

Occlusion rarely causes subsequent diplopia but care should be exercised in patients with a previous history of diplopia. In such cases the restoration of binocular vision is unlikely and there may be risk of reviving distressing diplopia.

The gravest hazard of amblyopia management is the erroneous assumption of functional amblyopia in a child whose binocular anomaly is secondary to active pathology, for example, the strabismus caused by retinoblastoma. This disastrous mistake can only be prevented by careful examination of the patient and continual reappraisal of diagnoses.

Conclusion

Amblyopia treatment remains dominated by occlusion. The effects of this primitive procedure are being systematically unravelled by neurophysiological research, while clinical observation slowly sifts out the more successful management strategies. There is progress and we are now in a better position to answer the basic questions, 'which of the two eyes should be occluded, and with what, and for how long?' (Tour, 1966).

Clinical management of the amblyope consists of a detailed investigation, exclusion of pathological causes, consideration of the implications of the history and of the probable effects of treating and of not treating, the initiation and monitoring of treatment as appropriate, and the acceptance of a long-term commitment to the patient's visual care.

Despite all efforts, many amblyopes do not respond to treatment. Treatment can be effective but, for the present, it can only realistically have the limited objectives of improvement of acuity rather than restoration of normal binocular function. The amblyopic child has a history of abnormal development and the crude techniques of clinical treatment cannot dismantle an anomalous visual system and flawlessly rebuild it.

References

ABRAHAMSSON, M., FABIAN, G. and SJÖSTRAND, J. (1988). Changes in astigmatism between the ages of 1 and 4 years: a longitudinal study. *British Journal of Ophthalmology, 72*, 145–149.

APPLEGATE, R.A., ADAMS, A.A., BRADLEY, A. and EISNER, A. (1986). Total occlusion does not disrupt photoreceptor alignment. *Investigative Ophthalmology and Visual Science, 27*, 441–443.

APPLEGATE, R.A. and BONDS, A.B. (1981). Induced movement of receptor alignment toward a new pupillary aperture. *Investigative Ophthalmology and Visual Science, 21*, 869–873.

ARCHER, S.M., HELVESTON, E.M., MILLER, K.K. and ELLIS, F.D. (1986). Stereopsis in normal infants and infants with congenital esotropia. *American Journal of Ophthalmology, 101*, 591–596.

ARRUGA, A. (1962). Effect of occlusion of amblyopic eye on amblyopia and eccentric fixation. *Transactions of the Ophthalmological Society of the UK, 82*, 45–61.

ASLIN, R.N. (1977). Development of binocular fixation in human infants. *Journal of Experimental Child Psychology, 23*, 133–150.

ASLIN, R.N. and JACKSON, R.W. (1979). Accommodative-convergence in young infants: development of a synergistic sensory-motor system. *Canadian Journal of Psychology, 33*, 222–231.

ATKINSON, J., ANKER, S., EVANS, C. *et al.* (1988). Visual acuity testing of young children with the Cambridge Crowding Cards at 3 and 6 m. *Acta Ophthalmologica, 66*, 505–508.

ATKINSON, J., BRADDICK, O., DURDEN, K. *et al.* (1984). Screening for refractive errors in 6–9 months old infants by photorefraction. *British Journal of Ophthalmology, 68*, 105–112.

ATKINSON, J., BRADDICK, O., WATTAM-BELL, J. *et al.* (1987). Photo-refractive screening of infants and effects of refractive correction. *Investigative Ophthalmology and Visual Science.*, Suppl 28, 399.

AWAYA, S. and VON NOORDEN, G.K. (1972). Visual acuity of amblyopic eyes under monocular and binocular conditions: further observations. *Journal of Pediatric Ophthalmology, 9*, 8–13.

BANKS, M. S. (1980). Infant refraction and accommodation. In *Electrophysiology and Psychophysics: Their Use in Ophthalmic Diagnosis* International Ophthalmology Clinics vol. 20, no. 1, edited by S. Sokol. Little, Brown & Co., Boston.

BANKS, M.S. and DANNEMILLER. J.L. (1987). Infant visual psychophysics. In *Handbook of Infant Perception*, vol. I, edited by P. Salapatek and L. Cohen. Academic Press, New York.

BARBEITO, R., BEDELL, H.E. and FLOM, M.C. (1988). Does impaired contrast sensitivity explain the spatial uncertainty of amblyopes? *Investigative Ophthalmology and Visual Science, 29*, 323–326.

BIRCH, E.E. and STAGER. D.R. (1985). Monocular acuities and stereopsis in infantile esotropia. *Investigative Ophthalmology and Visual Science, 26*, 1624–1630.

BIRNBAUM, M.H., KOSLOWE, K. and SANET, R. (1977). Success in amblyopia therapy as a function of age: a literature survey. *American Journal of Optometry and Physiological Optics, 54*, 269–275.

BLAKEMORE, C. and PRICE, D.J. (1987). Effects of dark-rearing on the development of area 18 of the cat's visual cortex. *Journal of Physiology, 384*, 293–309.

BLAKEMORE, C. and VITAL-DURAND, F. (1986). Effects of visual deprivation upon the development of the monkey's lateral geniculate nucleus. *Journal of Physiology, 380*, 493–511.

BOBIER, W.R. (1988). Quantitative photorefraction using an off-center flash source. *American Journal of Optometry and Physiological Optics, 65*, 962–971.

BOLTZ, R.L., MANNY, R.E. and KATZ. B.J. (1983). Effects of induced optical blur on infant visual acuity. *American Journal of Optometry and Physiological Optics, 60*, 100–105.

BRACK, B. (1976). Penalisation and prism. In *Orthoptics: Past, Present and Future*, edited by S. Moore, J. Mein and L. Stockbridge. Stratton Inter-Cont. Medical Book Corp., New York, pp. 99–103.

BRADDICK, O. and ATKINSON, J. (1984). Photorefractive techniques: applications in testing infants and young children. In *First International Congress of the British College of Ophthalmic Opticians* (Optometrists), Part II, edited by W.N. Charman, British College of Ophthalmic Opticians (Optometrists), London, pp. 25–34.

BRADLEY, A. and FREEMAN, R.D. (1985). Temporal sensitivity in amblyopia: an explanation of conflicting reports. *Vision Research,* **25**, 39–46.

BRADLEY, A., FREEMAN, R.D. and APPLEGATE, R. (1985). Is amblyopia spatial frequency or retinal locus specific? *Vision Research,* **25**, 47–54.

BRADLEY, A. and OHZAWA, I. (1986). A comparison of contrast detection and discrimination. *Vision Research,* **26**, 991–997.

BRODIE, S.E. (1987). Photographic calibration of the Hirschberg test. *Investigative Ophthalmology and Visual Science,* **28**, 736–742.

BROMLEY, J.M., JAVADNIA, A. and RUDDOCK, K.H. (1987). Visual spatial filtering and pattern discrimination are abnormal in strabismic amblyopia. *Clinical Vision Science,* **1**, 209–218.

BROOKMAN, K.E. (1983). Ocular accommodation in human infants. *American Journal of Optometry and Physiological Optics,* **60**, 91–99.

BROWN, A.M., DOBSON, V. and MAIER, J. (1987). Visual acuity of human infants at scotopic, mesopic and photopic luminances. *Vision Research,* **27**, 1845–1858.

BROWN, V.A. and WOODHOUSE, J.M. (1986). Assessment of techniques for measuring contrast sensitivity in children. *Ophthalmic and Physiological Optics,* **6**, 165–170.

DE BUFFON, G.L.L. (1743). Dissertation sur la cause du strabisme ou des yeux louches. Mémoires de l'Academie Royale des Sciences Paris, 231–248.

BUISSERET, P. and SINGER, W. (1983). Proprioceptive signals from extraocular muscles gate experience-dependent modifications of receptive fields in the kitten visual cortex. *Experimental Brain Research,* **51**, 443–450.

BURIAN, H.M. and VON NOORDEN, G.K. (1974). *Binocular Vision and Ocular Motility.* C.V. Mosby, St Louis.

CALOROSO, E. (1972). After-image transfer: a therapeutic procedure for amblyopia. *American Journal of Optometry and Archives of the American Academy of Optometry,* **49**, 65–69.

CAMPBELL, F.W., HESS, R.F., WATSON, P.G. and BANKS, R. (1978). Preliminary results of a physiologically based treatment of amblyopia. *British Journal of Ophthalmology,* **62**, 747–755.

CANNON, R.W. (1983). Contrast sensitivity: psychophysical and evoked potential methods compared. *Vision Research,* **23**, 87–95.

CANTOLINO, S.J. and VON NOORDEN, G.K. (1969). Heredity in microtropia. *Archives of Ophthalmology,* **81**, 753–757.

CANTONNET, A. and FILLIOZAT, J. (1938). *Strabismus,* 2nd edn, translated by M. Coque. M. Wiseman, London.

CHAVASSE, F.B. (1939). *Worth's Squint or The Binocular Reflexes and The Treatment of Strabismus,* 7th edn. Bailliere, Tindall and Cox, London.

CHELAZZI, L., MARZI, C.A., PANOZZO, G. *et al.* (1988). Hemiretinal differences in speed of light detection in esotropic amblyopes. *Vision Research,* **28**, 95–104.

CIUFFREDA, K.J. and FISHER, S.K. (1987). Impairment of contrast discrimination in amblyopic eyes. *Ophthalmic and Physiological Optics,* **7**, 461–467.

CLELAND, B.G., CREWTHER, D.P., CREWTHER, S.G. and MITCHELL, D.E. (1982). Normality of spatial resolution of retinal ganglion cells in cats with strabismic amblyopia. *Journal of Physiology,* **326**, 235–249.

COLLINGE, A. (1989). What is amblyopia ... can it be prevented? Owen Aves Memorial Lecture by Blakemore, C. *Optometry Today,* 4 December, 8.

COOPER, J. and FELDMAN, J. (1981). Depth perception in strabismus. *British Journal of Ophthalmology,* **65**, 510.

COOPER, J. and FELDMAN, J. (1978). Random-dot-stereogram performance by strabismic, amblyopic and ocular-pathology patients in an operant-discrimination task. *American Journal of Optometry and Physiological Optics,* **55**, 599–609.

COOPER, J. and WARSHOWSKY, J. (1977). Lateral displacement as a response cue in the Titmus stereo test. *American Journal of Optometry and Physiological Optics,* **54**, 537–541.

CRAWFORD, M.J.L., DE FABER, J-T., HARWERTH, R.S. *et al.* (1989). The effects of reverse monocular deprivation in monkeys. II Electrophysiological and anatomical studies. *Experimental Brain Research,* **74**, 338–347.

CRAWFORD, M.L.J., SMITH, E.L., HARWERTH, R.S. and VON NOORDEN, G.K. (1984). Stereoblind monkeys have few binocular neurons. *Investigative Ophthalmology and Visual Science,* **25**, 779–781.

CRAWFORD, M.J.L., VON NOORDEN., G.K., MEHARG, L. *et al.* (1983). Binocular neurons and binocular function in monkeys and children. *Investigative Ophthalmology and Visual Science,* **24**, 491–495.

CREWTHER, S.G., CREWTHER, D.P. and CLELAND, B.G. (1985). Convergent strabismic amblyopia in cats. *Experimental Brain Research,* **60**, 1–9.

CREWTHER, S.G., CREWTHER, D.P. and MITCHELL, D.E. (1983). The effects of short-term occlusion therapy on reversal of the anatomical and physiological effects of monocular deprivation in the LGN and visual cortex of kittens. *Experimental Brain Research,* **51**, 206–216.

DAY, S.H., OREL-BIXLER, D.A. and NARCIA, A.M. (1988). Abnormal acuity development in infantile esotropia. *Investigative Ophthalmology and Visual Science,* **29**, 327–329.

DELLER, M. (1979). Are amblyopic man and ape related? *Trends in Neuroscience,* **2**, 216–218.

DELLER, M. (1988). Why should surgery for early-onset strabismus be postponed? *British Journal of Ophthalmology,* **72**, 110–115.

DHOLAKIA, S. (1987). The application of a comprehensive visual screening programme to children aged 3–5 years. Can a modified procedure be devised for visual screening by ancillary staff? *Ophthalmic and Physiological Optics,* **7**, 469–476.

DICKEY, C.F. and SCOTT, W.E. (1987). Amblyopia – the prevalence in congenital esotropia versus partially accommodative esotropia – diagnosis and results of treatment. In *Orthoptic Horizons. Transactions of the 6th International Orthoptics Congress, Harrogate, UK,* edited by M. Lenk-Schafer, International Orthoptic Association, London, 107–112.

DOBSON, M. (1933). *Binocular Vision and the Modern Treatment of Squint.* Oxford University Press, Humphrey Milford, London.

DOBSON, V., HOWLAND, H.C., MOSS, C. and BANKS, M.S. (1983). Photorefraction of normal and astigmatic infants during viewing of patterned stimuli. *Vision Research,* **23**, 1043–1052.

DOBSON, V., SALEM, D., MAYER, D.L. *et al.* (1985). Visual acuity screening of children 6 months to 3 years of age. *Investigative Ophthalmology and Visual Science,* **26**, 1057–1063.

DOBSON, V. and SEBRIS, S.L. (1989). Longitudinal study of acuity and stereopsis in infants with or at-risk for esotropia. *Investigative Ophthalmology and Visual Science,* **30**, 1146–1158.

DOBSON, V. and TELLER, D.Y. (1978). Visual acuity in human infants: a review and comparison of behavioural and electrophysiological studies. *Vision Research,* **18**, 1469–1483.

DUKE-ELDER, S. (1973). Ocular motility and strabismus. In *System of Ophthalmology*, vol. VI, Henry Kimpton, London, 110–115.

ELLIOTT, R. (1985). A new linear picture vision test. *British Orthoptics Journal,* **42**, 54–57.

ELLIS, G.S., HARTMANN, E.E., LOVE, A. *et al.* (1988). Teller acuity cards versus clinical judgement in the diagnosis of amblyopia with strabismus. *Ophthalmology,* **95**, 788–791.

ENOCH, J.M. (1959). Receptor amblyopia. *American Journal of Ophthalmology,* **48**, 262–274.

ENOCH, J.M., BIRCH, D.G. and BIRCH, E.E. (1979). Monocular light exclusion for a period of days reduces directional sensitivity of the retina. *Science,* **206**, 705–707.

ENOCH, J.M., HAMER, R.D., LAKSHMINARAYANAN, V. *et al.* (1987). Effect of monocular light exclusion in the Stiles–Crawford function. *Vision Research,* **27**, 507–510.

FERN, K.D. and MANNY, R.E. (1986). Visual acuity of the preschool child: a review. *American Journal of Optometry and Physiological Optics,* **63**, 319–345.

FERN, K.D., MANNY, R.E., DAVIS, J.R. and GIBSON, R.R. (1986). Contour interaction in the preschool child. *American Journal of Optometry and Physiological Optics,* **63**, 313–318.

FLOM, M.C., KIRSCHEN, D.G. and BEDELL, H.E. (1980). Acuity in eccentrically fixating amblyopes. *American Journal of Optometry and Physiological Optics,* **57**, 191–194.

FLYNN, J.T. and CASSADY, J.C. (1978). Current trends in amblyopia therapy. *Ophthalmology,* **85**, 428–450.

FOX, R., PATTERSON, R. and FRANCIS, E.L. (1986). Stereoacuity in young children. *Investigative Ophthalmology and Visual Science,* **27**, 598–600.

FRANCE, T.D. (1984). Amblyopia update: diagnosis and therapy. *American Orthoptics Journal,* **34**, 4–12.

FULTON, A.B., DOBSON, V., SALEM, D. *et al.* (1980). Cycloplegic refractions in infants and young children. *American Journal of Ophthalmology*, **90**, 239–247.

GARZIA, R.P. (1987). Efficacy of vision therapy in amblyopia: a literature review. *American Journal of Optometry and Physiological Optics*, **64**, 393–404.

GLICKSTEIN, M. and MILLODOT, M. (1970). Retinoscopy and eye size. *Science*, **168**, 605–606.

GOTTLIEB, M.D., FUGATE-WENTZEK, L.A. and WALLMAN, J. (1987). Different visual deprivations produce different ametropias and different eye shapes. *Investigative Ophthalmology and Visual Science*, **28**, 1225–1235.

GREEN, D.G., POWERS, M.K. and BANKS, M.S. (1980). Depth of focus eye size and visual acuity. *Vision Research*, **20**, 827–835.

GROSE, J. (1988). The development of the visual system. *Optician*, **195**, (5131), 15 January, 18–21, 24–26.

GWIAZDA, J., BAUER, J., THORN, F. and HELD, R. (1986). Meridional amblyopia does result from astigmatism in early childhood. In *Clinical Vision Science*, **1**, 145–152.

HAASSE, W. (1976). Experiences with penalisation. In *Orthoptics: Past, Present and Future*, edited by S. Moore, J. Mein and L. Stockbridge. Stratton Inter-Cont. Medical Book Corp., New York, pp. 105–111.

HALLDEN, U. (1982). Suppression scotomata in concomitant strabismus with harmonious anomalous correspondence. *Acta Ophthalmologica*, **60**, 828–834.

HANSEN, R.H. and FULTON, A.B. (1989). Psychophysical estimates of ocular media density of human infant. *Vision Research*, **29**, 687–690.

HARWERTH, R.S., SMITH, E,L., CRAWFORD., M.J.L. and VON NOORDEN, G.K. (1989). The effects of reverse monocular deprivation in monkeys. I. Psychophysical experiments. *Experimental Brain Research*, **74**, 327–337.

HARWERTH, R.S., SMITH, E.L., DUNCAN, G.C. *et al.* (1986). Effects of enucleation of the fixing eye on strabismic amblyopia in monkeys. *Investigative Ophthalmology and Visual Science*, **27**, 246–254.

HELVESTON, E.M. and VON NOORDEN, G.K. (1967). Microtropia: a newly defined entity. *Archives of Ophthalmology*, **78**, 272–281.

HERON, G., DHOLAKIA, S., COLLINS, D.E. and MCLAUGHLIN, H. (1985). Stereoscopic threshold in children and adults. *American Journal of Optometry and Physiological Optics*, **62**, 505–515.

HESS, R.F. (1977a). On the relationship between strabismic amblyopia and eccentric fixation. *British Journal of Ophthalmology*, **61**, 767–773.

HESS, R.F. (1977b). The threshold contrast sensitivity function in stabismic amblyopia: evidence for a two type classification. *Vision Research*, **17**, 1049–1055.

HESS, R.F., BAKER, C.L., VERHOEVE, J.N. *et al.* (1985). The pattern evoked electroretinogram: its variability in normals and its relationship to amblyopia. *Investigative Ophthalmology and Visual Science*, **26**, 1610–1623.

HESS, R.F., BRADLEY, A. and PIOTROWSKI, L. (1983). Contrast coding in amblyopia. I. Differences in the neural basis of human amblyopia. *Proceedings of the Royal Society of London. Series B: Biological Sciences*, **217**, 309–330.

HESS, R.F., CAMPBELL, F.W. and GREENHALGH, T. (1978). On the nature of the neural abnormality in human amblyopia; neural aberrations and neural sensitivity loss. *Pflügers Archive European Journal of Physiology*, **377**, 201–207.

HESS, R.F., CAMPBELL, F.W. and ZIMMERN, R. (1980). Differences in the neural basis of human amblyopias: the effect of mean luminance. *Vision Research*, **20**, 295–305.

HESS, R.F. and POINTER, J.S. (1985). Differences in the neural basis of human amblyopia: the distribution of the anomaly across the visual field. *Vision Research*, **25**, 1577–1594.

HICKEY, T.L. and PEDUZZI, J.D. (1987). Structure and development of the visual system. In *Handbook of Infant Perception*, vol. I, edited by P. Salapatek and L. Cohen. Academic Press, New York.

HOKODA, S.C. and CIUFFREDA, K.J. (1986). Different rates and amounts of vision function recovery during orthoptic therapy in an older strabismic amblyope. *Ophthalmic and Physiological Optics*, **6**, 213–220.

HOWLAND, E.C., BRADDICK, O., ATKINSON, J. and HOWLAND, B. (1983). Optics of photorefraction: orthogonal and isotropic methods. *Journal of the Optical Society of America*, **73**, 1701–1708.

HOWLAND, H.C. and HOWLAND, B. (1974). Photorefraction: a technique for study of refractive state at a distance. *Journal of the Optical Society of America*, **64**, 240–249.

HOWLAND, H.C. and SAYLES, N. (1985). Photokeratometric and photorefractive measurements of astigmatism in infants and young children. *Vision Research*, **25**, 73–81.

HSU-WINGES, C., HAMER, R.D., NORICA, A.M. *et al.* (1989). Polaroid photorefractive screening of infants. *Journal of Pediatric Ophthalmology and Strabismus*, **26**, 254–260.

IKEDA, H. and TREMAIN, K.E. (1979). Amblyopia occurs in retinal ganglion cells in cats reared with convergent squint without alternating fixation. *Experimental Brain Research*, **35**, 559–582.

INGRAM, R.M. (1987). Screening by refraction to predict amblyopia and squint. *Research and Clinical Forums*, **9**, *New Perspective in Ophthalmology* (V), 39–41.

INGRAM, R.M., ARNOLD, P.E., DALLY, S. and LUCAS, J. (1990b). Results of randomised trial of treating abnormal hypermetropia from the age of 6 months. *British Journal of Ophthalmology*, **74**, 158–159.

INGRAM, R.M., HOLLAND, W.W., WALKER, C. *et al.* (1986b). Screening for visual defects in preschool children. *British Journal of Ophthalmology*, **70**, 16–21.

INGRAM, R.M., ROGERS, S. and WALKER, C. (1977). Occlusion and amblyopia. *British Orthoptics Journal*, **34**, 11–22.

INGRAM, R.M., WALKER, C., BILLINGHAM, B. *et al.* (1990a). Factors relating to visual acuity in children who have been treated for convergent squint. *British Journal of Ophthalmology*, **74**, 82–83.

INGRAM, R.M., WALKER, C., WILSON, J. (1985). A first attempt to prevent amblyopia and squint by spectacle correction of abnormal refractions from age 1 year. *British Journal of Ophthalmology*, **69**, 851–853.

INGRAM, R.M., WALKER, C., WILSON, J.M. (1986a). Prediction of amblyopia and squint by means of refraction at age 1 year. *British Journal of Ophthalmology*, **70**, 12–15.

JAY, B. and ELSTON, J. (1987). Genetic aspects of strabismus. In *Orthoptic Horizons, Transactions of the 6th International Orthoptic Congress Harrogate, UK*, edited by M. Lenk-Schafer, pp. 11–14.

JENKINS, T.C.A. and PICKWELL, L.D. (1982). Success rate in the treatment of amblyopia by conventional methods. *Ophthalmic and Physiological Optics*, **2**, 213–219.

KANDEL, G.L., GRATTAN, P.E. and BEDELL, H.E. (1977). Monocular fixation and acuity in amblyopic and normal eyes. *American Journal of Optometry and Physiological Optics*, **54**, 598–608.

KASAMATSU, T. and PETTIGREW, J.D. (1979). Preservation of binocularity after monocular deprivation in the striate cortex of kittens treated with 6-hydroxydopamine. *Journal of Comparative Neurology*, **185**, 139–162.

KAY, H. (1984). A new picture visual acuity test. *British Orthoptics Journal*, **41**, 77–80.

KIRSCHEN, D.G. and FLOM, M.C. (1978). Visual acuity at different retinal loci of eccentrically fixating functional amblyopes. *American Journal of Optometry and Physiological Optics*, **55**, 144–150.

LANG, J. (1969). Microstrabismus. *British Orthoptics Journal*, **26**, 30–37.

LANG, J. (1972). Therapeutic consequences of the analysis of simple forms of amblyopia. In *Orthoptics, Proceedings of the 2nd International Orthoptics Congress, Amsterdam*, edited by J. Mein, Excerpta Medica, Amsterdam.

LANG, J. (1984). The two-pencil test and the new Lang stereotest. *British Orthoptics Journal*, **41**, 15–21.

LARSON, J.S. (1971). The sagittal growth of the eye. IV. Ultrasonic measurement of the axial length of the eye from birth to puberty. *Acta Ophthalmologica*, **49**, 873–886.

LEPARD, C.W. (1975). Comparative changes in the error of refraction between fixing and amblyopic eyes during growth and development. *American Journal of Ophthalmology*, **80**, 485–490.

LEVENTHAL, A. (1984). Effects of monocular deprivation upon visual cortical areas 17, 18 and 19 in the cat. In *Neurology and Neurobiology*, vol. 9, *Development of Visual Pathways in Mammals*, edited by J. Stone, B. Dreher and D.H. Rapaport, Alan R. Liss, New York, pp. 347–361.

LEVI, D.M. and HARWERTH, R.S. (1982). Psychophysical mechanisms in humans with amblyopia. *American Journal of Optometry and Physiological Optics*, **59**, 936–951.

LEVI, D.M. and KLEIN, S.A. (1985). Vernier acuity, crowding and amblyopia. *Vision Research*, **25**, 979–991.

LEVI, D.M., YAP, Y.L. and GREENLEE, M.W. (1988). Is amblyopia an anomaly of photopic vision? *Clinical Vision Science*, **3**, 243–254.

LEVY, M.S. and GLICK, E.B. (1974). Stereoscopic perception and Snellen visual acuity. *American Journal of Ophthalmology*, **78**, 722–724.

LINKSZ, A. (1952). *Physiology of the Eye*, vol. 2, *Vision*. Grune and Stratton, New York.

LOTMAR, W. (1976). A theoretical model for the eye of new-born infants. *von Graefes Archives of Ophthalmology*, **198**, 179–185.

LYLE, T.K. and WYBAR, K.C. (1967). *Lyle and Jackson's Practical Orthoptics in the Treatment of Squint*, 5th edn. H.K. Lewis, London.

MACCANA, F., CUTHBERT, A. and LOVEGROVE, W. (1986). Contrast and phase processing in amblyopia. *Vision Research*, **26**, 781–789.

MCKEE, S.P. and MITCHISON, G.J. (1988). The role of retinal correspondence in stereoscopic matching. *Vision Research*, **28**, 1001–1012.

MALLETT, R.F.J. (1979). The use of prisms in the treatment of concomitant strabismus. *Ophthalmic Optician*, **19**, 27 October, 793–794, 797–798.

MALLETT, R.F.J. (1985). A unit for treating amblyopia and congenital nystagmus by intermittent photic stimulation. *Optometry Today*, **25**, (8), 260, 262–264.

MARG, E., FREEMAN, D.N., PELTZMAN. P. and GOLDSTEIN, P.H. (1976). Visual acuity development in human infants: evoked potential measurements. *Investigative Ophthalmology and Visual Science*, **15**, 150–153.

MAYER, D.L. and DOBSON, V. (1982). Visual acuity development in infants and young children, as assessed by operant preferential looking. *Vision Research*, **22**, 1141–1151.

MEHDORN, E. (1989). Suppression scotomas in primary microstrabismus – a perimetric artefact. *Documenta Ophthalmologica*, **71**, 1–18.

MITCHELL, D.E. (1988). The extent of visual recovery from early monocular or binocular visual deprivation in kittens. *Journal of Physiology*, **395**, 639–660.

MITCHELL, D.E. and MURPHY, K.M. (1984). The effectiveness of reverse occlusion as a means of promoting visual recovery in monocularly deprived kittens. In *Neurology and Neurobiology*, vol. 9, *Development of Visual Pathways in Mammals*, edited by J. Stone, B. Dieher and D.H. Rapaport, Alan R. Liss, New York, pp. 381–392.

MITCHELL, D.E., MURPHY, K.M. and KAYE, M.G. (1984). The permanence of the visual recovery that follows reverse occlusion of monocularly deprived kittens. *Investigative Ophthalmology and Visual Science*, **25**, 908–917.

MITCHELL, D.E., MURPHY, K.M., DZIOBA, H.A. and HORNS, J.A. (1986). Optimisation of visual recovery from early monocular deprivation in kittens: implications for occlusion therapy in the treatment of amblyopia. *Clinical Vision Science*, **11**, 173–177.

MOHINDRA, L., ZWAAN, J., HELD, R. *et al.* (1985). Development of acuity and stereopsis in infants with esotropia. *Ophthalmology*, **92**, 691–697.

MORLEY, J.W., LINDSEY, J.W. and JUDGE, S.J. (1988). Prism-adaptation in a strabismic monkey. *Clinical Vision Science*, **3**, 1–8.

MURPHY, K.M. and MITCHELL, D.E. (1987). Reduced visual acuity in both eyes of monocularly deprived kittens following short or long periods of reverse occlusion. *Journal of Neuroscience*, **7**, 1526–1536.

NAEGELE, J.R. and HELD, R. (1982a). Development of optokinetic nystagmus and effects of abnormal visual experience during infancy. In *Spatially Orientated Behaviour*, edited by Jeannerod and Hein. Springer, New York, pp. 155–174.

NAEGELE, J.R. and HELD, R. (1982b). The postnatal development of monocular optokinetic nystagmus in infants. *Vision Research*, **22**, 341–346.

NASTRI, G., CACCIA PERUGINI, G., SAVASTANO, S. *et al.* (1984). The evolution of refraction in the fixing and the amblyopic eye. *Documenta Ophthalmologica*, **56**, 265–274.

NAWRATSKI, I. (1976). Changing approaches to the treatment of amblyopia. In *Orthoptics: Past, Present and Future*, edited by S. Moore, J. Mein and L. Stockbridge. Stratton Inter-Cont. Medical Book Corp., New York, pp. 93–97.

NEUMANN, E., FRIEDMAN, Z. and ABEL-PELEG, B. (1987). Prevention of strabismic amblyopia of early onset with special reference to the optimal age for screening. *Journal of Pediatric Ophthalmology and Strabismus*, **24**, 106–110.

PALIAGA, G.P. (1989). Validity, sensitivity and specificity of the (Hirschberg) corneal light reflection test in 390 patients. *Binocular Vision*, **4**, 59-62.

PICKWELL, L.D. (1976). The management of amblyopia without occlusion. *British Journal of Physiological Optics*, **31**, 115–118.

PICKWELL, L.D. (1984). *Binocular Vision Anomalies: Investigation and Treatment*. Butterworths, London.

PRESSON, J. and GORDON, B. (1979). Critical period and minimum exposure required for the effects of alternating monocular occlusion in the cat visual cortex. *Vision Research*, **19**, 807–811.

QUICK, M.W. and BOOTHE, R.G. (1989). Measurement of binocular alignment in normal monkeys and in monkeys with strabismus. *Investigative Ophthalmology and Visual Science*, **30**, 1159–1168.

RAUSCHECKER, J.P., SCHRADER, W. and VON GRÜNAU, M.W. (1987). Rapid recovery from monocular deprivation in kittens after specific visual training. *Clinical Vision Science*, **1**, 257–268.

RAVIOLA, E.R. and WEISEL, T.N. (1985). An animal model of myopia. *New England Journal of Medicine*, **312**, 1609–1615.

REEVES, B.C. and HILL, A.R. (1987). Practical problems in measuring contrast sensitivity. *Optician*, **193**, Part I, (5085) 20 February, 29–30, 33–34; Part II (5086) 27 February, 32, 34.

REINEKE, R.D. (1986). Comment on Ingram *et al.* (1986b). Screening for visual defects in pre-school-children. *Survey of Ophthalmology*, **31**, 215–216.

REINEKE, R.D. and SIMONS, K. (1974). A new stereoscopic test for amblyopia screening. *American Journal of Ophthalmology*, **78**, 714–721.

REPKA, M.X., WELLISH, K., WISNICKI, H.J. and GUYTON, D.L. (1989). Changes in the refractive error of 94 spectacle-treated patients with acquired accommodative esotropia. *Binocular Vision*, 15–21.

ROBB, R.M. and PETERSEN, R.A. (1968). Cycloplegic refractions in children. *Journal of Pediatric Ophthalmology and Strabismus*, **5**, 110–114.

RODIER, D.W., MAYER, D.L. and FULTON, A.B. (1985). Assessment of young amblyopes – Arrays vs single picture acuities. *Ophthalmology*, **92**, 1197–1202.

ROGERS, G.L., BREMER, D.L. and LEGUIRE, L.E. (1987). The contrast sensitivity function and childhood amblyopia. *American Journal of Ophthalmology*, **104**, 64–68.

ROSE, D., BLAKE, R. and HALPERN, D.L. (1988). Disparity range for binocular summation. *Investigative Ophthalmology and Visual Science*, **29**, 283–290.

ROSS-DOMMASCH, E. and MORRIS, E. (1987). What are we doing when we occlude infantile esotropes? In *Orthoptic Horizons, Transactions of the 6th International Orthoptics Congress, Harrogate, UK*, edited by M. Lenk-Schafer, pp. 101–112.

RUBIN, G.S. (1988). Reliability and sensitivity of clinical contrast sensitivity tests. *Clinical Vision Science*, **2**, 169–177.

SARNIGUET-BADOCHE, J.M. and PINCON, F. (1982). The prevalence of strabismus in children born of squinters. In *Paediatric Ophthalmology*, edited by J. Francois and M. Maione. John Wiley, Chichester, pp. 375–377.

SATTERFIELD, D.S. (1989). Prevalence and variation of astigmatism in a military population. *Journal of the American Optometric Association*, **60**, 14–18.

SCHOR, C. (1978). A motor theory for monocular eccentric fixation of amblyopic eyes. *American Journal of Optometry and Physiological Optics*, **55**, 183–186.

SCHOR, C. and NARAYAN, V. (1981). The influence of field size upon the spatial frequency response of optokinetic nystagmus. *Vision Research*, **21**, 985–994.

SCHOR, C.M. and CIUFFREDA, K.J. (1983). *Vergence Eye Movements: Basic and Clinical Aspects*. Butterworths, Boston.

SETHI, B. (1986). Vergence adaptation: a review. *Documenta Ophthalmologica*, **63**, 247–263.

SHAPIRO, A., YANKO, L., NAWRATSKI, I. and MERIN, S. (1980). Refractive power of premature children at infancy and early childhood. *American Journal of Ophthalmology*, **90**, 234–238.

SILLITO, A.M. (1979). Pharmacological approach to the visual cortex. *Trends in Neuroscience*, **2**, 196–198.

SINGER, W. (1985). Central control of developmental plasticity in the mammalian visual cortex. *Vision Research*, **25**, 389–396.

SINGER, W., TRETTER, F. and YINON, U. (1982a). Central gating of developmental plasticity in kitten visual cortex. *Journal of Physiology*, **324**, 221–237.

SINGER, W., TRETTER, F. and YINON, U. (1982b). Evidence for long term functional plasticity in the visual cortex of adult cats. *Journal of Physiology*, **324**, 239–248.

SKOTTUN, B.C., BRADLEY, A. and FREEMAN, R.D. (1986). Orientation discrimination in amblyopia. *Investigative Ophthalmology and Visual Science*, **27**, 532–537.

SLATER, A.M. and FINDLAY, J.M. (1972). The measurement of fixation position in the newborn baby. *Journal of Experimental Child Psychology*, **14**, 349–364.

SLATER, A.M. and FINDLAY, J.M. (1975a). The corneal reflection technique and the visual preference method: sources of error. *Journal of Experimental Child Psychology*, **20**, 240–247.

SLATER, A.M. and FINDLAY, J.M. (1975b). Binocular fixation in the newborn baby. *Journal of Experimental Child Psychology*, **20**, 248–273.

SMITH, E.L., HARWERTH, R.S., CRAWFORD, M.L.J. and VON NOORDEN, G.K. (1987). Observations on the effects of form deprivation on the refractive status of the monkey. *Investigative Ophthalmology and Visual Science*, **28**, 1236–1245.

SOMERS, W.W., HAPPEL, A.W. and PHILLIPS, J.D. (1984). Use of a personal microcomputer for orthoptic therapy. *Journal of the American Optometric Association*, **55**, 262–267.

STEINBACH, M.J. (1987). Proprioceptive knowledge of eye position. *Vision Research*, **27**, 1737–1744.

STEINMAN, S.B., LEVI, D.M. and MCKEE, S.P. (1988). Discrimination of time and velocity in the amblyopic visual system. *Clinical Vision Science*, **2**, 265–276.

STIDWILL, D. (1985). The Lang stereopsis test. *Optician*, **190**, 23 August (5009) 11.

STREETEN, B.W. (1969). Development of the human retinal pigment epithelium and the posterior segment. *Archives of Ophthalmology*, **81**, 383–394.

THIBOS, L.N. and LEVICK, W.R. (1982). Astigmatic visual deprivation in cat: behavioural, optical and retinophysiological consequences. *Vision Research*, **22**, 43–53.

THOMAS, J., MOHINDRA, I. and HELD, R. (1979). Strabismic amblyopia in infants. *American Journal of Optometry and Physiological Optics*, **56**, 197–201.

THORN, F. and COMERFORD, J.P. (1983). Use of various measures of visual acuity and contrast sensitivity in the evaluation of monocular occlusion and active vision training of three adult amblyopes. *American Journal of Optometry and Physiological Optics*, **60**, 347–351.

TIMNEY, B. (1984). Monocular deprivation and binocular depth perception in kittens. In *Development of the Visual Pathways in Mammals*. Alan R. Liss, New York, pp. 405–423.

TOMMILA, V. and TARKKANEN, A. (1981). Incidence of loss of vision in the healthy eye in amblyopia. *British Journal of Ophthalmology*, **65**, 575–577.

TOUR, R.L. (1966). Strabismus – Annual Review. *Archives of Ophthalmology*, **76**, 293–306.

TUMOSA, N., NUNBERG, S., HIRSCH, H.V.B. and TIEMAN, S.B. (1983). Binocular exposure causes suppression of the less experienced eye in cats previously reared with unequal alternating monocular exposure. *Investigative Ophthalmology and Visual Science*, **24**, 496–506.

TYTLA, M.E., MAURER, D., LEWIS, T.L. and BRENT, H.P. (1988). Contrast sensitivity in children treated for congenital cateract. *Clinical Vision Science*, **2**, 251–264.

VAN HOF-VAN DUIN, J., HEERSEMA, D.J., GROENENDAAL, F. *et al.* (1989). Visual impairments in very low birth weight (VLBW) infants during the first year after term. *Ophthalmic and Physiological Optics*, **9**, 468.

VERBAKEN, J.H. and JOHNSTON, A.W. (1986). Clinical contrast senstivity testing; the current status. *Clinical and Experimental Optometry*, **69**, 204–212.

VEREECKEN, E.P. and BRABANT. P. (1984). Prognosis for vision in amblyopia after the loss of the good eye. *Archives of Ophthalmology*, **102**, 220–224.

VITAL-DURAND, F. (1989). Preferential looking in the clinic and eradication of functional amblyopia. *Ophthalmic and Physiological Optics*, **9**, 467.

VON NOORDEN, G.K. (1965). Occlusion therapy in amblyopia with eccentric fixation. *Archives of Ophthalmology*, **73**, 776–781.

VON NOORDEN, G.K. (1970). Etiology and pathogenesis of fixation anomalies in strabismus. IV: Roles of suppression scotoma and of motor factors. *American Journal of Ophthalmology*, **69**, 237–245.

VON NOORDEN, G.K. (1985a). Amblyopia: a multidisciplinary approach. *Investigative Ophthalmology and Visual Science*, **26**, 1704–1716.

VON NOORDEN, G.K. (1985b). Idiopathic amblyopia. *American Journal of Ophthalmology*, **100**, 214–217.

VON NOORDEN, G.K. (1988). A reassessment of infantile esotropia. XLIV Edward Jackson Memorial Lecture. *American Journal of Ophthalmology*, **105**, 1–10.

WALRAVEN, J. (1975). Amblyopia screening with random-dot stereograms. *American Journal of Ophthalmology*, **80**, 893–900.

WANGER, P. and WAERN, G. (1988). Instant photographic refractometry in children. *Acta Ophthalmologica*, **66**, 165–169.

WATTAM-BELL, J., BRADDICK, O., ATKINSON, K. and DAY, J. (1987). Measures of infant binocularity in a group at risk for strabismus. *Clinical Vision Science, 1*, 327–336.

WESTALL, C.A., WOODHOUSE, J.M. and BROWN, V.A. (1989). OKN asymmetries and binocular function in amblyopia. *Ophthalmic and Physiological Optics, 9*, 269–276.

WILDSOET, C.F. and PETTIGREW, J.D. (1988). Experimental myopia and anomalous eye growth patterns unaffected by optic nerve section in chickens: evidence for local control of eye growth. *Clinical Vision Science, 2*, 99–107.

WINN, B., ACKERLEY, R.G., BROWN, C.A. *et al.* (1988). Reduced aniseikonia in axial anisometropia with contact lens correction. *Ophthalmic and Physiological Optics, 8*, 341–344.

WINN, B. and HERON, G. (1990). The temporal accommodation response in amblyopia. *Clinical Vision Science, 5*, 157–166.

WORTH, C. (1905). *Squint: its Causes, Pathology and Treatment*, 2nd edn. J. Bale Sons & Danielsson, London.

WRIGHT, K.W., WEHRLE, M.J. and URREA, R.T. (1987). Bilateral total occlusion during the critical period of visual development. *Archives of Ophthalmology, 105*, 321.

YINON, U. and KOSLOWE, K.C. (1984). Eyelid closure effects on the refractive error of the eye in dark- and in light-reared kittens. *American Journal of Optometry Physiological Optics, 61*, 271–273.

YUODELIS, C. and HENDRICKSON, A. (1986). A qualitative and quantitative analysis of the human fovea during development. *Vision Research, 26*, 847–855.

7

The development of refractive errors

Michael Sheridan

Discussion of this subject often generates more heat than light. This is usually the result of conflicting views of the aetiology of refractive errors and particularly the question whether they are hereditarily determined or the result of environmental influences. This chapter will review the facts about the development and progress of refractive errors in children without commitment to any aetiological theories, though the nature of these and the clinical consequences of their adoption will also be considered.

The most striking fact about refractive errors is their relative rarity in the adult population. *Figure 7.1* shows the distribution of refractive errors in the eyes of 1033 men aged 17–27 years. Seventy-three per cent of these eyes had ocular refractions from 0 to +1.9 D and must be regarded as functionally normal, having regard to the amplitude of accommodation available at this age. Eighty-one per cent of eyes had ocular refractions lying between +2.0 D and −2.0 D, 4.5% had hypermetropia of more than +4.0 D and 1.8% myopia greater than −4.0 D. This last finding, which contradicts the conventional wisdom, is probably a result of the refractions having been carried out under cycloplegia and the results having been corrected for vertex distance to give ocular refraction.

At birth, the external axial length of the eye of a full-term male infant averages 17.9 mm (Sorsby and Sheridan, 1960). The axial length of the adult male eye is approximately 24 mm. If both the neonatal and the adult eye are assumed to be emmetropic, this increase in length implies a reduction in the power of the eye's optical system of at least 20 D. Most of this expansion occurs in the first 3 years of life, Sorsby, Benjamin and Sheridan (1961) having found a mean axial length of 23.2 mm in 3-year-old boys.

The distribution of refractive errors in the newborn has been the subject of many publications (Slataper, 1950; Cook and Glasscock, 1951; Mohindra *et al.*, 1978; Ingram, 1979). There is considerable divergence between the results of different investigators, which is not surprising considering the difficulty of measuring refraction accurately on neonates and the disparate techniques employed. Particularly worthy of note is the high incidence of astigmatism reported by Mohindra *et al.* (1978) which rapidly decreased over the first 2 years of life. By contrast, 81% of Sorsby's sample of adult males had astigmatism of 0.5 D or less.

Banks (1980), reviewing these results concluded that refractive error in the newborn appears to be normally distributed, with a mean of about +2.00 D and a standard deviation of 2.00 D. Sorsby, Benjamin and Sheridan (1961) found a mean refractive error of +2.33 D in a sample of 56 3-year-old boys with a standard error of ±0.24 (equivalent to a standard deviation of ±1.8 D) and a mean refractive error of

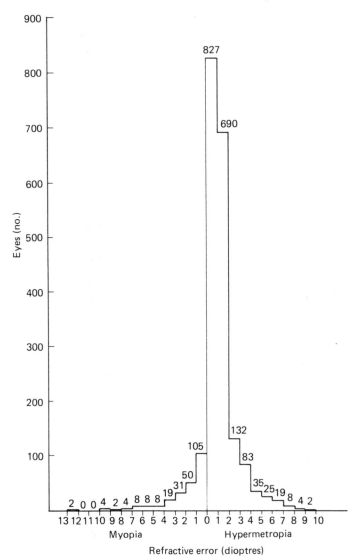

Figure 7.1. Distribution of ocular refraction in 2066 eyes of men aged 17–27 years. (After Sorsby *et al.*, 1960,)

+2.96 D in a sample of 39 3-year-old-girls, with a standard error of ±0.19 (equivalent to a standard deviation of ±1.19 D). By age 14, the mean refractive error in boys had declined to +0.93 D with a standard error of ±0.38 and that in girls to ±0.62 D with a standard error of ±0.26. The cross-sectional data of Sorsby *et al.* shows a steady decline in mean refractive error with age, the best fitting curves being:

$$\text{Ocular refraction} = \frac{1}{(0.2456 + 0.0521x)} \text{ for boys}$$

$$\text{Ocular refraction} = \frac{1}{(0.0778 + 0.0728x)} \text{ for girls}$$

where x = age in years. The 2066 adult male eyes examined by Sorsby *et al.* (1960) had a mean refractive error of $+0.92$ D with a standard deviation of ± 1.84 D which is not significantly different from that of the 14-year-old boys, although the standard error of the mean (0.04) is much smaller, reflecting the much larger number of observations.

In considering the results of cross-sectional studies, it should be borne in mind that, since the individuals in each age group are different, the results tend to smooth out individual variations in growth. For example, a graph of height in relation to age shows a steady increase from birth to maturity if based on cross-sectional data, while the growth of any individual child shows a marked spurt in growth at puberty. This effect is obscured in the cross-sectional data because puberty occurs at different chronological ages in different children. The girls examined by Sorsby, Benjamin and Sheridan (1961), for example, showed a range in age at menarche (first menstrual period) from 9 to 15 years. Sorsby *et al.* were unable to demonstrate any correlation between stature and refractive error or axial length. Indeed they found that girls had eyes that were on average 2% smaller than those of boys of the same age even in those age groups (from 10 to 14) in which the average girl is taller and heavier than the average boy. Their relatively small follow-up sample also showed no correlation between bodily growth and growth of either refractive error or axial length, although some of the children showed considerable ocular growth. Discussing these results they comment:

> First, it is clear that the averages obtained in the cross-sectional study cover considerable individual variations: in the follow up study some of the children showed no axial elongation at all (as against the expected 0.1 mm per annum); many showed elongation of 0.2 mm or 0.3 mm per annum, and a few had rates of 0.5 mm or more. Secondly, while the higher rates of axial elongation are potentially able to produce myopia, in actual fact myopia only develops in a few cases, for there is usually adequate compensation from changes in both the lens and cornea.

The picture which emerges from this evidence is of a pattern of growth of the eye which is more akin to that of the central nervous system than to that of the body as a whole. The eye at birth is about 75% of its adult size while the infant is less than 25% of its adult height. At birth there is a wide variation of refractive error, especially of astigmatism (Mohindra *et al.*, 1978), but the range of variation narrows rapidly. In this connection, it should be pointed out that although the standard deviation of the distribution of refractive error in adult eyes of ± 1.84 D is not very different from the ± 2.0 D suggested by Banks (1980) for the neonatal eye, the adult distribution is not a normal distribution but has a very high peak in the region from 0.00 to $+1.00$ D. In the distribution produced by Sorsby *et al.* (1960) the best fitting normal curve would predict only about half the number of eyes that actually fall into this group. It is therefore questionable whether the standard deviation is an appropriate statistic to describe this distribution. By the age of 3 years, the average eye has already attained about 96% of its adult size and the individual only about 58% of adult height. Between 3 and 14 years of age, there is a slow increase in the size of the globe, accompanied in most cases by compensating changes in the powers of the lens and cornea leading to a reduction of hypermetropia of about 1.00 D and leaving an essentially emmetropic eye.

Refractive errors arise therefore from a failure, in a minority of individuals, of coordinated growth. Spooner (1957a, b) has pointed out that expansion of the neonate globe in all dimensions will lead to flattening of the cornea and reduction of the power of the lens, whereas expansion along the axial direction at a greater rate than in transverse directions will tend to produce myopia, with the eye having a steeper cornea than would be found in an emmetropic eye with the same axial length. Conversely, transverse expansion at a greater rate than axial will lead to an eye with hypermetropia and a flatter cornea than would be found in an emmetropic eye with the same axial length. It has been known for many years that central corneal radius is related to refractive error, myopes having smaller and hyperopes larger radii than those found in emmetropes (Schiotz, 1886; Valk, 1897; Sulzer, 1904; Steiger, 1913; Cooper and Docrat, 1951; Sorsby et al., 1957). On this view, astigmatism results from differential growth of the transverse meridians, an interpretation which finds support from the commonplace observation during the fitting of scleral contact lenses that high corneal astigmatism is almost always accompanied by corresponding toricity of the sclera.

Deller, O'Connor and Sorsby (1947), measured the axial, transverse horizontal and transverse vertical diameters of 45 eyes using an X-ray method described by Rushton (1938). Their results tend to confirm the interpretation of the previous paragraph; with one exception the emmetropic eyes show transverse diameters which do not differ significantly from the axial length, while the myopic eyes are of greater volume and have proportionately longer axial length. The deviation from spherical shape is less in the hypermetropic eyes, which is not unexpected as the largest hypermetropic correction was + 3.00 D while the myopic eyes included four with refractive errors of − 10.00 D or more. Unfortunately Stenstrom (1946), who measured the axial length of 1000 eyes using a similar X-ray method, did not record the transverse measurements. The increased awareness of the dangers of ionizing radiation since the time these studies were carried out has led to this technique being abandoned and replaced first by ophthalmophakometry, as used by Sorsby et al. (1957, 1961, 1962) and later by A-scan ultrasound, used by almost all later investigators. Neither of these techniques produces results for the transverse dimensions of the globe, with the result that there has been a tendency to concentrate attention on the axial length to the detriment of consideration of the total architecture of the globe.

If refractive errors develop as a result of a failure of coordinated growth, the question arises as to the cause of this failure. Here attention has been concentrated on the development of myopia – most investigators seem to have been content tacitly to accept hypermetropia as a form of arrested development rather than to consider the possibility of disproportionate growth in the transverse dimensions, while there is no very obvious environmental influence which might be considered to produce hypermetropia. Myopia, on the other hand, tends to appear at a later stage in the growth process and is therefore more accesible to investigation. It is also a more obviously disabling condition, since even a small amount of myopia leads to an easily noticeable drop in distance visual acuity, while similar amounts of hypermetropia are compatible with normal visual acuity and usually symptom free.

The fact that the incidence of myopia is higher in some ethnic groups, especially Chinese (Edwards, 1990), Japanese, (Sato, 1957) and European Jews (Sourasky, 1928; Sorsby, 1933), suggests that there may be a genetic basis for refractive error. This view is reinforced by the findings of Sorsby, Sheridan and Leary (1962). They compared the results of measuring the ocular components in 78 pairs of uniovular twins with those of 40 pairs of like-sexed binovular twins and 48 pairs of unrelated persons of the same sex and age and with the same distribution of refractive errors as in the uniovular twins. The uniovular twins showed a much higher level of concordance not only in refractive error but also in the powers and dimensions of the components of the eye than did the binovular twins, while the control group showed the least concordance of all.

Although these results suggest that there is a strong genetic element in the development of refractive errors, they should not be interpreted as excluding environmental influences. Uniovular twins, except in those rare instances where they are separated at birth, share an almost identical childhood environment, as indeed do most like-sexed binovular twins. The greater discordance among the binovular twins indicates that essentially the same environment produces different results on persons with different genetic constitutions; only a study on the optical components in a series of uniovular twins reared apart would give an accurate estimate of the relative importance of genetic and environmental influences.

That the influence of environment is not negligible is shown by the work of Young *et al.* (Young *et al.*, 1954; Young, 1955, 1958, 1961a, b; Young, 1962; Young, Leary and Farrer, 1966; Young *et al.*, 1969; Young, Singer and Foster, 1975; Young, 1977; Young, 1981) on the development of myopia. Young points out that the incidence of myopia is associated with academic achievement, the proportion of myopes increasing steadily with higher levels of education so that in some American graduate schools as many as 50% of students may be myopic. Myopes are not, as is often supposed, more intelligent than non-myopes, their performance on standard IQ tests is not significantly different from non-myopes. They do however do better on tests of reading ability and of academic aptitude. It is significant that Douglas, Ross and Simpson (1967), studying a cohort of children all born in the same month, found that the children who became myopic showed a higher than average score on a standard test of academic ability at age seven, before most of them became myopic. The obvious environmental influence affecting the academically gifted is excessive close work. Young found that the incidence of myopia increased in Eskimo families in Alaska with the introduction of compulsory education. Few of the illiterate parents were myopic, but some 60% of the schoolchildren showed measurable myopia. This is a very much higher proportion than that found in young men by Sorsby *et al.* (1960) and it may be significant that Eskimos are Mongols – like the Chinese and Japanese who also show high incidence of myopia compared to Caucasians – so that the environmental influences may be enhanced by genetic predisposition. In Europe, there is little evidence that increased educational demands have led to an increase in myopia; the proportion of Danish conscripts with mild or moderate myopia was little changed in the 82 years between 1882 and 1964 (Goldschmidt, 1969).

Young attributes the development of myopia to high levels of accommodation particularly in low illumination. He was able to induce myopia in monkeys by keeping them in a restricted visual space. The amount of myopia developed was inversely related to the age of the animal at the start of the experiment and higher levels of myopia developed in the animals kept in an illumination of 4 ft/candles than in those in either higher or lower levels of illumination. Young suggests that prolonged demand for accurate accommodation leads first to spasm of accommodation and then to axial elongation due to increased pressure in the vitreous chamber. The fact that myopes show higher average intraocular pressure than non-myopes (Abdalla and Hamdi, 1970; Tomlinson and Phillips, 1970) would seem to lend support to this view. Young interprets the finding by Wiesel and Raviola (1977) that fusion of the eyelids in newborn macaque monkeys led to the development of myopia due to elongation of the vitreous chamber, the degree of myopia being proportional to the duration of lid fusion, as an extreme example of reduced fixation distance.

This discussion should be sufficient to show that, particularly in the case of myopia, there is strong evidence for environmental as well as genetic influences on the development of refractive errors. What are the consequences for clinical practice? Some authors (Sato, 1957; Bedrossian, 1966) have suggested atropinization as a means of preventing excessive accommodation in young myopes. A more popular, although less certain technique, is to prescribe a bifocal correction so that the demand for accommodation is reduced. The more variable results achieved with this method may be a result of some children failing consistently to use the bifocal segment for reading. The present author's personal practice is to prescribe bifocals for young myopes only when, as many do, they show convergence excess esophoria; in these circumstances a reading addition seems justified on all clinical grounds. It also seems rational to discourage extremely close working distances and to advise adequate illumination for close work.

If persistent accommodative effort is the cause of axial elongation, it would seem logical to refrain from correcting young hypermetropes, who far outnumber myopes (Sorsby *et al.*, 1960), unless they have asthenopia or binocular vision difficulties, since to do so would prevent the process of emmetropization. Although this course of action is never advocated, it is possible that it is indeed followed for many individuals since symptom-free hypermetropes seldom present for eye examination. A study on the effect of correction on the progress of hypermetropia would be welcome.

References

ABDALLA, M.I. and HAMDI, M. (1970). Applanation ocular tension in myopia and emmetropia. *British Journal of Ophthalmology*, **54**, 122.

BANKS, M.S. (1980). Infant refraction and accommodation. *International Ophthalmology Clinics*, **20**, 205.

BEDROSSIAN, R. (1966). Treatment of progressive myopia with atropine. *Proceedings of the XX International Congress on Ophthalmology, Munich*, 612.

COOK, R.C. and GLASSCOCK, R.E. (1951). Refractive and ocular findings in the newborn. *American Journal of Ophthalmology*, **34**, 1407.

COOPER, S.N. and DOCRAT, Y.A. (1951). Keratometry study in refractive conditions of the eye, particularly with reference to myopia. *Proceedings of the All-India Ophthalmological Society*, **12**, 27.

DELLER, J.F.P., O'CONNOR, A.D. and SORSBY, A. (1947). X-Ray measurement of the diameters of the living eye. *Proceedings of the Royal Society of London, Series B: Biological Sciences*, **134**, 456.

DOUGLAS, J.W.B., ROSS, J.M. and SIMPSON, H.R. (1967). The ability and attainment of short-sighted pupils. *Journal of the Royal Statistical Association A*, **130**, 479.

EDWARDS, M. (1990). An Investigation into the Refractive Status of Infants in Hong Kong. MPhil Thesis, University of Bradford.

GOLDSCHMIDT, E. (1969). Refraction in the newborn. *Acta Ophthalmologica (Kbh)*, **47**, 570.

INGRAM, R.M. (1979). Refraction of one year old children after atropine cycloplegia. *British Journal of Ophthalmology*, **63**, 343.

MOHINDRA, I., HELD, R., GWIAZDA, J. and BRILL, S. (1978). Astigmatism in infants. *Science*, **202**, 329.

RUSHTON, R.H. (1938). The clinical measurement of the axial length of the living eye. *Transactions of the Ophthalmological Society of the UK*, **58**, 136.

SATO, T. (1957). *The Causes and Prevention of Acquired Myopia*. Tanehara Shuppa, Tokyo.

SCHIOTZ, H. (1886). Ophthalmometrische und Optometrische Untersuchungen von 969 Augen. *Arch. Augenheilk.* **16**, 37.

SLATAPER, F.J. (1950). Age norms of refraction and vision. *American Medical Association Archives of Ophthalmology*, **43**, 466.

SORSBY, A. (1933). The normal refraction in infancy and its bearing on the development of myopia. *Annual Report of London County Council,* **4**, part 3, 55.

SORSBY, A., BENJAMIN, B., DAVEY, J.B. *et al.* (1957). *Emmetropia and its aberrations.* (Medical Research Council Special Report No. 293). HMSO, London.

SORSBY, A., BENJAMIN., B. and SHERIDAN, M. (1961). *Refraction and its Components During the Growth of the Eye from the Age of Three* (Medical Research Council Special Report No. 301).

SORSBY, A. and SHERIDAN, M. (1960). The eye at birth: measurement of the principal diameters in 48 cadavers. *Journal of Anatomy,* **94**, 193.

SORSBY, A., SHERIDAN, M. and LEARY, G.A. (1962). *Refraction and its Components in Twins* (Medical Research Council Special Report No. 303).

SORSBY, A., SHERIDAN, M., LEARY, G.A. and BENJAMIN, B. (1960). Vision, visual acuity and ocular refraction of young men: findings in a sample of 1033 subjects. *British Medical Journal,* **1**, 1394.

SOURASKY, A. (1928). Race, sex and environment in the development of myopia. *British Journal of Ophthalmology,* **12**, 197.

SPOONER, J.D. (1957a). Refractive errors as problems in growth and form. *British Journal of Physiological Optics,* **14**, 127.

SPOONER, J.D. (1957b). *Ocular Anatomy.* The Hatton Press, London, Chap. XVI.

STEIGER, A. (1913). *Die Entstehung der spharischen Refraktionen des menschlichen Auges.* Karger, Berlin.

STENSTROM, S. (1946). Untersuchengen uber die Variation und Kovariation der optischen Elemente des menschlichen Auges. *Acta Ophthalmologica,* (*Kbh*), Suppl. XXVI (English translation by Woolf, D. (1948). *American Journal of Optometry,* **25**, 218, reprinted as Monograph No 58).

SULZER, M. (1904). Les amétropies focales. In *Encyclopédie française d'Ophtalmologie* vol. III edited by F. Lagrange and E. Valude. Doin, Paris.

TOMLINSON, A. and PHILLIPS, C.I. (1970). Applanation tension and axial length of the eyeball. *British Journal of Ophthalmology,* **54**, 548.

VALK, F. (1897). The curvature of the cornea in reference to the refractive condition of the dioptric apparatus in the two principal meridians. *Ophthalmic Record,* **6**, 276, 329.

WIESEL, T.N. and RAVIOLA, E. (1977). Myopia and eye enlargement after neonatal lid fusion in monkeys. *Nature,* **266**, 66.

YOUNG, F.A. (1955). Myopes versus non myopes – a comparison. *American Journal of Optometry,* **32**, 180.

YOUNG, F.A. (1958). An estimate of the hereditary component of myopia. *American Journal of Optometry,* **35**, 337.

YOUNG, F.A. (1961a). The development and retention of myopia by monkeys. *American Journal of Optometry,* **38**, 545.

YOUNG, F.A. (1961b). The effect of restricted visual space on the primate eye. *American Journal of Ophthalmology,* **52**, 799.

YOUNG, F.A. (1962). The effect of nearwork illumination level on monkey refraction. *American Journal of Optometry,* **39**, 60.

YOUNG, F.A. (1977). The nature and control of myopia. *Journal of the American Optometric Association,* **48**, 451.

YOUNG, F.A. (1981). Primate myopia. *American Journal of Optometry and Physiological Optics,* **58**, 560.

YOUNG, F.A., BEATTIE, R.J., NEWBY, F.J. and SWINDAL, M.T. (1954). The Pullman study – a visual survey of Pullman school children. *American Journal of Optometry,* **31**, 111, 192.

YOUNG, F.A., LEARY, G.A. and FARRER, D.N. (1966). Ultrasound and phakometry measurements of the primate eye. *American Journal of Optometry,* **43**, 370.

YOUNG, F.A., LEARY, G.A., BALDWIN, W.R. *et al.* (1969). The transmission of refractive errors within Eskimo families. *American Journal of Optometry,* **46**, 676.

YOUNG, F.A., SINGER, R.M. and FOSTER, D. (1975). The psychological differentiation of male myopes and non myopes. *American Journal of Optometry and Physiological Optics,* **52**, 679.

8

Assessment of child vision and refractive error

Caroline Thompson

Visual assessment

Visual acuity tests have provided by far the most popular clinical means of assessing spatial visual performance for over a century. Accurate results may be obtained quickly from cooperative adult patients using simple equipment and, since the measure is particularly sensitive to optical defocus, letter visual acuity charts provide an ideal stimulus for subjective refraction purposes. Since pattern recognition skills are usually necessary letter charts enable some evaluation of the patients' reading abilities. However, visual acuity tests are not fully representative of everyday visual tasks as they provide only a measure of performance (i.e. the limit of resolution) at high contrast. An alternative measurement of visual performance that depends on determining patients' sensitivity to contrast is becoming increasingly popular, since it enables a more comprehensive assessment of visual function than provided by visual acuity alone. New methods have enabled determination of both visual acuity and contrast sensitivity in early infancy. This chapter reviews subjective and objective techniques for the assessment of visual acuity and contrast sensitivity, with particular emphasis on methods developed for use with children.

Visual acuity

Conventional, subjective methods for the clinical assessment of visual acuity in cooperative adults usually depend on the reading of letter charts. Such methods require literacy, which precludes their use with young children. For this reason various objective techniques and modified subjective tests have been developed for the assessment of visual acuity in preschool children. Only objective methods are applicable in the youngest age groups but subjective techniques become possible in some children from about 2 years. Numerous subjective tests have been developed for the visual assessment of preschool children (see reviews by Fern and Manny, 1986; McDonald, 1986) and, irrespective of method, most normal children respond well to subjective testing by about 4 years.

The practitioner attempting to select from the diverse range of available acuity tests the most appropriate method for a particular child is not faced with an easy task, particularly in the 3 to 4 year-old age group where the choice is largest. The magnitude of this problem was highlighted by a survey amongst UK district medical officers performing preschool vision screening. In total 13 different visual acuity methods (including both subjective and objective types) were used with more than one test being applied in some areas (Stewart-Brown, Haslum and Howlett, 1988).

An initial concern when selecting an appropriate acuity test for a child is that the assessment method is geared to the child's maturity, thereby increasing the likelihood of successful testing. The 'optimum' method will therefore vary according to the child's age and general level of development. Further requirements are that established acuity age norms should be available for the test which should be of fairly short testing duration and capable of providing repeatable results that are comparable to accepted standard measurements of visual acuity. The next section commences with consideration of general factors affecting visual acuity determination and therefore influencing the clinician's choice of test. This is followed by critical reviews of subjective tests devised for children and objective acuity methods which are, in some instances, applicable from birth. The latter intend to show what methods are practically possible as a function of age.

General considerations

Types of acuity

Several types of acuity may be measured depending on the stimulus presented to the patient. In literate adults *recognition* visual acuity is usually determined clinically, generally via reading from test charts having lines of different letters of graded size. Letters are particularly suitable targets for this purpose as they allow easy communication of results between patient and examiner. *Recognition* acuities may be obtainable from young children using modified subjective methods, but objective methods required during infancy depend upon *detection* or *resolution* acuity. Definitions of these types of visual acuity are given in *Table 8.1*.

Most test charts feature selections of different letters and therefore clearly fall into the category of recognition acuity tests. Several variables may affect the visibility of letters on such charts. These include letter contrast, construction, type, legibility and spacing as well as the progression of letter sizes (which is usually geometrical). The British Standard (1968 – No. 4274) for distance test charts stipulates that letters should be of 90% contrast, 5 by 4 sans serif construction and restricted to the following selection – D, E, F, H, N, P, R, U, V and Z – which are all of similar

TABLE 8.1. Definitions of types of visual acuity

Type of acuity	Definition
Detection	Ability to see whether or not an object, e.g. a circular target, is present in an otherwise empty visual field. Forms the basis of perimetric tests. Acuity is determined from the minimum size which permits visibility
Resolution	Ability to discriminate two or more spatially separated targets. The stimulus is often a black and white striped grating, which appears grey if not resolved. Acuity is recorded as the minimum separation which permits discrimination
Recognition	Ability to identify the shape of a target, e.g. letter, number, symbol. Acuity is recorded as the minimum size (of detail) which permits identification

legibility. The minimum luminance for internally illuminated charts should be 120 cd/m^2 and the minimum illuminance for externally illuminated charts should be 480 lux. Manufacturers of projected charts experience difficulty in achieving the British Standard level of contrast but this is of little practical significance providing it is not less than 84%.

Standard Snellen charts usually have a single 60-m letter and increasing numbers of letters on successive lines (*Figure 8.1(a)*). This traditional design is open to criticism since letter size is not the only variable between lines. The problem may be reduced by the use of improved charts (*Figure 8.1(b)*) which have been designed to minimize the effects of other variables, although these charts are somewhat less convenient in use owing to their bulky size (Lovie-Kitchin, 1988).

The problem of differing letter legibility may be avoided entirely by using charts which present a task depending solely on identification of the orientation of a known letter (e.g. Landolt C) rather than shape recognition. These tests technically fall into the resolution acuity category but they are sometimes classified erroneously (McDonald, 1986). Tests featuring black and white checkerboard or striped 'grating' targets (having a square wave luminance profile) also depend on resolution acuity. These types of stimuli are often used in objective methods. Reasonable performance on resolution (or detection) acuity tasks need not rule out the presence of moderate refractive error since target visibility is less influenced by optical defocus than are letters. Square wave grating targets are prone to a phenomenon termed spurious resolution. At its 'true' threshold stripe width (spatial frequency) a grating will appear a uniform grey but due to 'spurious resolution' a periodic pattern of reversed contrast may re-emerge as stripe width is reduced beyond this value. The phenomenon may lead to slight overestimation of resolution acuity but is unlikely to be observed using high spatial frequency gratings (for further discussion see Bennett and Rabbetts, 1989a).

Different threshold values will be found, for a given individual, depending on the type of acuity being measured. Of particular concern is the view that many amblyopic subjects (especially strabismics) show improved performance when tested with gratings rather than recognition acuity targets (*Figure 8.2*). The latter finding could be explained by assuming that the visual distortion reported by amblyopes produces a greater impairment in the recognition of shapes than in the perception of striped targets. Moseley and co-workers (1988), however, found a good correlation between grating and recognition acuities in their sample of young amblyopes, perhaps due to use of a strict criterion for their grating threshold.

Most clinicians are familiar with the Snellen fraction as a means of recording visual acuity level but some of the newer objective tests use different units. Results of tests which depend on finding resolution thresholds are generally expressed as the minimum angle of resolution (in minutes of arc) or spatial frequency (in cycles per degree) of the threshold pattern. It is recommended that these units are additionally converted to Snellen equivalents for ease of communication of test findings – using the mathematical equations below as a guide:

Suppose Snellen fraction $= D \div d$
Minimum angle of resolution $(MAR) = d \div D$ (minutes of arc)
Spatial frequency $= 30 \div MAR$ (cycles per degree)

Thus 6/12 (or 20/40) Snellen acuity converts to 2 minutes of arc or 15 cycles per degree (c.p.d. or cycles/degree).

H

60

P N

36

D Z U

24

F R V E

18

Z H N U D

12

V P D E F R

9

P R E U H D N Z

6

U V D H E N F P

5

R U Z P N H D F

4

(a)   E D N Z F H P U

3

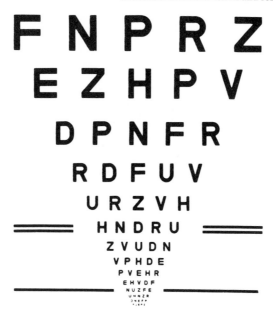

Figure 8.1. Visual acuity charts: (a) Snellen optotypes with BS 4274 (1968) letter selection; (b) Bailey-Lovie 'log MAR' design. (Reproduced from Bennett and Rabbetts, 1989a)

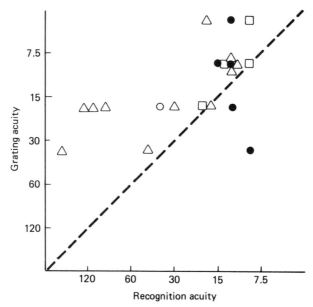

Figure 8.2. Comparison of grating and recognition acuity data (Snellen denominator) obtained from 21 amblyopic eyes. Points above the dotted 45° line indicate superior grating acuity. Symbols represent specific recognition acuity tests used: ●, Snellen; △, Allen pictures; □, Stycar; ○, linear E. (Adapted from Moskowitz, Sokol and Hansen, 1987, Rapid assessment of visual function in pediatric patients using pattern VEPs and acuity cards. *Clinical Vision Science*, **2**, 11–20 with kind permission from Pergamon Press Ltd, Headington Hill Hall, Oxford OX3 0BW, UK)

Contour interaction

The term contour interaction refers to the deleterious effect nearby contours have on the identification or recognition of letters or symbols. The phenomenon may also be described as visual crowding, separation difficulty or lateral masking. It can be measured by comparing acuity with single optotypes (sometimes termed 'angular acuity') and multiple optotypes ('linear' acuity) to produce a crowding ratio. Ratios greater than unity indicate that crowding is present. Precise measurement of contour interaction can only be achieved by using tests in which the spacing of optotypes is controlled to provide equivalent crowding for each optotype size, as in the Bailey-Lovie 'log MAR' design (Lovie-Kitchin, 1988). In adults a zone of interaction may be identified with the greatest visual impairment occurring when the adjacent contour is about twice the MAR from the optotype and maximal resolving power being obtained when the surround is separated from the target by at least five times the MAR (Flom, Weymouth and Kahneman, 1963). These values equate to about one half and one Snellen letter width respectively.

The crowding effect may be demonstrated in adults and children *with normal vision* but is most pronounced in amblyopic individuals (Hilton and Stanley, 1972) and in preschool rather than older children (*Figure 8.3*). The effect in young children appears genuine rather than an artifact of distraction by competing letters since it is still found when bar contours are used surrounding the central letter target (Fern *et al.*, 1986). Further research is necessary to properly explain the nature of contour interaction and to investigate the role of crowding ratio assessment in the early identification of amblyopia.

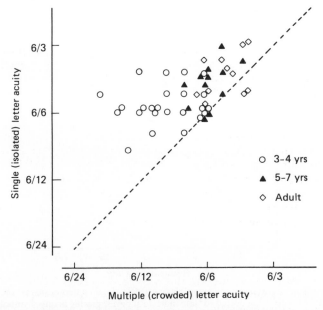

Figure 8.3. Comparison of single (isolated) and multiple (surrounded) letter acuity data obtained from young children and adults. Points above the 45° line indicate superiority of isolated letter acuity. Better performance for single optotypes is particularly noticeable in preschool children (○), whereas findings in 5 to 7 year olds (▲) and adults (◇) are similar. (After Atkinson *et al.*, 1988)

Practicalities of examining young children

Successful examination of young children depends as much on the examiner's experience and the provision of a suitable testing environment as it does on the selection of an appropriate test. The test room should be well illuminated, quiet and free from clutter which might otherwise distract the child, particularly in the case of an infant.

Adult subjective acuity tests usually depend on testing at 6 m. Children's attention on the task may be better maintained when a shorter testing distance is used. Whilst testing children at 3 m rather than 6 m produces little change in target vergence, several authors have noted shorter test durations. Overall testability is similar at both distances (Lippmann, 1969). Some authors have reported improved visual acuities when testing at 3 m but Atkinson and co-workers (1988) found no significant difference. Targets down to 6/3 Snellen size are required to provide adequate assessment at the 3 m distance.

Many vision tests for preschool children rely on the use of externally illuminated testing materials. Care should be taken to ensure that adequate illumination is provided when using such tests. This is particularly important when undertaking screening programmes in unfamiliar environments. Young children are often disturbed by wearing an eyepatch so it is often sensible to start testing binocularly so that at least one acuity value may be obtained before the child becomes unco-operative. This advice may be disregarded if the child is known to have amblyopia since monocular acuities are of more importance in such cases.

Subjective acuity methods

A vast array of subjective tests have been developed for assessment of distance visual acuity in preschool children. Detailed review of individual methods is outside the scope of this chapter. Two papers published in 1986 (Fern and Manny, 1986; McDonald, 1986) provide excellent sources of such material. This section will provide a summary and critical review of the main types of test available and give guidance on important factors which affect the suitability of various tests. Design of some recent tests will be described.

The tests described below have been categorized according to common features of their target construction. Alternative classifications can be made on the basis of the type of acuity (detection, resolution, recognition) measured (McDonald, 1986) or the child's method of responding to the stimuli presented (Blakey, 1988). The range of possible responses include naming, indicating stimulus orientation, matching or selecting the appropriate target from one or more presented. The latter method usually involves a two-alternative forced choice task.

Letter optotypes

Visual acuity tests using high-contrast letter optotypes fall into three main categories, being dependent respectively on correctly identifying Snellen letters (*Figure 8.1(a)*) or the orientations of either tumbling E or Landolt C targets. All of these optotypes can easily be constructed to Snellen principles (using either a 5 by 4 or 5 by 5 grid stroke widths of 1 unit). Clinically, letter optotypes are presented either as a single target on a flip card or ther face of a cube or as multiple targets on a chart or flip card. Many of the tests available for preschool children have been calibrated for use at both 6 m and shorter distances, typically 3 m.

Most of the letter optotype tests specifically developed for use with children are derivatives of those devised by Dr Mary Sheridan (Sheridan, 1976). The latter tests formed part of the *Stycar* vision testing methods (representing 'Sheridan tests – Young children and retardates'). During initial development work children responded by 'drawing out' letters in the air corresponding to a distant letter chart. This proved within the capabilities of most 5 year olds, though a tendency to draw letters smaller going down the chart made interpretation of the child's responses on the bottom row difficult. Younger children responded more successfully by pointing to letters which they matched on a key card, particularly when the testing distance was reduced and the letters were presented singly on 'flip cards'. Efforts were made to avoid letters which produced confusion in young children. A Stycar test chart and a single optotype letter matching test featuring nine letters (H, O, V, T, X, A, U, C and L) proved successful in testing older children but too complicated for preschool children. The latter could be tested by using restricted selections (see *Table 8.3* for details). Before 3 years children tend to confuse X and V so a minimum selection featuring four Stycar letters of varying shape is recommended. Several authors have subsequently used the selection (H, O, V, T) in their tests (Fern and Manny, 1986).

A direct derivative of the Stycar letter test is the more familiar *Sheridan–Gardiner* test. This uses the same distance test as the seven-letter Stycar test (in which all the letters are symmetrical about their vertical axis, thus avoiding any right-left confusion) and also includes a near visual acuity test developed by Peter Gardiner. Fern and Manny (1986) concluded that a well-designed preschool visual acuity test should consist of high-contrast Snellen optotypes without directional components that progress in 0.1 log unit steps down to a level of 6/3. A matching or forced-choice response was recommended to increase testability. They considered that the Sheridan–Gardiner (Stycar) came closest to meeting the criterion of the available tests.

Although highly successful from a practical point of view, a limitation of the Stycar and Sheridan–Gardiner letter tests is that they do not enable evaluation of the crowding effect since all testing is with widely spaced or completely isolated letters. This disadvantage may be offset by combining their use with other tests featuring the same letter selection but having surrounded optotypes. The *Cambridge crowding cards* (marketed by Clement Clarke International) appear particularly suitable for this purpose (Atkinson *et al.*, 1988). They are suitable for use at both 3 and 6 m and allow testing from 3/60 to 3/3. On each card the child has to identify a central letter which is surrounded by four others spaced at one half the overall letter width. The central letters are the same as in the five-letter Stycar test (H, O, V, T and X) but different surround letters are used to avoid confusion (e.g. L, U, A and C). The child merely has to identify the central letter from a selection of five large key letter cards which can be altered in position on a nylon loop board. Most children of 3½ years are able to perform the task satisfactorily. The *Sonksen–Silver acuity cards* also provide a method of determining linear acuities. They were designed for use from age 3 years, but this is probably slightly optimistic. The test comprises a flip-over chart displaying one line of standard spaced optotypes at a time. Optotype spacing is greater than in the Cambridge test, being equivalent to the overall letter width, and there is no vertical crowding. The child is asked to match the letters against a key card in which the six test letters (H, O, V, T, X and U) are placed on a curved line to improve the child's accuracy of pointing.

The *tumbling or illiterate E tests* predate the Stycar methods. The tests use Snellen E letter optotypes constructed on a 5 by 5 grid. The Es may be printed on or presented as rotatable letters on a chart, or may be presented individually, for example, on the face of a cube. In clinical use the open side of the E is presented either facing up, down, right or left. Testing success is dependent on the patient being able to accurately communicate the orientation of the symbol to the examiner. This can be by verbal report or more usually by the child pointing his fingers or turning a 'cut-off' E to the required orientation. Such orientation-based methods avoid any need for discrimination between different targets but require reasonable directional sense. Unfortunately, knowledge of spatial orientation is not well developed in the young child, particularly in distinguishing between right and left. Another disadvantage of these tests is their monotonous nature, particularly when using multiple optotypes. This may lead to boredom of both patient and examiner before completion and the examiner having difficulty in keeping in step with the child's responses. Attempts to design more interesting versions of the tumbling E test for children have been described by Fern and Manny (1986).

Landolt C or 'broken ring' tests have also been in use longer than the Stycar-based methods. The C target is based on a 5 by 5 Snellen grid construction. Generally the Landolt Cs are presented in the same four orientations used in the tumbling E test although four additional oblique presentations were included in the original test. The patient's task is to indicate the orientation of the gap in the ring. A two alternative forced choice test has also been developed in which the patient has to distinguish between a Landolt C and an O target presented simultaneously. An adaptation of this incorporates such targets as the wheels of a car and the child has to distinguish which car has 'broken wheels'. A slight drawback with Landolt C tests is that the gap will be recognized more easily in some directions than others when uncorrected astigmatism is present.

Picture and symbol optotypes

Picture optotype visual acuity tests usually depend on the child being able to correctly name familiar objects depicted on a chart or flip card. One problem resulting from the use of picture charts is the confusion caused by having two objects of greatly different size appearing on the same line. Many early tests were difficult to quantify because the optotypes used were not based on Snellen principles and often featured infilled (silhouette) figures. Attempts to calibrate such optotypes empirically included using trials with observers having known Snellen acuity or blurring lenses. In comparison with other tests the original picture charts, such as the Bealle Collins and Clement Clarke, gave unreliable acuity values (Keith, Diamond and Stansfield, 1972).

Recent examples of more satisfactory picture tests are the *Kay and Elliott* tests (Kay, 1983; Elliott, 1985). Both use pictures constructed on Snellen principles though the pictures in the Kay test are based on a 10 by 10 grid compared with a 7 by 7 grid in the Elliott test. The Kay test features 25 different optotypes presented singly on flip cards. The test is calibrated for use at either 3 or 6 m and the full set of cards cover the acuity range from 3/60 to 3/3. Picture recognition booklets are available so the child can be given some preliminary practice in picture naming at home or in the nursery school. Although the large range of optotypes may help maintain interest during testing the child's task becomes more demanding and the critical detail of some of the targets included, especially the duck, do not satisfy Snellen principles.

The Elliott test is perhaps more manageable as it features only eight different picture optotypes, presented in lines on a double-sided folding chart. The chart is designed for 6 m but could be used at shorter distances.

Complete standardization of picture optotypes is not possible even when their construction is based on Snellen principles. Accurate picture recognition is affected by other factors, for example, form interpretation, familiarity with the object and vocabulary, in addition to overall optotype size. Despite these criticisms data collated by Fern and Manny (1986) confirms the higher success rates attained using pictures (and symbols) rather than other optotypes in the 2- to 3-year age groups.

Tests using geometrical symbol optotypes generally depend on the child indicating their response by matching rather than giving a verbal report of the shape. Geometrical shapes can easily be constructed using Snellen principles. A popular test in this category is the *Ffooks* symbol test which uses three closed shapes – a square, triangle and a circle (Ffooks, 1965). The symbols may be presented singly on the face of a cube or as multiple optotypes on a flip card. The child is provided with three equivalent cardboard or plastic shapes which may be pointed to or held up. The restricted number of shapes may ease testing of young children but older children could lose interest in the test and there is a one in three chance of the child guessing correctly.

The *Sjögren hand test* is a picture test which depends on the child being able to accurately communicate the orientation of the symbol to the examiner. The symbols are usually printed singly on cards which can be rotated so that the figures of the hand point in different directions. The child has to turn their own hand to match that of the picture presented. This should be slightly easier for young children to understand than the similar Tumbling E test. A major limitation is that the optotypes are not Snellen based and the palm of the hand, being more distinct, gives a clue to the direction of the fingers.

The *Bailey–Hall cereal test* uses a two alternative forced choice testing method. It consists of six pairs of cards, featuring two pictures of comparable size, graded according to the distance at which adults with normal acuity can discriminate between them. One card of each pair shows a yellow cereal and the other a yellow square, each against a white background. The examiner holds up a pair of cards and the child's task is to indicate which depicts the cereal either by verbal report, pointing, reaching or preferential fixation. Each correct response is rewarded with a piece of cereal. The test was designed for use with children between 18 and 36 months. In older children a matching task has been recommended with the 6/60 test cards used as key cards (Livanes, Greaves and Bevan, 1986). The latter authors comment on several practical problems with the test.

Miniature toys

The *Stycar miniature toy* test was designed mainly for use with severely handicapped children. Although usually unable to match letters or name pictures such children can often recognize, match or sometimes name a variety of familiar objects. Miniature models of some of these objects (i.e. a car, aeroplane, doll, chair, knife, fork and spoon) were used as a means of testing visual function. The test requires the child to name a 'toy' held up by the examiner at a distance of about 3 m or match it with one from a selection in front of them. The test proved applicable from about 21 months mental age. One disadvantage with the test is that the child may prefer to play with the toys rather than pay attention to the examiner. It was claimed that ability to discriminate between the smallest fork and spoon objects represents a Snellen acuity of at least 6/6. The Stycar miniature toys test was largely superseded by the Stycar graded and mounted balls tests which were applicable over a wider age range (see later under objective methods). Better objective methods of assessing infant acuity are now available.

Objective acuity methods

A number of specific objective tests have been applied to the quantification of infant vision. In the absence of such tests, the practitioner may use simpler methods to provide some idea of visual status. These include evaluation of basic reflexes, for example, fixation and following or checking the child's response to alternate occlusion. The latter provides a gross test for the presence of amblyopia. It depends on the examiner covering each eye in turn (generally with a thumb) whilst noting any asymmetry in the child's resistance to occlusion. In theory the child should be more unhappy when its 'better' eye is covered; in practice the child is often equally resistant to either eye being occluded.

Although the results of objective tests may be converted to Snellen equivalents it is important to remember that they do not measure recognition acuity as in the Snellen letter test. Tests which use dot or spherical targets are really measuring detection or 'minimum visible acuity'. Many tests use high-contrast striped 'grating' targets which depend on resolution or 'minimum separable' acuity. The next section provides a summary of types of objective visual acuity test available. The following reviews are particularly recommended as sources of further information: Pearson (1966), Dobson and Teller (1978) and Teller and co-authors (1986).

Objective visual acuity tests for young children are often classified into three main groups being based respectively on optokinetic or visual evoked responses or preferential looking behaviour. Several of these methods are applicable from birth. An additional behavioural method (described below) does not fall easily into any of the aforementioned categories. It is based on the child's detection of stimuli which are either static or moving in a manner which may provoke visual interest but does not induce involuntary repetitive eye movements.

Voluntary target detection

The *Stycar graded and mounted balls* both involve successive presentation of white polystyrene spheres of graded size against a black background at a distance of 3 m. In the graded balls test the spheres are rolled across the child's field of view and the examiner watches for the presence of appropriate visual pursuit eye and/or head movements. The graded ball test is thus a derivative of the 'ivory balls test' devised, at the turn of the century, by a London ophthalmologist named Claude Worth. In the alternative test the spheres are mounted on rigid sticks, which are then introduced into the child's field of view (in varying positions) by an examiner who is hidden behind a screen but watching for appropriate fixation behaviour through a small aperture in the partition. The tests are applicable from about 6 months.

The *candy bead* or '*hundreds and thousands*' test described by Bock and others uses small spherical edible cake decorations as both stimulus and reward. The decorations are often held out in the examiner's palm. The child's ability to detect, pick up and subsequently eat these targets is monitored whilst using each eye in turn.

Ideally bead diameter and viewing distance should be carefully controlled to increase accuracy. Adequate hand–eye coordination is needed so the test cannot be used until this has been acquired. Successful testing is claimed to be possible from about 9 months. Technically this test could be classified as subjective since the child presumably makes a conscious decision to respond. However, because of other similarities with tests in this section, it has been included here for simplicity. The Dot visual acuity test is an adaptation of the method. It features a series of nine black dots which range from 1 to 40 minutes of arc angular subtense at the 25-cm viewing distance. Each dot may be positioned randomly on a white background within an aperture of 7-cm diameter. The child has to locate and touch each dot presented. The smallest dot correctly identified twice is recorded as the acuity level.

Optokinetic responses

Objective acuity tests based on optokinetic responses predate other methods. The techniques have declined in popularity so Pearson's review (1966) remains fairly comprehensive. The tests are dependent on the principle that contours moving across a subject's field of view will, if resolved, induce involuntary eye movements. Visual acuity is estimated either from the smallest moving stimulus (often a black and white striped field) which will induce or sustain reflex oscillatory eye movements or optokinetic nystagmus (OKN) or, more rarely, from the smallest stationary test object which, when superimposed on the moving test field, will consistently inhibit those eye movements. Eye movements may be observed directly or measured using electro-oculography, in which case a permanent record is obtained.

OKN may be elicited in newborns, so the method is applicable from birth. Several laboratory studies investigated newborn acuity by placing infants beneath a canopy of moving stripes (which could be varied in spatial frequency) and noting the narrowest stripe width which would induce or sustain OKN. As the viewing distance was fixed and only three or four stripe widths were available the method did not provide satisfactory individual acuity estimates. However, by pooling many infants' results and interpolation, an estimate of newborn acuity could be obtained. This mode of stimulation ensures that distractions are removed from the field of view but it is really only appropriate for very young infants, who are least likely to be distressed by the claustrophobic effect of a canopy of moving stripes.

Infant acuity has been assessed clinically using less cumbersome apparatus. Enoch and Rabinowicz (1976) successfully monitored the acuities of a young infant, before and after removal of a unilateral cataract, using a hand-held striped 'OKN' drum at variable distances. A disadvantage of this method is that the stimulus occupies less of the field of view as viewing distance increases, so a carefully controlled environment is necessary to eliminate room distractions. The commercially available Catford drum test alleviates this problem by providing a range of targets which unfortunately depend on stimulus visibility rather than resolution. The portable device uses black spots of various sizes (on a white background) which may be individually exposed through an aperture and moved by a small electric motor. These stimuli execute a slow movement across the aperture followed by a quick return. Since the targets measure minimum visible rather than minimum separable, the test overestimates visual acuity but unfortunately not in a systematic way, so the relationship of the measurement to visual acuity is doubtful (Atkinson *et al.*, 1981a).

Major limitations of methods based on eliciting optokinetic responses are that failure to do so may simply reflect poor cooperation with the test rather than inability to perceive the moving stripes and that acuity estimates are usually based on responses to moving stimuli. Both problems can be avoided by methods which depend on *arresting* of optokinetic responses by a stationary, preferably striped, test target as in a method devised by Voipio (1961). The author's attempts to develop such a method for use in infancy were, however, thwarted by technical difficulties (mainly in the photographic production of satisfactory stimuli) which may explain the absence of equivalent tests in the literature (Thompson, 1987).

Visual evoked responses

Visual evoked potential (VEP) recording techniques are usually confined to research units or hospitals. EEG-type scalp electrodes are worn during testing. Several electrophysiological methods of acuity determination have been devised. Variations in technique have included differences in stimuli (checks, sine waves or square waves), stimulation mode (pattern onset or contrast reversal) and temporal frequency (transient or steady state – sometimes with spatial frequency sweep), and signal analysis (conventional or Fourier). Each of the main methods has been successfully applied from early infancy. A summary of these is provided below. Detailed descriptions (and references) are provided in Chapter 17.

Theoretically the most accurate acuity method depends on extrapolating from electrophysiologically determined contrast sensitivity functions. Unfortunately this is very tedious using conventional transient stimulation as it requires several recordings with different contrasts and pattern sizes. The method is only feasible clinically when combined with a steady-state or preferably rapid electronic sweep technique which is not yet widely available. Although the latter reduce recording time, information about waveform configuration is lost. It is therefore important that confirmation of the genuineness of any response is based on analysis of VEP phase characteristics as well as amplitude.

Most clinical VEP acuity methods depend on finding the finest repetitive black and white checkerboard or striped 'grating' stimulus which will evoke a cortical response. The threshold pattern size may be located directly from the finest target to elicit a recognizable VEP (Marg *et al.*, 1976). This method may require lengthy recording and is limited by difficulty in establishing the endpoint due to contamination of the signal by noise sources originating outside the visual cortex. Recording time can be reduced by determining the threshold pattern indirectly by extrapolation from an amplitude versus spatial frequency function, particularly where this relies on a 'spatial frequency sweep' method. Despite several theoretical inadequacies the 'amplitude versus spatial frequency plot' method has proved fairly popular and appears to produce comparable normative data to other VEP techniques (Dobson and Teller, 1978).

All of the procedures outlined above use several pattern sizes to derive an acuity estimate. An alternative approach is to evaluate the monocular responses at one 'token' pattern size to identify any asymmetry or difference from predetermined age-related norms. This simplified procedure would not result in an acuity estimate but may be sufficient to identify amblyopia. Such methods could prove suitable for screening purposes in infancy because of reduced test duration (Moskowitz, Sokol and Hansen, 1987).

Compared with alternative objective tests, VEP-based methods show faster development of visual acuity and contrast sensitivity to adult levels. There is general agreement that an adult-like VEP contrast sensitivity function is attained by 6 to 10 months of age. However steeper VEP acuity growth functions are obtainable using pattern appearance rather than pattern reversal stimulation (Orel-Bixler and Norcia, 1987).

Preferential looking

Preferential looking (PL) techniques rely on the observation that infants will fixate patterned surfaces more than featureless surfaces (Berlyne, 1958; Fantz, 1958). During testing the infant is presented with a pattern paired with (or embedded within) a blank field of equivalent mean luminance. Although used to study other aspects of infant vision (e.g. stereoacuity, contrast sensitivity and colour vision), the most common application has been assessment of infant visual acuity using a series of black and white striped 'grating' stimuli paired with a grey surface. As the mean luminance of the grating and grey surface are matched both appear the same if the stripes are beyond the observer's resolution limit. During testing the grating is randomly presented either to the right or left on a particular trial and the infant's looking behaviour is simultaneously observed, by a concealed observer. As the standard grating stimuli are not very compelling viewing for older infants, specially constructed picture optotypes are used in the Cardiff acuity test (Woodhouse *et al.*, 1992). These optotypes are generated from alternate black and white bands and merge into their background above the resolution limit.

In the original procedure (Fantz, Ordy and Udelf, 1962), the observer is aware of the pattern location, whereas in a version known as forced-choice preferential looking (FPL) the observer judges the probable location of the pattern during each trial from cues given by the infant's looking behaviour and the response is scored as correct or incorrect (Teller, 1979). The latter method is preferable since it removes observer bias.

Initial studies suggested that PL was most effective between 1 and 6 months and not really possible beyond 1 year in normal children. Mayer and Dobson (1982) therefore introduced an 'operant' PL method in which reinforced conditioning was used to encourage infants of above 6 months to complete testing. The need for such formal conditioning has now been removed with the success of the acuity card method (described below) throughout the preschool age range. The original methods were less successful because they relied on lengthy psychophysical testing procedures such as the method of constant stimuli (Teller *et al.*, 1974; Gwiazda *et al.*, 1978) or formal staircase methods (Atkinson, Braddick and Pimm-Smith, 1982; Mayer, Fulton and Hansen, 1982). Responses were interpreted in terms of statistical probability to assess the threshold level. These methods provide accurate data for laboratory studies but are too time consuming for routine clinical use owing to the number of trials required.

Fewer trials are required for clinical use. The method of constant stimuli was adapted to provide a screening method as the diagnostic stripe width test. This uses repeated observations at one spatial frequency to screen out infants that fail to resolve stripes of the 'diagnostic' width for their age. The test was reasonably successful but not very popular, as it does not allow assessment of visual acuity. Further limitations include difficulties in screening high-risk premature infants at early ages (Manning *et al.*, 1982) and failure to establish a diagnostic width for 18 month olds (Dobson *et al.*, 1985).

Staircase procedures concentrate testing around the threshold level by selecting stimuli according to the response(s) on previous trials. Acuity estimates are thus obtained using fewer trials than required for the method of constant stimuli. Formal PL staircase methods were developed but still relied on far too many trials for routine clinical use. In contrast, the acuity card procedure has been shown to provide a fast and accurate method suitable for use in a variety of clinical settings (Teller *et al.*, 1986). A high percentage of children complete binocular and monocular tests at all ages. Average durations for individual acuity estimates range from 2 to 6 minutes, except in newborns where the average test time was 8 minutes.

Although based on the earlier staircase methods, the acuity card procedure does not require lengthy forced choice stimulus presentation because more information is gained on each trial. An integrated judgement of the child's acuity is made using information which is disregarded in traditional PL tests. Over a series of trials the observer evaluates both direction of gaze *and* quality of fixation responses. The latter information is very useful because infant's typically demonstrate strong, continual fixation of low spatial frequency gratings, only slight fixation preference just above and absence of differential fixation just below their acuity threshold. This extra qualitative information can readily indicate the infant's acuity limit using fewer trials.

Commercially available tests in the UK include the Teller acuity cards (*Figure 8.4(b)*) and the Keeler cards. Both are portable and relatively inexpensive. The cards

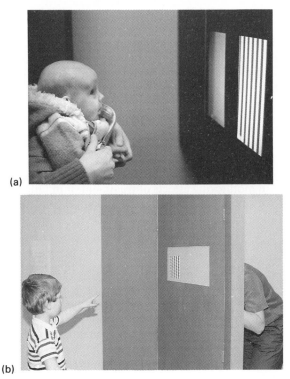

(a)

(b)

Figure 8.4. Visual (grating) acuity assessment using preferential looking procedures. (a) Three-month-old infant viewing a conventional, optically projected display. (b) Two-year-old responding (by pointing) to the grating on a Teller acuity card. Use of the partition screen is not essential so the latter commercially available test is more portable

may be obtained in sets featuring a series of gratings spaced in 0.5 octave intervals (an octave represents a doubling or halving of spatial frequency). They may be presented from behind an opening in a screen, although this is not essential. Testing distances of about 38 and 55 cm are used for infants and young children respectively. The acuity estimate is taken to be the finest grating the child is judged to see. Each card may be shown for as long as necessary and as many times as needed to make a decision. Between trials the observer is able to communicate with the child, which helps to retain older infants' interest in the test. The Teller cards each feature a grating embedded in a grey surround. Unfortunately this design causes an edge artifact to be seen at the border of the finer gratings which may allow correct identification of the grating position beyond the resolution limit (Robinson, Moseley and Fielder, 1988). Although this is only likely to be of importance in examination of older children, the Keeler cards eliminate the problem by adding a genuine edge around the grating and also on the blank side of the card.

The author's independent attempts to develop a clinically appropriate PL technique were based on a specially constructed optical projection system, used in a dark room (*Figure 8.4(a)*). The method commenced with a staircase procedure which rapidly provided an indication of the threshold location, testing continued using repeated trials around this level until sufficient information was available to make an acuity estimate. Acuity was defined as the finest spatial frequency (or interpolated frequency) for which 75% preference was shown for the grating rather than the homogeneous screen. The method proved clinically viable in normal infants and clinical patients between birth and 1 year (Thompson and Drasdo, 1988). Although several infants with very low acuity attended to the internally illuminated display more convincingly than to Teller acuity cards, older infants with better acuity seemed to resent the dark testing environment required. In most cases acuity card methods would appear to be particularly convenient in terms of their age range of application and portability.

PL methods are applicable from birth in both full-term and preterm infants. When comparing findings with age norms the child's post-term age should be used to correct for prematurity. The procedure has proven useful for assessing neurologically impaired individuals of any age and can greatly assist the paediatric ophthalmologist taking decisions regarding the management of young patients. Examples of this are in monitoring effects of treatment or in judging the need for or timing of surgery in certain cases such as partial unilateral congenital cataract.

Validity of acuity methods

Many factors should be considered when evaluating the clinical suitability of preschool acuity tests. Supporting data should demonstrate the appropriateness of the test procedure for the age group in question. Consistent acuity age norms should be available for the test. Evaluation should also include consideration of its reliability, the duration and success of testing and comparison of findings with other tests (McDonald, 1986). Unfortunately, most preschool acuity tests reported in the literature, including those which are commercially available, fall short of this ideal.

Mean acuity values as a function of age, obtained using objective tests, are summarized in *Figure 8.5(a)* whilst values derived from subjective testing are provided in *Figure 8.5(b)*. These figures illustrate the large variation in acuity age norms reported in the literature. Fern and Manny (1986) found subjective estimates

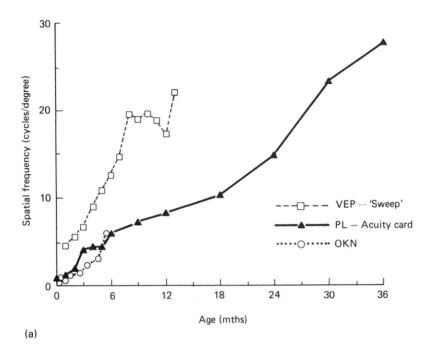

(a)

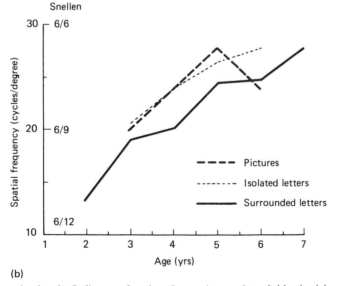

(b)

Figure 8.5. Mean visual acuity findings as a function of age, using a variety of objective (a) and subjective (b) procedures. In (a) VEP data is from Norcia and Tyler (1985), binocular preferential looking data is from Teller *et al.* (1986), and the OKN data represents the combined results of Fantz, Ordy and Udelf (1962) and Enoch and Rabinowicz, (1976). The recognition acuity curves (b) were adapted from Fern and Manny (1986)

of normal acuity varied between 6/6 and 6/18 at 3 years and between 6/5 and 6/11 at 6 years. Referral criteria for visual screening programmes showed a corresponding wide range, depending on the child's age, test used and presumably also professional opinion and local politics. The lack of close correspondence in average findings is not surprising given the presence of uncorrected refractive error in some of the samples, coupled with differences in optotype (design, sizes and contour interaction), methods of responding and threshold criteria. In general, acuity norms at any given age span an approximately one octave range, providing that one considers only binocular findings and ignores data obtained using sweep VEPs (higher values, *Figure 8.5(a)*) or tasks based on pursuit or OKN eye movement tasks (lower values). Teller acuity card findings in a sample of normal and monocularly deprived children are compared with published age norms for the test in *Figure 8.6*.

Reliability and comparability

Accuracy of acuity assessment can be evaluated by various statistical measures, for example, average test–retest differences, standard errors of estimates and test–retest reliability coefficients. However, these measures have not been reported frequently enough to enable meaningful comparison of procedures. This is particularly true of preschool tests of a subjective nature, whereas various PL methods, including acuity card procedures, have been rigorously evaluated (Teller *et al.*, 1986; Preston *et al.*, 1987; Birch and Hale, 1988).

Despite the lack of appropriate data regarding the validity of subjective preschool acuity tests, some general points can be made based on findings in adults (for more details see Bennett, 1965). Landolt C and in particular illiterate E targets are known to be easier to see than Snellen letters of the same size. In preschool children, Livanes, Greaves and Bevan (1986) found use of the standard Landolt C chart more

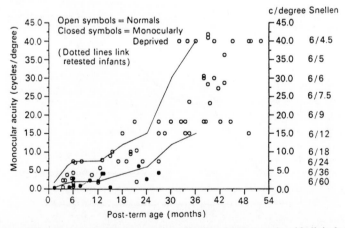

Figure 8.6. Comparison of monocular Teller acuity card findings in 61 normal and 9 clinical patients (data from deprived eye). The clinical sample had variously suffered unilateral deprivation from cataract (five cases), Sturge–Weber syndrome, ptosis, vitreous opacity or convergent squint. Most of the normal childrens' data falls within the expected ranges (denoted by the solid lines) whereas most of the patients' data is at the low end of the normal range or falls below the minimum expected. Open symbols, normals; closed symbols, monocularly deprived. Dotted lines link retested infants. (From Thompson and Drasdo, 1988)

difficult than the illiterate E test with the former tending to produce different results compared with other tests. Also of interest is the observation that several letters used in the Stycar tests (L, T, U, V, C) are amongst the ones which (in serif form) adults find easiest to recognize, though the letter H falls within the most difficult group.

Some studies have compared adults' (or older childrens') acuities on specific preschool tests with their findings on standard Snellen charts. Much of the available data relates to picture tests. Faye (1968) specifically modified her Lighthouse picture designs so that in normal and subnormal adults measured picture acuities were comparable to Snellen test type findings. The Kay and Elliott picture tests tend to produce slightly lower acuity findings compared with Snellen letters. Exact agreement between picture and Snellen acuity has been claimed in 67% of individuals tested with Elliott pictures (Elliott, 1985) and 45% of those tested with Kay pictures (Kay, 1983). With either test, acuity differences rarely exceeded one line although recorded acuity was one line worse than Snellen in 40% of individuals tested using Kay pictures. Control trials indicate that all three non-letter Stycar tests (miniature toys, graded and mounted balls) which are not based on conventional optotypes, often considerably overestimate acuity in children (>6 years) and adults (Hall, Pugh and Hall, 1982).

In theory, the reliability of PL acuity estimates will be greatly reduced by using fewer trials, especially if measurement is based on less than 60 trials (Teller, 1983). One might expect that this would limit the usefulness of the acuity card procedure, in which each estimate is based on relatively few trials (generally not exceeding 20). Studies have, however, demonstrated relatively high intra- and inter-observer reliability of acuity card findings and generated age norms and population standard deviations similar to those reported for lengthier PL techniques (Teller *et al.*, 1986; Preston *et al.*, 1987). In the first year of life, it appears that cross-sectional variability in acuity findings is lower for data obtained via the sweep VEP method (s.d. ≈ 0.4 octaves; Norcia and Tyler, 1985), rather than with acuity cards (s.d. ≈ 0.7 octaves; Teller *et al.*, 1986). Some of this difference is caused by using cards spaced in 1.0 octave spatial frequency steps in early studies. Average population standard deviations of around 0.4–0.5 octaves have been reported in toddlers, when using acuity cards spaced in 0.3- (Heersema and van Hof-van Duin, 1988) or 0.5-octave steps.

Considering acuity cards spaced in spatial frequency steps of 0.5 octaves, repeated estimates typically fall within a 1.0-octave range and observers can mostly agree to within ± 1.0 octave on the magnitude and direction of any interocular acuity difference. Most results obtained via acuity card and formal PL testing methods agree to within 1 octave. Although encouraging, these findings do not indicate that acuity card procedures allow very precise estimates of acuity to be made with great certainty. In fact the procedure has lower test retest reliability and larger confidence intervals than other methods (*Table 8.2*). As a rough rule an accuracy of about ± 1 octave can be expected with acuity cards, so an estimate of 10 c.p.d. (6/18) should really be interpreted as indicating a value between 5 c.p.d. (6/36) and 20 c.p.d. (6/9). Variability might be reduced using finer gradations of card or interpolation of test findings. Intersubject variability is lower for interocular grating acuity differences than for binocular and monocular grating acuity norms, so the former offers a more sensitive measure for identifying monocular acuity deficits (Birch and Hale, 1988). Nevertheless, interocular acuity differences (mostly below 1.5 octaves) are frequently encountered in normal infants (e.g. Thompson and Drasdo, 1988), so a policy of repeat testing is advisable in doubtful cases.

TABLE 8.2. Success rate, variability and reliability statistics for several acuity tests, administered to young children and adults

Test	Sample age	Success rate (%)	s.d. (octave)	Test – retests		
				'r'	% within ± 0.5 octave	95% confidence interval (octave)
Acuity cards	2 years	90 (80)	0.59	– 0.06	75	1.19
	3 years	95 (95)	0.48	0.08	83	0.90
	Adult	—	0.25	—	—	—
Dot test	2 years	60 (40)	0.32	0.47	100	0.46
	3 years	92 (85)	0.24	0.52*	100	0.32
	Adult	—	0.47	—	—	—
Broken wheel	2 years	43 (—)	0.49	– 0.24	83	1.07
	3 years	92 (80)	0.47	0.62*	89	0.57
	Adult	—	0.43	—	—	—
AO pictures	2 years	40 (—)	0.38	—	100	—
	3 years	90 (80)	0.25	– 0.12	94	0.52
	Adult	—	0.36	—	—	—
Snellen chart	Adult	—	0.29	—	—	—

Data is from McDonald and Chaudry (1989) and is all based on binocular testing, except that success rate data is also provided for monocular testing (figures in brackets). The spread of acuity findings for each test and age group are indicated by population standard deviations (s.d.). Test–retest correlation coefficients ('r') which reached statistical significance are denoted by asterisks. The final column represents the range in which a child's true acuity will fall 95% of the time (given the estimated acuity). An octave represents a doubling or halving of spatial frequency. Acuity cards were spaced in approximately 0.5 octave steps.

Testability

Evaluation of the suitability of any test method must include consideration of the success rate in testing. A number of direct comparison studies of clinical preschool acuity tests have been conducted (Keith, Diamond and Stansfield, 1972; Fern *et al.*, 1986; Livanes, Greaves and Bevan, 1986; McDonald and Chaudry, 1989). Further data has been assembled in review articles (Fern and Manny, 1986; McDonald, 1986; Teller *et al.*, 1986; Blakey, 1988). Unfortunately interpretation of findings is complicated by differences in sample ages in various investigations. Despite this, several general observations can be made. The most obvious of these are that, regardless of technique, the numbers of children that can be successfully tested increases with age. Secondly, success rates for monocular testing are poorer than equivalent findings binocularly. It should also be noted that another important variable – testing duration – is often inversely related to the test success rate.

Before about 24 months of age, objective acuity methods are really the only practical testing option. Of these, the only test to be widely clinically validated is the acuity card PL procedure, which has consistently provided impressive success rate data throughout infancy. A single check size VEP method offers a reasonably (77%) successful means of detecting unequal vision below 2 years (Moskowitz, Sokol and Hansen, 1987), but the rapid sweep VEP acuity method (see Chapter 17) has not yet been fully clinically validated. Even at 2 years it is clear that children respond more favourably to an acuity card procedure than to subjective testing methods (*Table 8.2*).

Performances of 2–3 year olds on *subjective* acuity tests vary considerably according to the method. In many children naming of simple pictures is first achieved between 20 and 30 months, whereas the ability to match simple shapes or point to forms that are like a model, develops around 3 years (McDonald, 1986). It is claimed that preliminary practice at home or in the nursery school can greatly enhance performance on matching tests (Sheridan, 1976). It is generally believed that 2 year olds respond best for picture naming tests, but as is evident from *Table 8.2* this is very dependent on the particular version used. From 3 years reasonable (>60%) success is obtained on single letter matching tests, such as the Stycar 5 letter test, but initially performance may be very poor (≈25%) for tests either having a directional component or requiring letter naming. It has been claimed that 3 year olds respond better to both the Bailey–Hall cereal test and Stycar letter tests compared with lighthouse pictures (Livanes, Greaves and Bevan, 1986).

Pickert and Wachs (1980) studied the independent effect of changes in stimulus targets and response methods on testability of preschool and primary school children (mean ages 4.75 and 6.75 years respectively). Stimuli including a directional component proved more difficult than others and verbal report was easier than matching. The latter finding is presumably owing to the relatively mature preschool sample possessing appropriate language skills. The finding of poorer performance for tests relying on a directional component (e.g. tumbling E, Landolt C) is consistent with many other studies. Such tests are almost completely ineffective before age 3 and success rates lag behind those of alternative tests throughout the preschool years. Although the conventional Snellen chart remains beyond the capabilities of many 4 year olds, from this age children respond to most tests whether requiring a directional, matching or naming response. Use of the standard (6 m) Snellen letter test chart with unmodified procedure becomes appropriate at school age.

Contrast sensitivity

Theoretical aspects

A series of innovative experiments by Cambell and his associates, using sine wave grating stimuli (*Figure 8.7*), first drew attention to the possibilities of contrast sensitivity measurement at different spatial frequencies and initiated a wealth of studies applying Fourier principles to the visual system (Campbell and Robson, 1968). In basic investigations stimuli viewed on an oscilloscope screen may be used to define a subject's contrast thresholds (minimum contrast for detection) at different spatial frequencies (grating bar width). If the sensitivity (reciprocal of threshold) data thus derived is plotted versus spatial frequency a curve known as the contrast sensitivity function (CSF) is generated. The function (*Figure 8.8*) is an inverted 'U' shape with a peak at intermediate spatial frequencies.

Visual acuity, the limit of resolution at maximum contrast, is represented by only a single, high frequency 'cut-off' point on the CSF (typically between 30 and 40 c.p.d.). The CSF can provide a detailed description of an individual's visual function which is more relevant, since visual environments are not usually restricted to small targets of high contrast. An obvious application is in evaluation of the quality of vision in patients with developing cataract, since opacities causing generalized loss (*Figure 8.9(e)* are more devastating than those resulting in only high spatial frequency deficits (*Figure 8.9(a)*). The test is valuable as a means of monitoring subtle changes in visual performance and provides a useful method for assessing glare disability in patients with cataracts and other media abnormalities such as

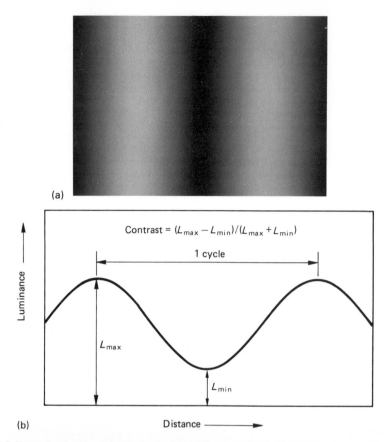

Figure 8.7. Example of a sinusoidal grating and the definition of its contrast. About two cycles of the grating are shown (a), with the luminance profile of one cycle drawn below (b). (After Levi and Harwerth, 1982, American Academy of Optometry, reproduced from Edwards and Llewellyn, 1988)

corneal oedema (Elliott, Gilchrist and Whitaker, 1989). Research has also identified a number of disorders (e.g. multiple sclerosis, optic neuritis, glaucoma, diabetes and Parkinson's disease) which may produce contrast sensitivity losses at medium and/or low spatial frequencies in patients with normal visual acuity (see Regan, 1988, for details of individual studies). In fact a wide range of abnormal CSFs may be obtained (*Figure 8.9*). The sharp notch deficit (*Figure 8.9(d)*) may be associated with reports of monocular diplopia. Strabismic amblyopia may result in only high frequency loss (*Figure 8.9(a)*) or generalized loss (*Figure 8.8(e)*). Care is required in interpretation since several conditions may result in similar patterns of loss. Contrast sensitivity loss, in certain conditions, may be affected by stimulus temporal frequency and orientation as well as spatial frequency (Regan, 1988).

Contrast sensitivity data is greatly influenced by the conditions of measurement, for example, sensitivity increases with the stimulus field size until a certain critical number of bars in a grating are reached (Rovamo and Virsu, 1979). This finding indicates that contrast sensitivity tests sample over an extended retinal area which depends on the spatial frequency. A contrast sensitivity determined with gratings having this critical number of bars has the same value as if the grating were presented

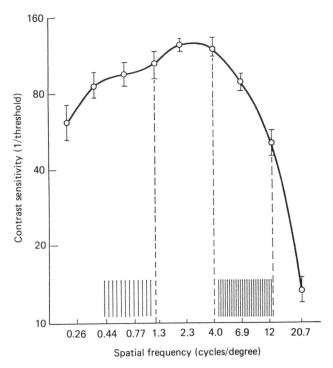

Figure 8.8. The contrast sensitivity function represents the reciprocal of the minimal contrast that can be perceived for a range of spatial frequencies. The curve shows the average data obtained from 12 normal subjects, error bars = ± 1 standard error. (Reproduced from Drasdo, 1988)

across the entire visual field and this sensitivity is therefore the contrast sensitivity of the complete visual field (Drasdo, 1988). From a practical viewpoint these findings emphasize the need for careful evaluation and consideration of stimulation conditions when developing new methods. Sine wave gratings provide the most appropriate test stimuli since they allow measurement at one specific spatial frequency. According to Fourier theory any other stimulus is composed of a series of sine waves of different spatial frequencies and contrasts. A square-wave consists of a fundamental frequency at high contrast and harmonics at successively higher frequencies and lower contrasts. Sinusoidal gratings are not easily reproduced photographically and square wave-based stimuli (e.g. bar grating or letters) may be used as a cheaper or more convenient option. The latter produce similar sensitivity findings to sine waves, providing their fundamental spatial frequency exceeds about 2 c.p.d.

Subjective assessment techniques

The earliest popular contrast sensitivity test was the George Young threshold test which was introduced in 1918 and involved a visual search task. This featured a series of grey circular patches, produced using successive dilutions of ink, which were presented in a test booklet. Although the test had several inadequacies, notably the small retinal area which could be sampled by the stimuli and an inappropriate range of ink densities, Drasdo (1988) recalls its value in one clinical case.

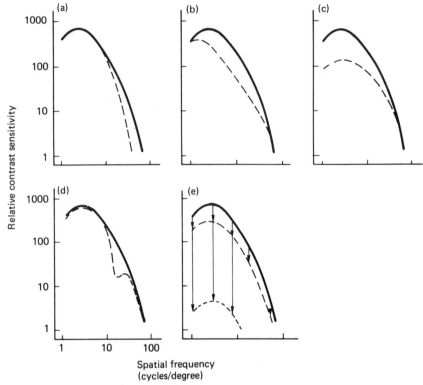

Figure 8.9. Several types of abnormal contrast sensitivity function. The continuous curve is a normal function, the non-continuous curves represent: selective contrast sensitivity loss for high (a) or intermediate spatial frequencies (b), loss for low and intermediate frequencies (c), a sharp notch deficity (d) or generalized uniform losses of sensitivity (e). (Adapted from Regan, 1988, low-contrast letter charts and sinewave grating tests in ophthalmological and neurological disorders. *Clinical Vision Science*, **2**, 235–250 with kind permission from Pergamon Press Ltd, Headington Hill Hall, Oxford OX3 0BW, UK)

In research laboratories contrast sensitivity determinations typically employ expensive computer-based equipment coupled with time-consuming psychophysical methods. Such sophisticated systems enable computer control of stimulus presentation (usually electronically generated sinusoids) and data analysis. The experimenter has great scope in selection of stimulus parameters. Although some systems have become commercially available (e.g. Nicolet CS 2000; Nicolet Biomedical Instruments, Wisconsin, USA and the currently available CRS visual stimulus generator VSG 2/2 with psycho software from Cambridge Research Systems, Rochester, Kent, UK), they are not appropriate for general use in clinical practice. Several cheaper and simpler methods have been devised for clinical use. The initial methods were based on grating stimuli but recent attempts to produce more convenient tests have led to the introduction of low-contrast letter charts. Some of the commercially available clinical tests are discussed below.

Arden gratings test

The test is often described as the Arden 'plates' since it comprises a series of photographic plates featuring sine wave gratings each of constant spatial frequency but increasing in contrast from top to bottom. Six spatial frequencies are available from 0.2 to 6.4 c.p.d. The practitioner slowly withdraws each plate from its case whilst noting the point at which the patient first sees the grating by reference to a scale on the side. The results are usually presented as the sum of scores from individual gratings. This 'Arden score' will be raised by a defect in contrast sensitivity. According to Arden's scoring criteria, abnormalities are indicated by any eye scoring more than 82, interocular differences exceeding 10 or individual plates scoring above 16. Unfortunately, test results are influenced by several factors including the speed of movement of the plate and the criterion used by the patient to determine threshold. For these reasons use of a forced choice testing protocol has been advocated. Some disadvantages have been noted with the test. Although children may be tested from about 4 years, Arden's original abnormality criteria are too strict for them (Brown, Doran and Woodhouse, 1987). The range of spatial frequencies appears inadequate for monitoring amblyopia therapy but this could be remedied by doubling the viewing distance. The test, which is marketed by the American Optical Company, has been used in optometric practice (Yap *et al.*, 1985), but is not widely available.

Vistech contrast sensitivity system

This widely promoted test is based on a chart featuring circular photographic plates arranged in five rows and nine columns. The plates contain a sine wave grating, oriented vertically or 15° to the right or left. Each row has a different spatial frequency (1.5–18 c.p.d. range) and contrast decreases (30–0% range) from left to right across the columns. The patient is asked to look along each row in turn, indicating the grating orientations. When in doubt the patient should be encouraged to guess, as this increases measurement accuracy. Results (last stimulus on each row correctly identified) are transferred to a simple recording chart, which shows the normal expected range of findings. The distance version of the chart is designed for use at 3 m and a near version is also available. The test is marketed by Vistech Consultants Inc. (Dayton, Ohio, USA).

The test has been criticized in terms of its poor repeatability, use of a constant stimulus size rather than one dependent on the critical grating bar number, difficulty in illuminating the distance chart evenly and accommodative problems experienced with the near test. Although it is debatable whether the high spatial frequency results provide any additional information over acuity, it certainly offers the most rapid way of obtaining a CSF curve. The test is applicable in young children from about 4 years (Mantyjarvi *et al.*, 1989). In visually impaired children, testing at two grating orientations (vertical and horizontal) is recommended (Woodhouse and Westall, 1989).

Cambridge low contrast gratings

The Cambridge test (Wilkins *et al.*, 1988) was designed as a screening method for patients with normal acuity. It comprises a series of pairs of plates within a spiral bound A4 size booklet. One plate of each pair features a square wave grating, the other is a uniform grey. The patient's task on each presentation is to indicate which page contains the grating. The first pair of plates is for demonstration purposes and includes a grating of good (13%) contrast. Grating contrast successively declines from 5% to 0.14% within the test series of 10 plate pairs. A strict two alternative forced choice testing method is used involving four series of presentations per eye. Each series ends by recording the plate number on which an error is first made. These numbers are totalled and converted to a contrast sensitivity value. The test is available from Clement Clarke International Ltd (London).

Advantages of the test are its cheapness and compactness coupled with use of a good psychophysical method. However, the latter could prove tedious and this coupled with use of a long viewing distance may explain why 4–9 year olds expressed preference for alternative tests such as low contrast picture charts or Vistech charts (Mantyjarvi *et al.*, 1989). Only a single frequency near the peak of the CSF is used, so pathologies solely affecting low frequencies could be missed. As each grating is of 4 c.p.d. at the recommended 6 m viewing distance, halving the distance enables additional measurement at 2 c.p.d. without interference from harmonics.

Regan low contrast acuity charts

This testing system comprises three letter charts of high, medium and low contrasts (96%, 7% and 4% respectively). The first two are recommended for general use (usually at 3 m but this could be doubled or halved); it is suggested that the latter may be helpful for detailed testing in certain cases. Charts feature Snellen-type letters progressing in 11 lines down to 6/3 size. Each line usually has eight letters. Letter size halves every third line. The high and medium contrast charts are read in the usual manner and the 'acuity' threshold results are transferred to a nomogram which may be used to indicate whether Snellen acuity or intermediate contrast vision are outside normal limits and whether there is a visual pathway abnormality. A Sheridan–Gardiner type version of the low-contrast vision test proved effective from about 3 years (Regan, 1988).

Pelli–Robson low contrast letter sensitivity chart

This test requires only a single chart, which features letters of constant size but decreasing in contrast (by a factor of $1/\sqrt{2}$) after each block of three. There are eight lines of six letters. Contrast sensitivity (CS) is derived from the contrast of the last block on which the patient is able to read at least two letters correctly. Test instructions have caused some confusion in respect of appropriate viewing distance, since the 1 m recommendation differs from first suggestions of 3 m (Pelli, Robson and Wilkins, 1988). Evaluation of the chart in visually impaired children suggests the need for testing at both distances since data obtained at 1 m appears to indicate the location of the peak of the CSF and at 3 m a high frequency CS measure is obtained (Woodhouse and Westall, 1989). When viewed from 1 m each letter subtends 3°, the fundamental spatial frequency is about 1 c.p.d. and there is some contribution from higher harmonics around 3 and 5 c.p.d. At 3 m, the fundamental is at about 4 c.p.d. and higher harmonics do not contribute much. The test is marketed by Keeler Instruments. Although further evaluation of the Pelli–Robson charts is required, initial reliability and repeatability data seems encouraging (Rubin, 1988).

Objective and other specific paediatric assessment techniques

CS in infancy has been investigated using some of the objective methods described earlier for measurement of visual acuity. In common with many other laboratory CS studies, sine wave gratings have usually been generated electronically on oscilloscopes or monitors. These enable presentation of static, drifting or contrast reversing gratings and easy alteration of stimulus parameters including contrast and spatial frequency. Electrophysiological assessment of the CSF in infancy is discussed in Chapter 17; the electronic rapid sweep method offers the only possibility for clinical testing, although the technology is not widely available. Behavioural assessment of infant CS has involved lengthy PL testing even when modified staircase procedures are used, since separate contrast thresholds must be determined for several spatial frequencies.

Maturation of the CSF in early infancy is discussed in Chapter 17. An overview is provided here. Newborns and 1 month olds do not show low-frequency attenuation and their overall sensitivity is greatly reduced. The CSF shape is similar to that of adults, from 2 to 3 months, although shifted to lower spatial frequencies and sensitivities, particularly when obtained via behavioural means. At this time, rapid sweep VEP methods indicate adult-like sensitivity below about 1 c.p.d., the relative immaturity of the foveal (cf. extrafoveal) retinal projection being considered responsible for lower sensitivity at high spatial frequencies (*Figure 8.10(a)*). It appears that there are two phases in the development of contrast sensitivity (and acuity), with improvement occurring at all frequencies until 9 weeks and only at higher spatial frequencies thereafter (Norcia, Tyler and Hamer, 1990). Spatial frequency selective mechanisms with narrower bandwidths than the CSF are present in adults, and have been noted during infancy from 6 weeks using VEP (Fiorentini, Pirchio and Spinelli, 1983) and 12 weeks using PL methods (Banks and Stephens, 1982). An adult-like function is attained by 6–10 months using VEPs but behavioural methods, including those of a subjective nature, suggest sensitivities are similar to adults' by about 3 years (*Figure 8.10(b)*), although subsequent gradual improvement may be noted during the following few years, no doubt due as much to non-visual as neural factors (Bradley and Freeman, 1982).

Several novel methods have been applied to contrast sensitivity assessment in preschool and older children. Atkinson and French (1983) conducted a preliminary study, relying on 7 to 10-month-old infants reaching for cylindrical 'rattles' displaying grating stimuli (of 3 c.p.d.) in preference to similar cylinders with uniform fields but no auditory reinforcement when picked up. The task was affected by the development of hand preferences and could not be considered clinically useful.

Atkinson, French and Braddick (1981) devised an 'alley running' task which provided a simple means of measuring contrast sensitivity from about 3 years of age. Stimuli comprised photographically produced sinusoidal gratings of various contrasts and high-contrast square wave gratings (to obtain the acuity point on the CSF). These stimuli were mounted on the inner surfaces of transparent acrylic cubes. Each cube was packed with polyurethane foam, apart from a small cavity in the base where a reward could be concealed. On each trial two cubes were presented one on either side of a vertical barrier (*Figure 8.11*). Before the trial the child was instructed whether a present would be placed under the striped box with the 'standing up' or 'lying down' stripes on it. Their task was to run to the correct cube to get the present. Stimulus spatial frequency was varied by adjusting the barrier length to produce different viewing distances. The method depended on multiple trials at each of four spatial frequencies. Three or four testing sessions were usually required per child.

Brown and Woodhouse (1986), using oscilloscope generated sinusoidal gratings, compared four psychophysical techniques for assessing contrast sensitivity in 3 to 11-year-old children, concluding that a staircase method was the most appropriate clinically. Below 4 years only two or three spatial frequencies could be measured due

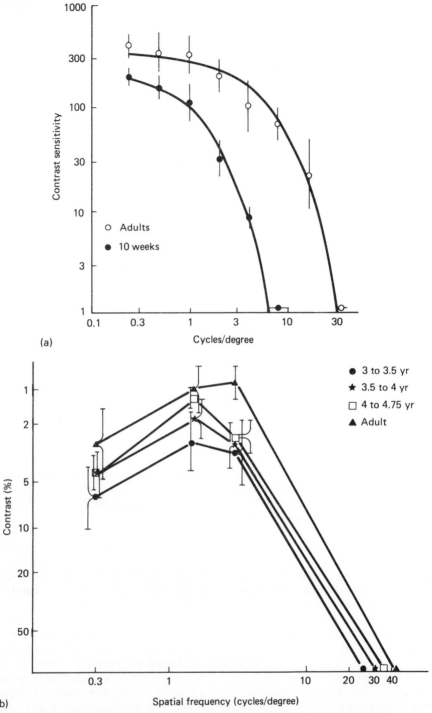

Figure 8.10. Development of the contrast sensitivity function. (a) Group data obtained using electrophysiological means, showing remarkably high sensitivity in 10-week-old infants; error bars indicate 95% confidence limits. ○, Adult; ●, 10 weeks old (From Norcia, Tyler and Hamer, 1988.) (b) Group data obtained behaviourally, showing improvement between 3 and 5 years; error bars represent standard deviations. ●, 3–3.5 years; ★, 3.5–4 years; □, 4–4.5 years; ▲, adult. (From Atkinson, French and Braddick, 1981)

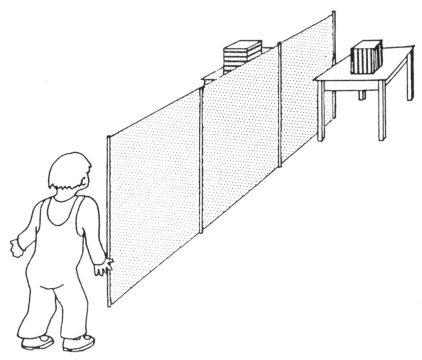

Figure 8.11. Alley running task devised for measuring contrast sensitivity in young children. Two cubes were randomly placed either to the right or left side of a central barrier. Children had to correctly discriminate between the cubes in order to locate a reward hidden beneath one. (From Atkinson, French and Braddick, 1981)

to limited cooperation, suggesting that a monitoring regimen may require several sessions to establish a baseline CSF prior to any treatment, followed by assessment at two or three frequencies chosen where curves of the two eyes are initially the same (to check against occlusion amblyopia) and where one eye is initially worse (to check for improvement).

Hainline and co-workers (1987) devised an indirect 'eye movement voting' CSF technique for use with subjects having limited cooperation. Eye movements in response to drifting gratings are used as the basis for an observer's forced choice vote on stimulus direction. Although this produced slightly lower estimates of CS in adult subjects also tested directly, the shape of the function was maintained, thereby providing useful data on the relative sensitivity to various spatial frequencies. Meijler and Van den Berg (1982) previously applied an objective CS method, based on measuring pursuit eye movements synchronized to the motion of low contrast gratings. The report was poorly documented and the method not apparently very successful in infancy.

Refractive assessment

In cooperative subjects, refractive assessment is generally based on subjectively refining the initial estimate obtained using an objective method. Where cooperation is limited, refractive determination may be based solely on the results of an objective procedure. During infancy refraction has generally been assessed directly using clinical objective methods – primarily retinoscopy, although occasionally reports of indirect, experimental methods have appeared in the literature. The latter have included use of VEPs (Harter, Deaton and Odom, 1977; Regan, 1977) and mathematical calculation using ultrasonographic measurement of axial length combined with other biometric data (Belkin *et al.*, 1973; Gordon and Donzis, 1985).

Before retinoscopy became generally available, direct ophthalmoscopy was sometimes used as a simple method for estimating a subject's mean refractive error (from the power of the sight-hole lens giving the clearest view of the fundus). Although greatly limited in accuracy (Borish, 1970c) and its ability to measure astigmatism, the method was particularly popular with German ophthalmologists interested in newborn refraction (see Goldschmidt, 1969). More recently auto-refractors and photorefractors have emerged as alternative procedures for objective refraction. The following review will emphasize clinically appropriate objective refractive techniques especially those specifically developed for use with children. Readers requiring a more general historical review covering the development of refractive procedures may find an article by Bennett (1986) of interest.

Objective refraction techniques

Retinoscopy

Retinoscopy is essentially a nulling method in which trial lenses are positioned before the subject's eye in order to neutralize movement of a reflex seen within the pupil. Various standard texts provide detailed descriptions of the optical principles and clinical use of these instruments (e.g. Borish, 1970a; Bennett and Rabbetts, 1989b; Taylor, 1988).

Static methods

Retinoscopic techniques may be subdivided into static methods in which efforts are made to ensure that the patient's accommodation is relaxed and dynamic procedures which involve investigation of the accommodating eye. Adult's accommodation can be relaxed by asking them to view a large distant object and adding plus power to the eye not under examination. In infants and young children the same effect is usually achieved by instilling a cycloplegic drug to temporarily paralyse the ciliary muscle. A significantly higher incidence of myopia is noted in newborn samples if cycloplegics are not used. This finding is consistent with much recent evidence confirming that young infants are capable of adjusting their accommodation (Braddick *et al.*, 1979; Banks, 1980b; Howland, Dobson and Sayles, 1987). As pupil dilation accompanies the cycloplegic effect spherical aberration may be observed and care must be taken to neutralize the centre of the reflex. When examining young children, rather than using a trial frame or phoropter head, trial lenses (sometimes in lens bar form) are typically hand held making the use of an artificial pupil impractical.

Mohindra (1977a) introduced an apparently reliable form of static retinoscopy which enables refractive assessment of infants without requiring cycloplegia. Unlike dynamic retinoscopy, Mohindra's 'near retinoscopy' technique does not depend on active accommodation. It is conducted in a totally darkened room with the patient's non-examined eye occluded and a distance of 50 cm between the patient and a low intensity retinoscope light (the only stimulus). An adjustment factor of $-1.25\,\mathrm{D}$ is algebraically added to the sphere component when computing the final results. This value was initially arrived at empirically (Mohindra, 1977b), although it was found to be similar to the *average* adjustment factor required – presumably due to 'inadequate stimulus myopia' – in a group of adults under the conditions of near retinoscopy (Owens, Mohindra and Held, 1980). The appropriate correction factor varies to some extent between individuals, this being a source of error in the method.

Dynamic methods

In dynamic retinoscopy methods the subject binocularly fixates a finely detailed and well-illuminated near target specifically designed to stimulate accommodation, whereas the retinoscope beam is kept as dim as possible. The test is performed through the distance-correcting lenses and the retinoscope beam is moved in a continuous path to rapidly investigate the horizontal meridians of each eye in turn. Many different procedures have been described, details of specific methods being provided by Borish (1970b), and useful summaries by Bennett and Rabbetts (1989b) and Taylor (1988). The main differences in procedure relate to the positioning of the fixation target and whether or not trial lenses are required to neutralize the reflex.

In the most frequently reported method the subject views a fixation target located within the plane of the retinoscope mirror. The level of accommodation is measured using trial lenses, often placed in lens racks for convenience, positioned close to the subject's eyes. An initial 'with' movement is observable, followed by a range of neutrality as positive lenses are added (denoted by 'low' and 'high' neutral points and assumed to correspond to negative relative accommodation). An alternative procedure involves use of a separate fixation object, held in the median line with the retinoscope behind it. By gradually moving the fixation target towards the patient an objective measurement of accommodation amplitude may be obtained. Initially an 'against' movement is seen, which changes to a 'with' movement. At the latter point the dioptric distance of the retinoscope sighthole from the spectacle plane represents the estimate of accommodation.

Dynamic retinoscopy techniques do not enjoy current popularity, no doubt connected with their limited value in determining distance refractive error, confusion regarding terminology and controversy in interpreting findings. The methods do, however, offer a means of objectively evaluating near-vision requirements and the accommodation–convergence relationship.

Theoretical sources of error

Several factors may limit the accuracy of retinoscopy, although some of the difficulties may be avoided by good technique. As detailed discussions of these points may easily be found in earlier texts (e.g. Henson, 1983; Taylor, 1988; Bennett and Rabbetts, 1989a), only a brief outline will be provided.

Induced astigmatic errors may be avoided by ensuring that retinoscopy is conducted on or close to the visual axis and also by refraining from applying excess pressure on the globe when manual lid retraction is required (e.g. in sleeping infants). Careful control of working distance is needed (especially when shorter distances are used), otherwise errors in the spherical component of the refraction will be introduced. Bracketing of the neutral point is helpful, particularly in the presence of irregular media which may produce a 'split' reflex. Whenever large pupils are encountered care should be taken to neutralize the central part of the reflex, perhaps with the aid of a 3-mm aperture pinhole disc if appropriate, to avoid errors due to spherical aberration. Even with a perfect technique, slight differences may be anticipated between objective and subjective refractive findings. These are most likely related to variation in accommodative tonus during the procedures. Alternative hypotheses include the possibility of an artifact due to the retinoscopy reflex originating from a surface other than the receptor layer (Glickstein and Millodot, 1970). If this is true larger errors would be anticipated in smaller eyes such as those of newborns. Later evidence indicates that chromatic aberration (due to the red fundus reflex) could explain a slightly more hyperopic retinoscopy result in human eyes (Nuboer and Van Genderen-Takken, 1978).

Autorefractors

The group of refraction instruments which have collectively become known as autorefractors are automated or semi-automated electronic objective optometers. The first electronic objective optometer was designed over 50 years ago and like its successors used infrared radiation rather than visible light (Collins, 1937). Latterly, with the advent of the microchip, a large number of computerized electronic infrared optometers have become commercially available. A useful review of such instruments has recently been provided by Wood (1988).

Current infrared autorefractors fall into three groups. These are variously dependent on retinal image quality, the coincidence 'Scheiner double pinhole' method or retinoscopy (either by neutralizing the retinal reflex with lenses or measuring the reflex speed). Most autorefractors measure the refraction in any particular meridian by determining the 'endpoint' position of the instrument's servo-controlled lenses with respect to a dioptrically calibrated scale. All currently available instruments allow measurement within the refractive ranges ±15 DS, ±6 DC and 0–180° axis (in 1° intervals). The type of instrument which is completely automated can be considered truly objective, as neither the patient's or the operator's judgement is required. In addition to providing a rapid objective estimation of the refraction (within a second in some modern autorefractors), some instruments enable subjective checking of the visual acuity through the objective findings and may also incorporate facilities to allow subjective modification of both the spherical and cylindrical components of the refraction.

Difficulties

Several difficulties may be encountered using autorefraction, these are briefly outlined below (see Woods, 1988, for elaboration of these points). An *empirical* correction factor must be incorporated within the autorefractor calibration system to compensate for the use of infrared radiation rather than visible light. This is likely to vary according to whether the instrument uses polarized or non-polarized radiation (Charman, 1980). In addition the distance between the patient's eye and the instrument must be controlled or taken into account to avoid introducing errors due to the effectivity of the prescription. Eye movements should be minimized so that the patient's eye is accurately aligned in a transverse direction. These requirements of accurate alignment are the most limiting in terms of assessing young infants. Adequate reflected light must be received by the autorefractor's photodetectors. This may create difficulties with small pupils (below 3 mm), irregular media

(Wesemann and Rassow, 1987) or retinal changes. At the other extreme, a blink of the patient's eyelids will saturate the infrared signal. Proximal accommodation can affect the accuracy of autorefractor measurements. The incorporation of fogged targets or allowing of distance viewing appears to overcome this difficulty in older age groups. However up to 8 D of proximal accommodation may be induced in young children (Helvaston *et al.*, 1984).

Evaluation in paediatric samples

One research group has recently undertaken the arduous task of using a modified (Canon) autorefractor to measure refractive errors (under cycloplegia) and accommodative responses in early infancy (Aslin, Shea and Metz, 1990). Data collection involved three experimeters. The holder viewed an extra video monitor and thereby aligned the infant's eye with the instrument's alignment ring. An experimenter (holding a fixation object) helped minimize the infant's eye and head movements by attracting their gaze. An operator viewed the original video monitor and triggered the autorefractor whenever the infant's eye was successfully aligned. Alert 1 to 4 month olds, the age group participating in the study, are relatively cooperative and less affected by distractions than are older infants (particularly toddlers). Even so only 30% of the readings were satisfactory and laborious post-test processing of the video-recording and autorefractor output were needed to remove unwanted measurements.

Photorefraction

Photorefractive techniques are objective methods of refraction specifically designed for *screening* very young children, although they may also prove useful in other circumstances, for example, when examining mentally handicapped individuals. All methods involve delivering a flash of light to the subject's eyes from a small source set in front of a camera lens and photographing the light returning to the camera. The sizes of the observed light patches depend both on the defocus of each eye relative to the camera distance and on the pupil diameter. In fact the term 'photorefraction' covers three distinctly different techniques, namely orthogonal, isotropic and eccentric methods depending on the type and arrangement of optical components. In orthogonal and isotropic photorefractors the flash source is located along the optical axis of the camera lens, whereas in the eccentric method it is paraxial and often displaced outside the camera lens aperture. Young children usually sit on a parent's lap during the examination and their attention is directed towards the camera by the operator waving a brightly coloured rattle, etc. The immediate source is typically the end of a fibreoptic bundle which is linked to a standard camera flash unit. The distribution of light returning from the subject's retina may be captured on high speed 35-mm photographic film or stored as a video image.

The original technique, a form of orthogonal photorefraction, was developed by Howland and Howland (1974). It was based on modification of a standard single lens reflex camera, as were all of the earliest methods reported. More recently photorefractors depending on video recording and computer analysis have been developed, some becoming commercially available. The optics of various photorefractive methods have been outlined by Bennett and Rabbetts (1989c) and described in detail in specific reports (Howland *et al.*, 1983; Bobier and Braddick,

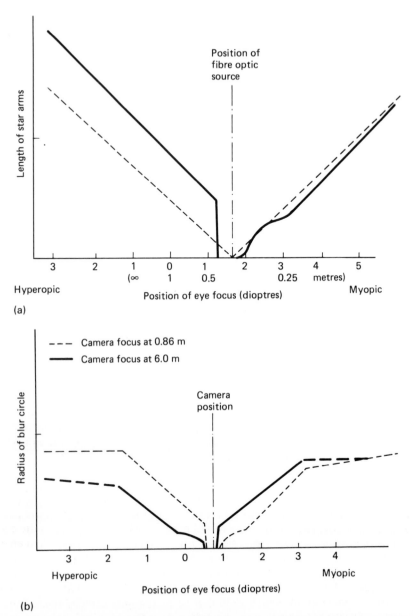

Figure 8.12. Functions relating image size at the film plane to the refractive state of the eye for various photorefractive methods and 6-mm pupil. (a) + 1.50 D orthogonal photorefractor (75 cm camera to subject distance). (b) Isotropic photorefractor (1.5 m camera to subject distance). The solid line in (a) denotes values obtained from computer ray tracing and is the more correct function. The dashed line represents the imprecise linear function derived from simple calculation (equation 3, Howland and Howland, 1974). In (b) the camera lens is focused 0.50 D behind the eye (at 6.0 m, solid line) and 0.50 D in front of the eye (at 0.86 m, dotted line). The functions were obtained by computer ray tracing, the linear portions can be explained by geometrical optics, whereas a more complex function is found in the vicinity of the camera plane. The nearly horizontal outer portions arise from the finite diameter of the camera lens aperture. (After Howland *et al.*, 1983)

1985; Howland, 1985; Crewther *et al.*, 1987). Detailed discussions of the relative merits of each technique have been provided by Braddick and Atkinson (1984).

Orthogonal photorefraction

Orthogonal photorefractors feature a point light source centred in a camera lens and surrounded by four cylindrical lens segments arranged in two pairs with their axes at right angles. The resultant photograph from which measurements are made shows a star or cross image centred on each eye. The length of the star arms indicate the defocus in two orthogonal directions and increase with increasing defocus relative to the camera working distance. At least one more photograph must be taken, without the cylindrical lens segments, to determine pupil diameter. Further photographs may reveal additional information on the refractive state (Howland and Howland, 1974). More useful information on astigmatism may be gained by orienting the photorefractor cylindrical lenses both vertically and obliquely. The presence of hyperopia and presbyopia may be identified by use of supplementary positive lenses and reduced viewing distances. Owing to the effects of chromatic aberration use of both red and blue probe lights may enable inferences on the sign of error. The photorefractive image is usually processed as a photographic slide and then projected at around ×25 to 29 magnification, although an enlarged photographic print could be used. The length of the star arms are measured and corresponding values for the dioptric defocus relative to the camera are determined according to a theoretical curve for the appropriate pupil size and camera to subject distance (*Figure 8.12(a)*).

Isotropic photorefraction

Isotropic photorefraction is conducted using apparatus identical to that used for orthogonal photorefraction except there are no cylindrical lens segments surrounding the central fibreoptic probe on the camera lens. The blur circle of the fundus reflex does not have a star pattern. This adaptation was devised by Howland working in collaboration with Atkinson and associates (1981b). Three photographs (*Figure 8.13(a)–(c)*) are taken while the subject looks in the direction of the camera. An initial photograph (*Figure 8.13(a)*) is taken with the lens focused in the plane of the pupil to determine pupil size. Additional photographs are taken with the camera defocused a fixed number of dioptres posteriorly (*Figure 8.13(b)*) and then an equal amount anteriorly (*Figure 8.13(c)*). Values of 0.50 and 0.67 D defocus and camera to subject distances of between 75 and 150 cm are typical.

   The diameter of the blur circles obtained increases with the defocus of the eye relative to the camera distance. When astigmatism is present a blur ellipse is produced – the long and short axes being related to the eye's axes of maximum and minimum optical power (*Figure 8.13(d)*). If colour film is used a reddish component of the image may appear elongated in the direction of a hyperopic meridian while a bluish component appears elongated in the direction of a myopic meridian. When the subject's eye is myopically focused relative to the camera the blur circle is greater with the camera focused behind rather than in front of the subject. The converse is true if the subject's eye is hypermetropic relative to the camera. Hence the sign of the defocus (myopic or hypermetropic) can be determined by comparing the size of blur circle in the photographs taken at the two focal distances (*Figure 8.12(b)*).

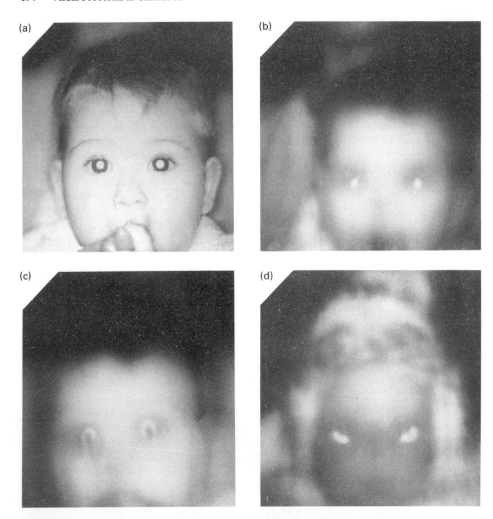

Figure 8.13. Isotropic photorefraction. An initial in-focus photograph (a) is used to determine pupil size. Subsequent photographs are taken with the camera focused a fixed amount (0.67 D) posteriorly (b) and the same amount anteriorly (c). The camera was focused at 75, 150 and 50 cm respectively in these photographs. Refractive error is calculated by comparing the blur circle sizes in (b) and (c) with the known pupil size. Larger more diffuse images in (c) indicate a hyperopic focus with respect to camera distance. (d) Elliptical blur images obtained from an infant with (oblique) astigmatism, enabling determination of direction and power of the principal meridians. (Material reproduced from Clement Clarke International Ltd advertising brochure)

Eccentric photorefraction

The essential feature of eccentric photorefractors is the off-centre position of the flash source. The camera is adjusted to provide a clearly focused image of the pupil and red reflex (as well as a sharply focused corneal reflex). Kaakinen (1979) introduced this form of photorefraction, referring to the method as photographic static skiascopy due to its analogy with retinoscopy. Other authors have used the terms 'photoretinoscopy' or paraxial photorefraction. If the subject's eyes are focused on the camera, light reflected from their eyes will, in theory, be returned along its original path to the source. No light will be visible in a subject's pupil until the defocus of the eye exceeds a minimum amount which varies according to the eccentricity of the flash source. When the 'threshold' refractive error is exceeded a crescent will first become visible in the pupil. The crescent appears on the same side

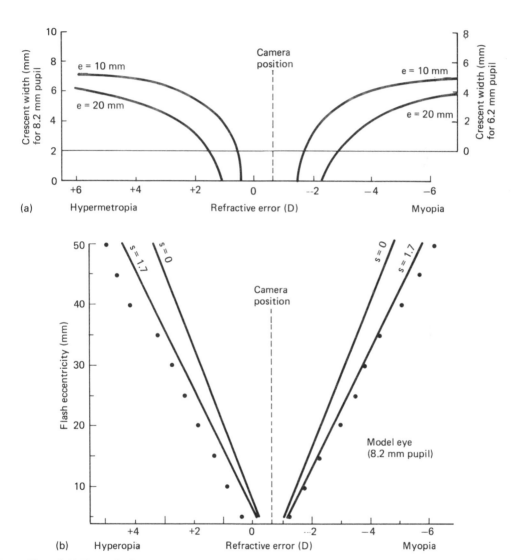

Figure 8.14. Eccentric photorefractor calibration functions. (a) Theoretical curves relating crescent width to optical defocus for two different eccentricities of the flash source and two pupil diameters. (From Bobier, 1990). (b) Theoretical (—) and empirical (●) data on the critical refractive error required for the formation of a visible crescent (width = s). A closer agreement between theoretical and empirical data is found when crescent width is a finite value of 1.7 mm rather than zero. (From Bobier and Braddick, 1985)

of the pupil as the source for myopic errors and on the opposite side if the error is hypermetropic. Above threshold crescent width increases as refractive error increases. This effect saturates about 2 D above threshold so the method is most sensitive for refractive errors just greater than the threshold (*Figure 8.14(a)*).

As refractive power is only measured along the axis parallel to the flash axis, the source orientation has to be adjusted to refract along other meridians. Kaakinen (1981) adapted the original method by adding a second flash source perpendicular to the first so that refraction could be simultaneously conducted in two meridians. Kaakinen's original method was unable to detect refractive errors of less than 2 to 3 D. Improved sensitivity (detection of errors exceeding 0.75 D) may be attained using a catadioptric lens and longer working distance to reduce the angle between the flash source and the entrance pupil of the photorefractor (Norcia, Zadnik and Day, 1986). Chromatic aberration may be used to classify refractive errors within the initial null zone (Crewther *et al.*, 1988). Bobier (1988) has developed and calibrated an instrument in which the position of the flash source can be varied. This modification produces an extended measuring range. As eccentricity increases a proportionately larger refractive error is required to produce a crescent (*Figure 8.14(b)*). The refraction can therefore be calculated from the maximum eccentricity at which a crescent is still visible. A point spread retinoscope, constructed from a disposable penlight and paper shield (Howland *et al.*, 1987), applies similar principles. The latter cannot, however, provide any permanent record of the measurement and appears less accurate than Bobier's more sophisticated method.

Schaeffel, Farkas and Howland (1987) introduced another video-based version of eccentric photorefractor, which has become known as an infrared 'photoretinoscope'. The method uses infrared LEDs to prevent pupillary constriction (thereby increasing sensitivity) and allow measurement without alerting the subject. These sources, which are fixed and flash sequentially producing an apparent motion of the reflex, are set at different eccentricities to extend the instrument measuring range. The method copes well with very small eyes, and it is claimed that even tadpoles may be refracted!

Comparison of photorefractive techniques

A summary of the essential features of various photorefractive procedures is provided in *Table 8.3*. Each method has certain advantages and limitations, so that photorefraction is most useful if a combination of methods is used (e.g. Aslin and Dobson, 1983; Howland and Sayles, 1985). The main limitation of the methods is in the measurement range.

Isotropic photorefraction is the only method allowing direct assessment of the axis of astigmatism, but the magnitude of this error may be estimated more accurately using orthogonal photorefraction providing its axis is known in advance. Isotropic and eccentric photorefraction enable the sign of the refractive error to be easily determined, the latter requiring only a single photograph rather than the three necessary in the isotropic technique. Eccentric photorefraction allows measurement of refractive errors beyond the vignetting limit imposed by the finite size of the camera aperture in the orthogonal and isotropic methods. The latter methods do not allow accurate measurement of large errors since, for typical values of working distance, lens aperture and pupil size, the cone of rays returning to the camera fills the lens plane at about 4 D of ametropia. There is also an initial small null zone due to the vignetting effect of the fibreoptic tip obstructing some of the rays returning to

TABLE 8.3. Comparison of refractive information derived using various photorefractive methods

			Refractive information obtained		
Specific method	Blur shape	Minimum number of photographs	Sign	Axis	Measurement range (Dioptres)
Orthogonal	Star	Two	No	No	Initial small null area then ≤ ≈ 4 D. Ametropia
Isotropic	Circle or ellipse	Three	Yes	Yes	Similar to orthogonal but slightly reduced range
Eccentric	Crescent	One	Yes	No	Dependent on source eccentricity; extends ≈ 2 D beyond generally large initial null area*

More information may be gained about refractive state using the orthogonal method providing additional photographs are taken (see text). The initial small null area in the orthogonal and isotropic photorefraction measuring range is due to the vignetting effect of the fibreoptic tip obstructing some of the rays returning to the camera. The upper limit of measurement (for a particular pupil size and camera–subject distance) is determined by the finite size of the camera lens aperture (entrance pupil). Quoted values indicate the range of accurate measurement.
* Assumes source eccentricity is constant.

the camera. Although the eccentric method (coupled with adjustable flash source) provides the greatest dioptric range of measurement, it fails to eliminate a 'dead zone' in which refractive error cannot be measured (*Figure 8.14(b)*) and is also limited by its inability to specify the axes of astigmatism.

Photorefractive screening programmes, reported in the literature, have generally depended on either isotropic (Atkinson and Braddick, 1983a,b) or eccentric methods (Kaakinen, Kaseva and Kause, 1986; Duckman and Meyer, 1987). In each case the methods appear well suited to refractive screening of infants and young children and can be easily taught to unskilled personnel. Due to the limitations discussed earlier, eccentric photorefraction is probably more suitable for subsequent assessment of individuals having ametropia exceeding the accurate measuring range of the isotropic method. There remains some controversy regarding the importance of examination under cycloplegia during refractive screening. If cycloplegic agents are not used underestimation of spherical hypermetropia must be accepted (Day and Norcia, 1986; Kaakinen and Ranta-Kemppainen, 1986) and photorefractions must be conducted in a darkened room as the sensitivity of the method depends on pupil size (Howland, 1980). Following recent work, Atkinson *et al.* (1989) are, however, of the opinion that a single video-refraction measurement without cycloplegia will identify 80% of infants having ≥4 D of hypermetropia under cycloplegia and give high predictive values for amblyopia and strabismus.

The presence of clearly visible corneal reflexes in eccentric photorefraction photographs may be helpful in the detection of strabismus. Examination of the positions of such reflexes (Hirschberg test) suggests that individuals having at least 2° (Abrahamsson, Fabian and Sjostrand, 1986) or 5 Δ (Griffin, McLin and Schor, 1986) of strabismic deviation may be reliably identified. However, this method may be less reliable when examining mentally retarded children (Philipsen and Hobolth, 1985). Although the other methods have been used (e.g. Braddick *et al.*, 1979), eccentric photorefraction is the most appropriate for studying accommodation since all the

TABLE 8.4. Summary of several studies that have provided statistical information on the reliability of certain refraction techniques in child samples

Technique	Study	Age (years)	Dioptric power ranges			Correlations (with CR)	
			Spherical	Cyl	n	Sphere power	Cyl power
Retinoscopy							
Near	1 Mohindra (1977a)	'Infant'	−2.5 − +2.0	≤2.0	29 (24)	0.88	0.85
	2 Mohindra and Molinari (1979)	5–7	−1.0 − +3.0	—	62	0.80	—
				≤2.5	31	0.83	0.67
					31	0.75	0.27
Cycloplegic	3 Thompson (1987)	0.0	−3.25 − +8.25	≤5.0	70 (35)	0.94	0.61
			−1.0 − +3.0	≤2.5	31	0.80	0.43
			0.0 − +7.0	—	50	0.84	—
	2 Mohindra and Molinari (1979)	5–7	−1.0 − +3.0	≤2.5	31	0.92	0.07
Photorefraction							
Isotropic	4 Atkinson *et al.* (1984)	0.5–0.75	≈ −5 − +6.0	—	1532	0.77	—
	5 Bobier (1988)	0.6–4.1	+0.5 − +7.5	—	48	0.73	—
Eccentric	5 Bobier (1988)	0.6–4.1	+0.5 − +7.5	—	50	0.82	—
Autorefraction							
Canon R1	6 Aslin, Shea and Metz (1990)	0.15–0.25	−0.5 − +4.5	≤1.0	34	0.83*	−0.35

In each case estimates of refractive power were compared with cycloplegic retinoscopy (CR) findings. Data was from right eyes only in studies 1–3, and otherwise from both eyes. Dioptric range information is based on the CR findings, 'n' values represent numbers of data (figures in brackets relate to cylindrical data) and for study 1 these were estimated directly from published graphs. In study 2 separate and combined data of two examiners are presented and CR data (1% tropicamide and 10% phenylephrine) was adjusted for tonus allowance. The full sample of study 3 has been variously reduced and the data reanalysed in order to correspond with the refractive range and numbers of studies 2 and 5.
* SER (spherical equivalent refraction) not sphere.

necessary information (pupil size, width of photorefractive pattern and direction of defocus) is provided in one photograph. Bobier (1990) successfully investigated the accommodative abilities of a group of highly hyperopic infants using the eccentric method.

Validity of infant refraction methods

There are, unfortunately, no simple means of evaluating the true precision of any objective refraction procedure. Although not possible in young children, in older subjects findings are often compared with subjective results, as an individual's 'true' refractive error remains undefined. Useful data may be derived by considering the repeatability of a particular procedure. There are, however, surprisingly few reports of such studies in the published literature. Typically refractive estimates derived from newer objective procedures are directly compared with measurements from an established method (generally retinoscopy following cycloplegia). Relevant data from child studies have been summarized in *Table 8.4* and *Figure 8.15*. Often analysis involves determination of correlation coefficients, rather than slope and intercept (which ideally should be close to 1 and 0, respectively), but these can be markedly affected by the numbers of readings and the dioptric range of the data (as demonstrated by the individual analyses of study 3, *Table 8.4*). Consideration of the dioptric differences between successive measurements can avoid this problem (*Figure 8.15*).

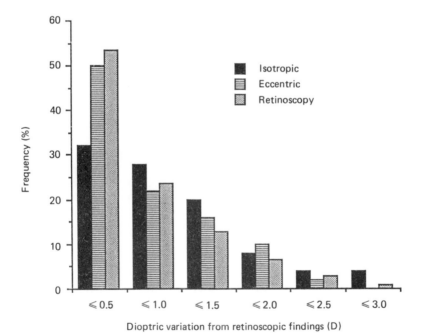

Figure 8.15. Precision of various refractive methods in comparison with cycloplegic retinoscopy findings in infants and young children. Isotropic and 'variable source' eccentric photorefractive data (after Bobier, 1988) are from a sample aged 7 to 48 months. Retinoscopy findings are from 35 newborn infants (after Thompson, 1987). More details of these studies are provided in Table 8.4. In each case data is presented from both eyes and examinations were performed following instillation of 1% cyclopentolate

Retinoscopy

It is well recognized amongst clinicians that retinoscopy can, with experience, provide very valuable estimates of refraction, even with patients having limited cooperation. Bennett and Rabbetts (1989b) note that a skilled examiner, examining a cooperative patient, having a medium sized pupil and normal ocular media would expect to *easily* achieve an accuracy of better than 0.50 D on the (subjectively determined) ametropia in either meridian and within 15° on the astigmatic axis (of a 1.00 DC).

On purely mathematical grounds one might expect the cylindrical component to show more variation than other power findings because it is based on the difference between two readings rather than their mean (e.g. SER) or an isolated measurement (e.g. sphere). This prediction, which assumes that accommodation is stable during measurement and that meridians are neutralized independently, appears not to be supported by current evidence from repeat retinoscopy studies. In ten cooperative young adults (having ametropia ≤ 3.00 D and ≤ 2.00 DC), repeatedly examined (without cycloplegia) by five ophthalmologists (Safir *et al.*, 1970; Hyams, Safir and Philpot, 1971), greater sensitivity was noted in defining cylindrical rather than spherical power. There was a 50% probability of two consecutive measures of the sphere power differing by ≥ 0.40 D. The standard deviation for determination of astigmatic axis was 12.1°. A three-fold difference in reliability was noted between the least and most precise practitioners. The same ranking of sensitivities was observed by Thompson (1987) in newborns examined under cycloplegia, although the more hyperopic meridian provided the most stable power measure. Measurements of sphere power were rather less precise in this 'more difficult to examine' sample, around half of second estimates being within 0.50 D of the initial result (*Figure 8.15*), however the standard deviation for cylinder axis was lower (4.9°) presumably in consequence of the higher levels of astigmatism encountered.

Initial evaluations of the 'near retinoscopy' procedure indicated that valid, reliable refractive measurements could be obtained from adults (Mohindra, 1977b) and young children (Mohindra and Molinari, 1979). In the latter study, correlations between near and cycloplegic retinoscopic data were better for spherical (note: slope = 0.99, intercept = -0.02) than cylindrical power findings, although this was also true of other procedures, to some extent reflecting the refractive ranges of the data (*Table 8.4*). A tendency was also noted for 'near' retinoscopy to give higher estimates of astigmatism. Evidence from independent studies indicates that near retinoscopy may reveal less positive power than retinoscopy under cycloplegia (Borghi and Rouse, 1985) and greater variability (Kohl, Samek and Coffey, 1987).

Autorefraction

Wood (1988) has assembled and compared reliability and accuracy (validity) statistics for a variety of autorefractors and conventional refractive methods. It was clear that, with cooperative adults, some autorefractors produce a result which is more repeatable than measures obtained using retinoscopy or subjective examination. Independent and emphatic confirmation of this point has been provided by a recent study (Adams, Zadnik and Mutti, 1990). In Wood's comparisons each autorefractor showed at least 90% agreement between repeated spherical power findings, although the reliability statistics for cylinder power and axis measurements differed greatly between instruments. There was over 60% agreement between the sphere and cylindrical power components of infrared autorefractors and conventional (subjective) refraction measurements. However, there was a much lower level of agreement for the axis of astigmatism, presumably explained by the inability (of any method) to precisely specify the axis of low-powered cylindrical components.

Aslin, Shea and Metz (1990) reported a good correspondence between autorefractive and retinoscopic spherical equivalent (i.e. mean sphere) findings in a sample of young infants (*Table 8.4*, but autorefraction revealed higher estimates of cylindrical power (mean differences being 0.13 and 1.97 D respectively). In older children (Evans, 1984), autorefractive results do not correspond well with retinoscopic findings, mostly due to poor control of accommodation. Discrepancies particularly affect spherical power data and do not appear to be adequately alleviated by examination under cycloplegia.

Photorefraction

Despite the scarcity of supporting evidence in the published literature photorefractive techniques have typically been credited with a precision in the order of ± 0.5 D within their measuring ranges. It appears that results correspond well with retinoscopy findings providing that the photorefractor is calibrated against empirical values rather than the theoretical results predicted from computer ray tracing (Atkinson *et al.*, 1984). This discrepancy is probably due to the visible blur image being smaller than the calculated value, for example, in the eccentric method (*Figure 8.14(b)*) the crescent must be a finite size to be detected (Bobier, 1990). Howland and Howland (1974) quoted a standard deviation of 0.6 D for the difference between their subjects' orthogonal photorefractive estimates and current optical corrections. In humans a sensitivity of ± 0.3 D or better, over a range of ± 5 D, is claimed using the infrared photoretinoscopy method at a distance of 1.5 m (Schaeffel, Farkas and Howland, 1987). In monkeys examined under cycloplegia, using Norcia and co-workers' eccentric photorefraction method, an accuracy within 1 D has been reported (Crewther *et al.*, 1988). Comparing photorefractive measurements with retinoscopic data, Bobier (1988; *Table 8.4*) noted an improved correlation for estimates derived using the eccentric ($r = 0.82$, slope $= 0.80$, intercept $= 0.74$) rather than the isotropic method ($r = 0.73$, slope $= 0.61$, intercept $= 0.37$). The eccentric method appeared to provide data which was comparable to the precision of retinoscopy in newborns (*Figure 8.15*).

Concluding remarks

Child vision testing

Clinical testing should ideally include determination of recognition acuity using targets with a surrounding contour, otherwise some amblyopia may escape detection. Separate measurement of acuities for both isolated and surrounded optotypes may assist in differential diagnosis, a large discrepancy being suggestive of strabismic amblyopia (Mallett, 1988). It is clearly not always possible to obtain such measurements from patients having limited cooperation. The information provided in *Table 8.5* is an attempt to indicate suitable visual acuity tests for differing levels of child development. Since absolute acuity values are partly dependent on the test

TABLE 8.5. Summary of recommended acuity testing methods and ages of application

Age	Quantitative method	Response	Specific tests
From birth	Acuity card PL procedure	Direction of gaze	Teller, Keeler
≥2.5 years	Snellen-based pictures	Verbal report	
	Isolated		Kay
	Surrounded		Elliott
	Snellen-based symbols	Matching	
	Isolated		Ffooks* – cube
	Surrounded		Ffooks* – flip cards
From ≈ 3 years	2 AFC Landolt C procedure	Pointing/gazing	Broken wheel
≥3 years	Isolated Snellen letters	Matching	Stycar based:
	5 letter (for 3 year olds)		HOVTX†
	7 letter (for 4 year olds)		HOVTXAU
			(Sheridan Gardiner)
	9 letter (for 5 year olds)		HOVTXAUCL
≥3.5 years	Surrounded Snellen letters	Matching	Cambridge crowding cards
			Sonksen–Silver acuity cards

Only tests considered both theoretically and clinically appropriate have been included (the list of specific tests is not intended to be comprehensive). The ages specified are the minima commensurate with reasonable expectations of success. Note 2AFC = two alternative forced-choice.
* Claimed to be easily performed by children of ≤3 years but no documented reports.
† Omit the X, and cover this option on the key card to adapt test for younger children.

method, any statement of visual acuity should be accompanied by a comment on the exact method used.

If an individual's lack of maturity prevents appropriate cooperation with subjective tests an objective acuity method based on determining resolution (rather than detection) threshold should be selected. Where such a technique is adopted for vision screening purposes care should be taken to ensure that it is not conducted in isolation (Katz and Sireteanu, 1989). Important additional information can be gained using the cover test (Stager and Birch, 1986) and refractive assessment should be performed as target visibility is less affected by optical blur than is the case with Snellen letters. The acuity card PL procedure offers the most clinically suitable of currently available objective tests and appears to be the method of choice for at least the first 2 years of life. Toddlers are particularly difficult to assess, being bored with methods used for infant assessment and not capable of responding to tests designed for older children and adults. Consequently there is currently no widely preferred standard acuity test for this age group, though a new method which combines 'vanishing' picture optotypes with a preferential looking procedure appears promising (Woodhouse et al., 1992). The clinician should ideally have a battery of tests available from which to select one best geared to the child's abilities. The latter increase rapidly with age and more demanding (and scientifically preferable) tests should be applied as competence improves. Although not the most reliable method, high success rates and short test durations of acuity card procedures support their use in 2 year olds. From around 2.5 years some measure of recognition acuity should be obtainable. Initially Snellen-based picture or symbol tests may prove more successful but from 3 years children should respond well to specially adapted Landolt C or Snellen letter tests. The most widely applied adaptation is the use of matching responses (as in the Sheridan–Gardiner and Cambridge crowding card tests).

Subjective two alternative forced choice procedures also prove successful for testing young childrens' visual acuity (Broken wheel test) and contrast sensitivity. Tests requiring directional responses should be avoided.

Rapid sweep VEP methods currently offer the best possibility for clinically assessing infant contrast sensitivity, but the technology is not widely available and sensitivity estimates are much higher than corresponding behavioural data. Although Regan (1988) has claimed that a Sheridan–Gardiner-type version of low-contrast vision test is effective from about 3 years, other authors using behavioural techniques (e.g. Mantyjarvi et al., 1989) have expressed difficulty in successfully investigating contrast sensitivity below about 4 years.

Child refractive assessment

Three types of objective technique have been applied to the clinical assessment of children's refraction in recent years. These are photorefraction, autorefraction and conventional or modified methods of retinoscopic assessment. Each of these has various advantages and limitations.

Autorefractors enable measurement of refractive error over a wide range. Although the instruments are relatively expensive, a highly skilled operator is not required to obtain the results. Developments in instrumentation have resulted in autorefractors capable of rapidly providing estimates of refractive error, in cooperative adults, which are at least as reliable as other *objective* refractive techniques. Despite the rapidity and precision of measurement in adults, the need for precise alignment of the subject's eye with the instrument head presents a major difficulty limiting the use of autorefractors in young children. In infants adequate data collection may remain a problem, even with the assistance of three experimenters (Aslin, Shea and Metz, 1990). If undertaken, examination of young children should be conducted under cycloplegia to avoid problems of proximal accommodation, and if possible repeated readings should be obtained to indicate measurement accuracy and provide an average. However, young children, particularly of preschool age, may find the instrument intimidating and refuse to sit with their heads restrained for long enough to complete the test.

In addition to research studies in human infants, photorefractive techniques have been applied to other species including chickens (Schaeffel and Howland, 1988) and monkeys (Crewther et al., 1988). In humans, particular interest has been directed to evaluating the techniques' usefulness in screening for refractive error and to the study of infant astigmatism (Howland et al., 1978; Atkinson, Braddick and French, 1980) and accommodation. Howland and Sayles (1985) applied photokeratometry and photorefractive techniques in combination to compare corneal and total astigmatism in children.

Three distinct photorefractive techniques have been developed (orthogonal, isotropic and eccentric). Even when used in combination they cannot provide measurement of absolute refractive error across the entire spectrum. Measurement limits provided by the methods would not, for example, encompass the range of refractions encountered in a newborn population. Although efforts are being made to extend the measurement range of the eccentric technique, photorefraction is currently really only appropriate as a screening method to be backed up by conventional (retinoscopic) assessment. Despite these limitations certain advantages are evident. Photorefractive assessments can be performed relatively quickly and do not require a highly skilled operator. An instantaneous (and permanent) measure of the refractive state of each eye may be obtained simultaneously which should be of advantage in identification of anisometropia. The isotropic photorefractor image can be used to demonstrate the presence (and axis) of astigmatism to an infant's parents, which may assist in their acceptance of the need for optical correction. The infant may be more cooperative as photorefraction enables a remote method of examination and does not require lenses to be held close to the subject's eye. Unfortunately photorefractor results cannot be completely predicted from optical theory and computer ray tracing. Anyone wanting to construct their own instrument would, therefore, need to conduct laborious initial studies using individuals having a range of refractive errors to empirically calibrate the photorefractor before use. This work can be avoided by purchasing a commercially available instrument such as the 'Cambridge video-refractor'. The latter is an isotropic photorefractor system developed by Atkinson and Braddicks' group (marketed by Clement Clarke International), which is, as its name suggests, video based. Very few photorefractor systems have become commercially available. Instruments that have been marketed are sophisticated, video based and relatively expensive, but have the advantage of allowing instant retrieval and analysis of photorefractive images.

Since retinoscopy is based on a nulling method it provides equal accuracy of measurement throughout the range of possible refractive errors. This gives the method a clear advantage compared with photorefraction. The equipment required is also much less expensive. However, retinoscopy requires a skilled examiner especially when assessing young children who may rapidly become intolerant of having trial lenses held close to their eyes. Unlike photorefractive methods, retinoscopy enables assessment of only one eye (and one meridian) at a time, which may be a slight limitation when quantifying anisometropia or astigmatism. Although Mohindra's 'near retinoscopy' technique (Mohindra, 1977b) does not require use of cycloplegia, review of the literature suggests that it is not widely used and examination of infants under cycloplegia is to be recommended. Many studies of infant refraction have applied static retinoscopy techniques (reviewed by Banks, 1980a; Thompson, 1987), whereas dynamic methods have occasionally been used to assess accommodative ability and accuracy (Haynes, White and Held, 1965; Banks, 1980b; Brookman, 1983).

In conclusion, it appears therefore that autorefractive techniques have not yet proven sufficiently robust (when applied in isolation) for routine clinical use in young children. Photorefraction appears to offer a useful option for screening purposes, although conventional retinoscopic assessment currently remains the method of choice prior to prescribing. Whatever the method of assessment, accurate objective measurements of refraction are dependent on the presence of regular media and adequate control of the subject's accommodation and fixation. This implies that examination of young children should preferably be conducted under cycloplegic conditions, particularly when an optical correction is to be prescribed on the basis of the findings. However *initial* examinations, undertaken without cycloplegia, may provide useful information, for example on whether a child is overcoming their hyperopia (Atkinson *et al.*, 1989).

References

ABRAHAMSSON, M., FABIAN, G. and SJOSTRAND, J. (1986). Photorefraction: a useful tool to detect small angle strabismus. *Acta Ophthalmologica*, **64**, 101–104.

ADAMS, A.J., ZADNIK, K. and MUTTI, D.O. (1990). The reliability and validity of measurements of the ocular components of refraction. *Investigative Ophthalmology and Visual Sciences* (Suppl.), **31**, 417.

ASLIN, R.N. and DOBSON, V. (1983). Dark vergence and dark accommodation in human infants. *Vision Research*, **23**, 1671–1678.

ASLIN, R.N., SHEA, S.L. and METZ, H.S. (1990). Use of the Canon R-1 autorefractor to measure refractive errors and accommodative responses in infants. *Clinical Vision Science*, **5**, 61–70.

ATKINSON, J., ANKER, S., EVANS, C. *et al.* (1988). Visual acuity testing of young children with the Cambridge Crowding Cards at 3 and 6 m. *Acta Ophthalmologica*, **66**, 505–508.

ATKINSON, J. and BRADDICK, O. (1983a). Vision screening and photorefraction – the relation of refractive errors to strabismus and amblyopia. *Behavioural Brain Research*, **10**, 71–80.

ATKINSON, J. and BRADDICK, O. (1983b). The use of isotropic photorefraction for vision screening in infants. *Acta Ophthalmologica Supplementum*, **157**, 36–45.

ATKINSON, J., BRADDICK, O.J., AYLING, L. *et al.* (1981b) Isotropic photorefraction: a new method for refractive testing of infants. *Documenta Ophthalmologica Proceedings Series*, **30**, 217–223.

ATKINSON, J., BRADDICK, O.J., DURDEN, K. *et al.* (1984). Screening for refractive errors in 6–9 month old infants by photorefraction. *British Journal of Ophthalmology*, **68**, 105–112.

ATKINSON, J., BRADDICK, O. and FRENCH, J. (1980). Infant astigmatism: its disappearance with age. *Vision Research*, **20**, 891–893.

ATKINSON, J., BRADDICK, O., PIMM-SMITH, E. *et al.* (1981). Does the Catford Drum give an accurate assessment of acuity? *British Journal of Ophthalmology*, **65**, 652–656.

ATKINSON, J., BRADDICK, O. and PIMM-SMITH, E. (1982). Preferential looking for monocular and binocular acuity testing of infants. *British Journal of Ophthalmology*, **66**, 264–268.

ATKINSON, J., BRADDICK, O., WATTAM-BELL, J. *et al.* (1989). The prediction and prevention of strabismus and amblyopia achieved in the Cambridge infant photorefraction screening programme. *Ophthalmic and Physiological Optics*, **9**, 467.

ATKINSON, J. and FRENCH, J. (1983). Reaching for rattles: a preliminary study of contrast sensitivity in 7–10 month old infants. *Perception*, **12**, 323–329.

ATKINSON, J., FRENCH, J. and BRADDICK, O. (1981). Contrast sensitivity function of preschool children. *British Journal of Ophthalmology*, **65**, 525–529.

BANKS, M.S. (1980a). Infant refraction and accommodation. *International Ophthalmology Clinics*, **20**, (1), 205–232.

BANKS, M.S. (1980b). The development of visual accommodation during early infancy. *Child Development*, **51**, 646–666.

BANKS, M.S. and STEPHENS, B.R. (1982). The contrast sensitivity of human infants to gratings differing in duty cycle. *Vision Research*, **22**, 739–744.

BELKIN, M., TICHO, U., SUSAL, A. and LEVINSON, A. (1973). Ultrasonography in the refraction of aphakic infants. *British Journal of Ophthalmology*, **57**, 845–848.

BENNETT, A.G. (1965). Ophthalmic test types. *British Journal of Physiological Optics*, **22**, 238–271.

BENNETT, A.G. (1986). An (sic) historical review of optometric principles and techniques. *Ophthalmic and Physiological Optics*, **6**, 3–21.

BENNETT, A.G. and RABBETTS, R.B. (1989a). Visual acuity and contrast sensitivity. In *Clinical Visual Optics*, 2nd edn. Butterworth, London, pp. 23–72.

BENNETT, A.G. and RABBETTS, R.B. (1989b). Retinoscopy (skiascopy). In *Clinical Visual Optics*, 2nd edn. Butterworth, London, pp. 393–419.

BENNETT, A.G. and RABBETTS, R.B. (1989c). Objective optometers. In *Clinical Visual Optics*, 2nd edn. Butterworth, London, pp. 421–442.

BERLYNE, D.E. (1958). The influence of albedo and complexity of stimuli on visual fixation in the human infant. *British Journal of Psychology*, **49**, 315–318.

BIRCH, E.E. and HALE, L.A. (1988). Criteria for monocular acuity deficit in infancy and early childhood. *Investigative Ophthalmology and Visual Science*, **29**, 636–643.

BLAKEY, J. (1988). A review of children's test charts. *Optician*, 24 June, 17–25.

BOBIER, W.R. (1988). Quantitative photorefraction using an off-center flash source. *American Journal of Physiological Optics*, **65**, 962–971.

BOBIER, W.R. (1990). Eccentric photorefraction: a method to measure accommodation of highly hypermetropic infants. *Clinical Vision Science*, **5**, 45–60.

BOBIER, W.R. and BRADDICK, O.J. (1985). Eccentric photorefraction: optical analysis and empirical measures. *American Journal of Optometry and Physiological Optics*, **62**, 614–620.

BORGHI, R.A. and ROUSE, M.W. (1985). Comparison of refraction obtained by 'near retinoscopy' and retinoscopy under cycloplegia. *American Journal of Optometry and Physiological Optics*, **62**, 169–172.

BORISH, I.M. (1970a). Retinoscopy. In *Clinical Refraction*, 3rd edn, The Professional Press, Chicago, pp. 659–695.

BORISH, I.M. (1970b). Dynamic skiametry. In *Clinical Refraction*, 3rd edn. The Professional Press, Chicago, pp. 697–713.

BORISH, I.M. (1970c). Ophthalmoscopy. In *Clinical Refraction*, 3rd edn. The Professional Press, Chicago, pp. 501–525.

BRADDICK, O. and ATKINSON, J. (1984). Photorefractive techniques: applications in testing infants and young children. In *The Frontiers of Optometry, Transactions of the First International Congress, The British College of Ophthalmic Opticians*, vol. 2, edited by W.N. Charman, British College of Ophthalmic Opticians, London, 26–34.

BRADDICK, O., ATKINSON, J., FRENCH, J. and HOWLAND, H.C. (1979). A photorefractive study of infant accommodation. *Vision Research*, **19**, 1319–1330.

BRADLEY, A. and FREEMAN, R.D. (1982). Contrast sensitivity in children. *Vision Research*, **22**, 953–959.

BS 4274 (1968). Specification for Test Charts for Determining Distance Visual Acuity. British Standards Institution, London.

BROOKMAN, K.E. (1983). Ocular accommodation in human infants. *American Journal of Optometry and Physiological Optics*, **60**, 91–99.

BROWN, V.A., DORAN, R.M.L. and WOODHOUSE, J.M. (1987). The use of computerized contrast sensitivity, Arden gratings and low contrast letter charts in the assessment of amblyopia. *Ophthalmic and Physiological Optics*, **7**, 43–51.

BROWN, V.A. and WOODHOUSE, J.M. (1986). Assessment of techniques for measuring contrast sensitivity in children. *Ophthalmic and Physiological Optics*, **6**, 165–170.

CAMPBELL, F.W. and ROBSON, J.G. (1968). Application of Fourier analysis to the visibility of gratings. *Journal of Physiology (London)*, **197**, 551–566.

CHARMAN, W.N. (1980). Reflection of plane-polarized light by the retina. *British Journal of Physiological Optics*, **34**, 34–49.

COLLINS, G. (1973). Electronic refractionometer. *British Journal of Physiological Optics*, **11**, 30–42.

CREWTHER, D.P., KIELY, P.M., McCARTHY, A. and CREWTHER, S.G. (1988). Evaluation of paraxial photorefraction in screening a population of monkeys for refractive errors. *Clinical Vision Science*, **3**, 213–220.

CREWTHER, D.P., McCARTHY, A., ROPER, J. and COSTELLO, K. (1987). An analysis of eccentric photo-refraction. *Clinical and Experimental Optometry*, **70**, 2–7.

DAY, S.H. and NORCIA, A.M. (1986). Photographic detection of amblyogenic factors. *Ophthalmology*, **93**, 25–28.

DOBSON, V., SALEM, D., MAYER, D.L *et al*. (1985). Visual acuity screening of children 6 months to 3 years of age. *Investigative Ophthalmology and Visual Science*, **26**, 1057–1063.

DOBSON, V. and TELLER, D.Y. (1978). Visual acuity in human infants: a review and comparison of behavioral and electrophysiological studies. *Vision Research*, **18**, 1469–1483.

DRASDO, N. (1988). Patterns and contrasts in ophthalmic investigation. *Ophthalmic and Physiological Optics*, **8**, 3–13.

DUCKMAN, R.H. and MEYER, B. (1987). Use of photoretinoscopy as a screening technique in the assessment of anisometropia and significant refractive error in infants/toddlers/children and special populations. *American Journal of Optometry and Physiological Optics*, **64**, 604–610.

EDWARDS, K. and LLEWELLYN, R. (1988). *Optometry*. Butterworths, London.

ELLIOTT, D.B., GILCHRIST, J. and WHITAKER, D. (1989). Contrast sensitivity and glare sensitivity changes with three types of cataract morphology: are these techniques necessary in a clinical evaluation of cataract? *Ophthalmic and Physiological Optics*, **9**, 25–30.

ELLIOTT, R. (1985). A new linear picture vision test. *British Orthoptics Journal*, **42**, 54–57.

ENOCH, J.M. and RABINOWICZ, I.M. (1976). Early surgery and visual correction of an infant born with unilateral eye lens opacity. *Documenta Ophthalmologica*, **41**, 371–383.

EVANS, E. (1984). Refraction in children using the R × 1 auto-refractor. *British Orthoptics Journal*, **41**, 46–52.

FANTZ, R.L. (1958). Pattern vision in young infants. *Psychological Record*, **8**, 43–47.

FANTZ, R.L., ORDY, J.M. and UDELF, M.S. (1962). Maturation of pattern vision in infants during the first six months. *Child Development*, **46**, 3–18.

FAYE, E.E. (1968). A new visual acuity test for partially-sighted non readers. *Journal of Pediatric Ophthalmology*, **5**, 210–212.

FERN, K.D. and MANNY, R.E. (1986). Visual acuity of the preschool child: a review. *American Journal of Optometry and Physiological Optics*, **63**, 319–345.

FERN, K.D., MANNY, R.E., DAVIS, J.R. and GIBSON, R.R. (1986). Contour interaction in the preschool child. *American Journal of Optometry and Physiological Optics*, **63**, 313–318.

FFOOKS, O. (1965). Vision test for children: use of symbols. *British Journal of Ophthalmology*, **49**, 312–314.

FLORENTINI, A., PIRCHIO, M. and SPINELLI, D. (1983). Electrophysiological evidence for spatial frequency selective mechanisms in adults and infants. *Vision Research*, **23**, 119–127.

FLOM, M.C., WEYMOUTH, F.W. and KAHNEMAN, D. (1963). Visual resolution and contour interaction. *Journal of the Optical Society of America*, **53**, 1026–1032.

GLICKSTEIN, M. and MILLODOT, M. (1970). Retinoscopy and eye size. *Science*, **168**, 605–606.

GOLDSCHMIDT, E. (1969). Refraction in the newborn. *Acta Ophthalmologica*, **47**, 570–578.

GORDON, R.A. and DONZIS, P.B. (1985). Refractive development of the human eye. *Archives of Ophthalmology*, **103**, 785–789.

GRIFFIN, J.R., McLIN, L.N. and SCHOR, C.M. (1986). Photographic method for strabismus detection – effectiveness of Bruckner and Hirschberg testing. *American Journal of Optometry and Physiological Optics*, **63**, (10), 110P.

GWIAZDA, J., BRILL, S., MOHINDRA, J. and HELD, R. (1978). Infant visual acuity and its meridional variation. *Vision Research*, **18**, 1557–1564.

HAINLINE, L., BIE, J.D., ABRAMOV, I. and CAMENZULI, C. (1987). Eye movement voting: a new technique for deriving spatial contrast sensitivity. *Clinical Vision Science*, **2**, 33–44.

HALL, S.M., PUGH, A.G. and HALL, D.M.B. (1982). Vision screening in the under-5s. *British Medical Journal*, **285**, 1096–1098.

HARTER, M.R., DEATON, F.K. and ODOM, J.V. (1977). Maturation of evoked potentials and visual preference in 6–45 day-old infants: effects of check size, visual acuity and refractive error. *Electroencephalography and Clinical Neurophysiology*, **42**, 595–607.

HAYNES, H., WHITE, B.L. and HELD, R. (1965). Visual accommodation in human infants. *Science*, **148**, 528–530.

HEERSEMA, T. and VAN HOF-VAN DUIN, J. (1988). Age norms for visual acuity at toddler age using the acuity card method in a clinical setting. *Investigative Ophthalmology and Visual Science*, **29**, 436.

HELVASTON, E.M., PACHTMAN, M.A., CADERA, W. *et al.* (1984). Clinical evaluation of the Nidek AR auto refractor. *Journal of Pediatric Ophthalmology and Strabismus*, **21**, 227–230.

HENSON, D.B. (1983). Retinoscopes. In *Optometric Instrumentation*, 1st edn. Butterworths, London, pp. 14–24.

HILTON, A.F. and STANLEY, J.C. (1972). Pitfalls in testing children's vision by the Sheridan Gardiner single optotype method. *British Journal of Ophthalmology*, **56**, 135–139.

HOWLAND, H.C. (1980). The optics of static photographic skiascopy; comments on a paper by K. Kaakinen. *Acta Ophthalmologica*, **58**, 221–227.

HOWLAND, H.C. (1985). Optics of photoretinoscopy: results from ray tracing. *American Journal of Optometry and Physiological Optics*, **62**, 621–625.

HOWLAND, H.C. and HOWLAND, B. (1974). Photorefraction: a technique for study of refractive state at a distance. *Journal of the Optical Society of America*, **64**, 240–249.

HOWLAND, H.C., ATKINSON, J., BRADDICK, O. and FRENCH, J. (1978). Infant astigmatism measured by photorefraction. *Science*, **202**, 331–333.

HOWLAND, H.C., BRADDICK, O., ATKINSON, J. and HOWLAND, B. (1983). Optics of photorefraction: orthogonal and isotropic methods. *Journal of the Optical Society of America*, **73**, 1701–1708.

HOWLAND, H.C., DOBSON, V. and SAYLES, N. (1987). Accommodation in infants as measured by photorefraction. *Vision Research*, **27**, 2141–2152.

HOWLAND, H.C. and SAYLES, N. (1985). Photokeratometric and photorefractive measurements of astigmatism in infants and young children. *Vision Research*, **25**, 73–81.

HOWLAND, H.C., SAYLES, N., CACCIOTTI, C. and HOWLAND, M. (1987). Simple pointspread retinoscope suitable for vision screening. *American Journal of Optometry and Physiological Optics*, **64**, 114–122.

HYAMS, L., SAFIR, A. and PHILPOT, J. (1971). Studies in refraction. ii. Bias and accuracy of retinoscopy. *Archives of Ophthalmology*, **85**, 33–41.

KAAKINEN, K. (1979). A simple method for screening of children with strabismus, anisometropia or ametropia by simultaneous photography of the corneal and the fundus reflexes. *Acta Ophthalmologica*, **57**, 161–171.

KAAKINEN, K. (1981). Simultaneous two flash static photoskiascopy. *Acta Ophthalmologica*, **59**, 378–386.

KAAKINEN, K., KASEVA, H. and KAUSE, E.R. (1986). Mass screening of children for strabismus or ametropia with two-flash photoskiascopy. *Acta Ophthalmologica*, **64**, 105–110.

KAAKINEN, K. and RANTA-KEMPPAINEN, L. (1986). Screening of infants for strabismus and refractive errors with two flash photorefraction with and without cycloplegia. *Acta Ophthalmologica*, **64**, 578–582.

KATZ, B. and SIRETEANU, R. (1989). The Teller acuity card test: a useful method for the clinical routine? *Ophthalmic and Physiological Optics*, **9**, 469.

KAY, H. (1983). New method of assessing visual acuity with pictures. *British Journal of Ophthalmology*, **67**, 131–133.

KEITH, C.G., DIAMOND, Z. and STANSFIELD, A. (1972). Visual acuity testing in young children. *British Journal of Ophthalmology*, **56**, 827–832.

KOHL, P., SAMEK, B.M. and COFFEY, B. (1987). Reliability of Mohindra's 'near retinoscopy' in human infants (0–2 yrs). *Investigative Ophthalmology and Visual Science*, (Suppl.), **28**, 394.

LIPPMANN, O. (1969). Vision of young children. *Archives of Ophthalmology*, **81**, 763–775.

LIVANES, A., GREAVES, D. and BEVAN, J. (1986). Pre-school visual acuity tests. *Clinical and Experimental Optometry*, **69**, 145–148.

LOVIE-KITCHIN, J.E. (1988). Validity and reliability of visual acuity measurements. *Ophthalmic and Physiological Optics*, **8**, 363–370.

MALLETT, R. (1988). Techniques of investigation of binocular vision anomalies. In *Optometry*, edited by K. Edwards and R. Llewellyn. Butterworths, London, pp. 238–269.

MANNING, K.A., FULTON, A.B., HANSEN, R.M. *et al.* (1982). Preferential looking vision testing: application to evaluation of high-risk, prematurely born infants and children. *Journal of Pediatric Ophthalmology and Strabismus*, **19**, 286–293.

MANTYJARVI, M.I., AUTERE, M.H., SILVENNOINEN, A.M. and MYOHANEN, T. (1989). Observations on the use of three different contrast sensitivity tests in children and young adults. *Journal of Pediatric Ophthalmology and Strabismus*, **26**, 113–119.

MARG, E., FREEMAN, D.N., PELTZMAN, P. and GOLDSTEIN, P.J. (1976). Visual acuity development in human infants: evoked potential measurements. *Investigative Ophthalmology and Visual Science*, **15**, 150–153.

MAYER, D.L. and DOBSON, V. (1982). Visual acuity development in infants and young children, as assessed by operant preferential looking. *Vision Research*, **22**, 1141–1151.

MAYER, D.L., FULTON, A.B. and HANSEN, R.M. (1982). Preferential looking acuity obtained with a staircase procedure in pediatric patients. *Investigative Ophthalmology and Visual Science*, **23**, 538–543.

McDONALD, M.A. (1986). Assessment of visual acuity in toddlers. *Survey of Ophthalmology*, **31**, 189–210.

McDONALD, M.A. and CHAUDRY, N.M. (1989). Comparison of four methods of assessing visual acuity in young children. *American Journal of Optometry and Physiological Optics*, **66**, 363–369.

MEIJLER, A.P. and VAN DEN BERG, T.J.T.P. (1982). High contrast sensitivity in babies, found using an eye movement reflex. *Documenta Ophthalmologica Proceedings Series*, **31**, 229–235.

MOHINDRA, I. (1977a). A non-cycloplegic refraction technique for infants and young children. *Journal of the American Optometric Association*, **48**, 518–523.

MOHINDRA, I. (1977b). Comparison of 'near retinoscopy' and subjective refraction in adults. *American Journal of Optometry and Physiological Optics*, **54**, 319–322.

MOHINDRA, I. and MOLINARI, J.F. (1979). Near retinoscopy and cycloplegic retinoscopy in early primary grade school children. *American Journal of Optometry and Physiological Optics*, **56**, 34–38.

MOSELEY, M.J., FIELDER, A.R., THOMPSON, J.R. *et al.* (1988). Grating and recognition acuities of young amblyopes. *British Journal of Ophthalmology*, **72**, 50–54.

MOSKOWITZ, A., SOKOL, S. and HANSEN, V. (1987). Rapid assessment of visual function in pediatric patients using pattern VEPs and acuity cards. *Clinical Vision Science*, **2**, 11–20.

NORCIA, A.M. and TYLER, C.M. (1985). Spatial frequency sweep VEP: visual acuity during the first year of life. *Vision Research*, **25**, 1399–1408.

NORCIA, A.M., TYLER, C.W. and HAMER, R.D. (1988). High visual contrast sensitivity in the young human infant. *Investigative Ophthalmology and Visual Science*, **29**, 44–49.

NORCIA, A.M., TYLER, C.W. and HAMER, R.D. (1990). Development of contrast sensitivity in the human infant. *Vision Research*, **30**, 1475–1486.

NORCIA, A.M., ZADNIK, K. and DAY, S.H. (1986). Photorefraction with a catadioptric lens improvement on the method of Kaakinen. *Acta Ophthalmologica*, **64**, 379–385.

NUBOER, J.F.W. and VAN GENDEREN-TAKKEN, H.V. (1978). The artifact of retinoscopy. *Vision Research*, **18**, 1091–1096.

OREL-BIXLER, D.A. and NORCIA, A.M. (1987). Differential growth of acuity for steady-state pattern reversal and transient pattern onset-offset VEPs. *Clinical Vision Science*, **2**, 1–9.

OWENS, D.A., MOHINDRA, I. and HELD, R. (1980). The effectiveness of a retinoscope beam as an accommodative stimulus. *Investigative Ophthalmology and Visual Science*, **19**, 942–949.

PEARSON, R.M. (1966). The objective determination of vision and visual acuity. *British Journal of Physiological Optics*, **23**, 107–128.

PELLI, D.G., ROBSON, J.G. and WILKINS, A.J. (1988). The design of a new letter chart for measuring contrast sensitivity. *Clinical Vision Science*, **2**, 187–199.

PHILIPSEN, A. and HOBOLTH, I. (1985). Photographic screening for strabismus among mentally retarded children. *Acta Ophthalmologica*, **63**, 268–273.

PICKERT, S.M. and WACHS, H. (1980). Stimulus and communication demands of visual acuity tests. *American Journal of Optometry and Physiological Optics*, **57**, 875–880.

PRESTON, K.L., McDONALD, M.A., SEBRIS, S.L. et al. (1987). Validation of the acuity card procedure for assessment of infants with ocular disorders. *Ophthalmology*, **94**, 644–653.

REGAN, D. (1977). Rapid methods for refracting the eye and for assessing visual acuity in amblyopia using steady-state visual evoked potentials. In *Visual Evoked Potentials in Man: New Developments*, edited by J.E. Desmedt. Clarendon Press, Oxford, pp. 418–426.

REGAN, D. (1988). Low-contrast letter charts and sinewave grating tests in ophthalmological and neurological disorders. *Clinical Vision Science*, **2**, 235–250.

ROBINSON, J., MOSELEY, M.J. and FIELDER, A.R. (1988). Grating acuity cards: spurious resolution and the 'edge artifact'. *Clinical Vision Science*, **3**, 285–288.

ROVAMO, J. and VIRSU, V. (1979). An estimation and application of the human cortical magnification factor. *Experimental Brain Research*, **37**, 495–510.

RUBIN, G.S. (1988). Reliability and sensitivity of clinical contrast sensitivity tests. *Clinical Vision Science*, **2**, 169–177.

SAFIR, A., HYAMS, L., PHILPOT, J. and JAGERMAN, L.S. (1970). Studies in refraction. i. The precision of retinoscopy. *Archives of Ophthalmology*, **84**, 49–61.

SCHAEFFEL, F., FARKAS, L. and HOWLAND, H.C. (1987). Infrared photoretinoscope. *Applied Optics*, **26**, 1505–1509.

SCHAEFFEL, F. and HOWLAND, H.C. (1988). Visual optics in normal and ametropic chickens. *Clinical Vision Science*, **3**, 83–98.

SHERIDAN, M.D. (1976). *Manual for the Stycar Vision Tests*, revised 1976 edn. NFER Publishing Co. Ltd, Windsor, Berks.

STAGER, D.R. and BIRCH, E.E. (1986). Preferential-looking acuity and stereopsis in infantile esotropia. *Journal of Pediatric Ophthalmology and Strabismus*, **23**, 160–165.

STEWART-BROWN, S.L., HASLUM, M.N. and HOWLETT, B. (1988). Preschool vision screening: a service in need of rationalisation. *Archives of Diseases in Childhood*, **63**, 356–359.

TAYLOR, S. (1988). Retinoscopy. In *Optometry*, 1st edn, edited by K. Edwards and R. Llewellyn, Butterworths, London, pp. 81–91.

TELLER, D.Y. (1979). The forced-choice preferential looking procedure: a psychophysical technique for use with human infants. *Infant Behaviour and Development*, **2**, 135–153.

TELLER, D.Y. (1983). Measurement of visual acuity in human and monkey infants: the interface between laboratory and clinic. *Behavioural Brain Research*, **10**, 15–23.

TELLER, D.Y., McDONALD, M.A., PRESTON, K. *et al.* (1986). Assessment of visual acuity in infants and children: the acuity card procedure. *Developmental Medicine and Child Neurology*, **28**, 779–789.

TELLER, D.Y., MORSE, R., BORTON, R. and REGAL, D. (1974). Visual acuity for vertical and diagonal gratings in human infants. *Vision Research*, **14**, 1433–1439.

THOMPSON, C.M. (1987). Objective and Psychophysical Studies of Infant Visual Development. Unpublished PhD thesis, University of Aston.

THOMPSON, C. and DRASDO, N. (1988). Clinical experience with preferential looking acuity tests in infants and young children. *Ophthalmic and Physiological Optics*, **8**, 309–321.

VOIPIO, H. (1961). The objective measurement of visual acuity by arresting optokinetic nystagmus without change in illumination. *Acta Ophthalmologica Supplementum*, **66**, 1–70.

WESEMANN, W. and RASSOW, B. (1987). Automatic infrared refractors – a comparative study. *American Journal of Optometry and Physiological Optics*, **64**, 627–638.

WILKINS, A.J., DELLA SALA, S., SOMAZZI, L. and NIMMO-SMITH, I. (1988). Age-related norms for the Cambridge low contrast sensitivity gratings, including details concerning their design and use. *Clinical Vision Science*, 2, 201–212.

WOOD, I. (1988). Computerized refractive examination. In *Optometry*, 1st edn, edited by K. Edwards and R. Llewellyn. Butterworths, London, pp. 92–110.

WOODHOUSE, J.M., ADOH, T.O., ODUWAIGE, K.A. *et al.* (1992). New acuity test for toddlers. *Ophthalmic and Physiological Optics*, **12**, 249–251.

WOODHOUSE, J.M. and WESTALL, C.A. (1989). Clinical contrast sensitivity evaluation in visually impaired children. *Ophthalmic and Physiological Optics*, **9**, 469.

YAP, M., GREY, C., COLLINGE, A. and HURST, M. (1985). The Arden gratings in optometric practice. *Ophthalmic and Physiological Optics*, **5**, 179–183.

Refractive routines in the examination of children

Terry Buckingham and A.R. Shakespeare

Introduction

Increased interest in health care will almost certainly mean a rise in the number of children seen by optometrists. Parents may simply seek reassurance that their child's vision is normal following something which they have observed, or that the child has reported. There may be a family history of eye problems and it is valuable if the optometrist has ready access to records of other family members.

The incidence of visual disorders amongst infants is not insignificant. About 3.7% of 1-year-old children have been found to have a highly abnormal refraction (Ingram *et al.*, 1986), whilst photorefractive studies estimate that significant refractive errors were present in over 11% of 6 to 9 month-old infants (Atkinson *et al.*, 1984). Amongst this latter group 4.6% were estimated to have hypermetropia over 3.50 D, 4.5% appeared mildly myopic, 0.5% had myopia greater than 3.00 D, and 0.6% had anisometropia over 1.00 D. Whilst there are obvious difficulties in correcting refractive errors in young infants an early correction of them not only improves vision but reduces the likelihood of amblyopia and strabismus.

The nature of the optometric investigation will depend on the developmental level of the child, as well as signs and symptoms, rather than their chronological age. For older children the composition, if not the order of the routine, is identical to that for an adult. Rather more specialized techniques are required for infants and the mentally retarded. For many children the routine may take the form of a screening examination, but there may be indications for more detailed investigation including a cycloplegic refraction. These include unequal or poor acuities, significant hypermetropia, reduced accommodation, significant differences between objective and subjective findings, large heterophorias, manifest or intermittent squint, relevant immediate family history and unexplained signs or symptoms.

It is within the controlled environment of the optometric practice that the relatively sophisticated tests necessary in the ocular assessment of infants and young children are best conducted. If possible a particular session should be allocated for young children's appointments each week and a toy box made available in the waiting room. A child who has had to wait for some time prior to the examination, and who finds the procedure difficult as well as dull, is unlikely to cooperate in an objective assessment let alone give valuable subjective responses. The young child should be accompanied into the consulting room by a parent and ideally a toy should be brought. The presence of distracting brothers and sisters should be discouraged. Reference has been made to a 'parent' accompanying the child, but this is not always the case. If in doubt, it is wise to establish the relationship of the accompanying adult to avoid embarrassment.

It is important to consider beforehand what type of routine would be most appropriate, assuming that the child's date of birth is known. The capabilities of children of similar ages can vary markedly and their level of cooperation can vary by the hour. The practitioner, therefore, needs to be very flexible about the nature of the routine undertaken, modifying it even as it progresses depending upon the level of cooperation of the child.

Children are rarely typical of their age and the following routines have been suggested as an appropriate starting point in their examination.

Routine for an infant (between 2.5 and 5 years of age)

Young infants are easily overawed by unfamiliar faces and places. If possible it is a good idea for the child to accompany a parent to an appointment a few days beforehand. On the first visit it is advisable that the child should be given time to familiarize themselves with their surroundings and build up confidence, while the practitioner speaks briefly to the parent. The practitioner should make eye contact with the child and call them by their name. It is perhaps worth establishing the name by which the child is habitually known – this is not necessarily their formal first name. In discussions with the parent the practitioner should establish the following:

(1) *Visual status*. Does the child appear to see well at distance and at near? Does the young child reach out for small objects and appear to judge distances well? Do the eyes appear straight? Has the parent ever noticed one eye drifting into the corner or out? If so, under what conditions – when tired or looking at books? Is the child good at recognizing colours? The child's mother is generally a very good judge of their visual capability, since they will have observed the child for some time in many practical situations.
(2) *Ocular history*. Has the child been examined before and with what result? If not, have any problems arisen? Does the child appear to rub his/her eyes excessively? Does the child appear to be uncomfortable in bright light?
(3) *Family history*. Is there any history of visual defects in the rest of the family? What is the child's birth order – does he/she have any older/younger brothers or sisters?
(4) *General health*. Is the child in good health? Has the child had any of the childhood diseases? Was the child's birth normal and did pregnancy follow its normal course?
(5) *Developmental status*. At what age did the child start to walk, talk and develop handedness? This can have particular relevance when considering children exhibiting specific learning disorders (see Chapter 16).

Examination

The span of concentration of a young child is extremely limited. The main areas of concern should be done at the start of the examination and these, to some extent, determine the outline of the examination. Much of the routine may have to be omitted and the first result, however inadequate, may be the only one available to the practitioner. The child should be positioned where they are most comfortable, either on a parent's knee, or with the parent sitting next to them. The practitioner should take care to explain to the child what is being done. This puts them at their ease and encourages their cooperation.

The pen torch may be held up in order for the examiner to assess the appearance of the eyes together with the corneal reflections. Ocular motility can be assessed by asking the child to follow the pen torch bulb with their eyes. The cover test can be performed at near using the pen torch bulb as the fixation target, but with a cooperative child a small target, for example, one on a children's near fixation bar, will provide a better accommodative target. It is probably less disturbing for the child if the practitioner uses his hand, or a thumb, as a cover rather than an opaque occluder. The cover test itself can be a useful screening procedure; Graham (1974) found that 7% of children exhibited abnormal cover test movements. It is probably better not to startle the child by directing bright light into their eyes at the start of the examination. Pupil reactions are probably better assessed later during ophthalmoscopy.

An assessment of refractive error can be made with retinoscopy, although this may have to be performed fairly quickly because of the child's short span of attention. It is possible that only a limited number of lens changes can be made and adjusting the working distance may help in assessing the refractive error. During retinoscopy a pair of trial case lenses are held in one hand, so that one lens is in front of each eye (*Figure 9.1(a)*). The first pair of lenses may be around $+2.50\,D$, this allows for a small degree of hypermetropia and a shorter working distance than normal. The fingers of the hand are extended so that they rest on the child's forehead. Ideally some interesting distance fixation target should be provided, such as a mobile, although the red and green bichromatic plate may have to suffice. Assuming the latter to be the case, explain to the child that the lenses will make the red and green lights appear foggy. The child should be encouraged to keep their attention on the duochrome plate, to assist in obtaining an accurate retinoscopy result and reduce the likelihood of accommodation. The child's attention should be continually directed towards the target by asking what colours they see, which appears the brightest and whether they ever disappear. The child can also be asked if they see any rings on the red or green. Initially the practitioner has to assess the refractive error in four meridians of both eyes working from one side, usually the right. The practitioner has to consider the possibility of significant astigmatism, high hypermetropia or (less commonly) myopia. Ideally the practitioner should swap over to the left side in order to make a more accurate assessment of the refractive error of the left eye. If a significant amount of astigmatism is present the practitioner may have to hold a spherocylindrical combination in front of one eye in order to assess the cylindrical power and axis (*Figure 9.1(b)*). Under such circumstances, and if a high degree of hypermetropia is present, a further appointment for a cycloplegic refraction would be advisable. During retinoscopy the practitioner needs to pay particular care to his working position. This is especially true of his height relative to the patient. Children have very steep corneas, and the penalties for being off-axis are much greater than for an adult. It has been observed that 48% of children, aged 1 year, with a refraction of $+3.50\,D$ or greater in one meridian have amblyopia and 45% have squint (Ingram *et al.*, 1986).

Some practitioners prefer to use near-fixation retinoscopy for young children (Mohindra, 1977), which ideally is performed in a totally darkened room. However, this can be frightening for some children. The eye not under examination is occluded and the child views the low-intensity retinoscope light. Although the usual working distance is about 50 cm, $+1.25\,D$ is deducted from the retinoscopy result. This figure, having been established empirically, may vary between individuals. The use of dynamic retinoscopy in young children, although limited, is described in Chapter 8.

The basic assumption for children within this group is that they can match letters

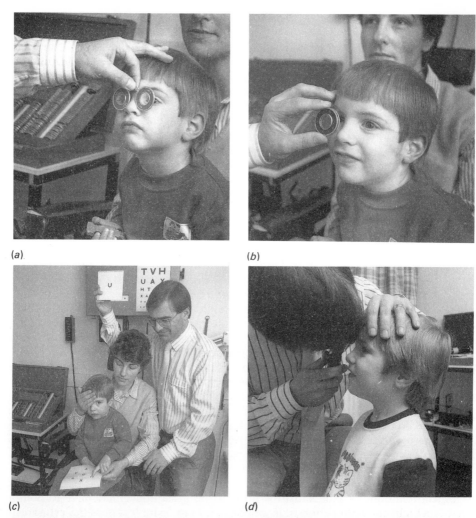

Figure 9.1. (a) Lenses are held before both eyes during retinoscopy to reduce accommodation. If a cycloplegic refraction is being performed the child may fixate the retinoscope light rather than a distance fixation target. (b) A sphero-cylindrical combination may have to be held before one eye when assessing an astigmatic correction. (c) A letter matching test to establish acuity may be performed directly at 3 m or at a distance of 6 m with the child looking through the mirror. It is important to maintain eye contact with the child. (d) Ophthalmoscopy may be more easily performed with the child standing and the practitioner seated.

with greater accuracy than they can name them. A number of techniques are available to assess visual acuity. It should be remembered that these are very dependent upon the level of cooperation given by the child. Only brief reference will be made to those tests commonly encountered, since detailed description is contained in Chapter 8. The test most commonly used is the Sheridan–Gardiner test, in which symmetrical letters are printed on a keycard. This is held by the child, who points to the letters matching those indicated by the practitioner on an internally illuminated chart or ring-bound booklet. Originally published as part of the STYCAR vision test (STYCAR is an acronym for Screening Test for Young Children And Retardates), it is available in three versions of five-, seven- and nine-letter sets. The five-letter sets contain the letters HOTVX, to which the letters AU are added for the seven-letter and AUCL for the nine-letter sets. The seven-letter sets are the ones most commonly used. The practitioner should explain to the child how the test is to be performed beforehand. Sometimes it is better to explain it in terms of a game which the child can play with the examiner. The practitioner should sit about 1 m away from the child and show them a letter and ask them to point to one which exactly matches it on the keycard which they are holding. Once the child has understood the purpose of the test the Sheridan–Gardiner letters can be held at 3 or 6 m. It is sometimes said that children have difficulty in identifying letters at 6 m through a mirror. If the test is to be performed at 6 m the practitioner should position himself slightly behind the child, so that he is visible in the mirror holding the Sheridan–Gardiner letters (*Figure 9.1(c)*). The child should be asked if they can see the practitioner clearly in the mirror – if possible eye contact should be made and maintained. Obviously, if the child repeatedly turns round to look at the letters which the practitioner is holding a shorter, direct-viewing approach may have to be adopted. The Sheridan–Gardiner test can also be performed at near, when the child holds the chart containing reduced Snellen letters. The examiner holds the keycard and asks the child to find the matching letters on the near chart. The practitioner should assess the likely impact of the refractive error upon the visual acuity beforehand. The child's parent may occlude one eye, by holding a folded tissue in the palm of their hand over it, and prescription lenses before the other eye if necessary (*Figure 9.1(c)*).

The advantage of viewing a single optotype, as in the Sheridan–Gardiner test, is that the child is not faced with the difficulty of understanding what is required of him and with losing his place in a line of letters. Single letter acuity tends to be slightly better than line acuity. Interestingly, amblyopes have greater difficulty in identifying letters arranged in rows than single, isolated optotypes. This is known as the crowding effect and may be more useful than single optotypes in identifying amblyopes. This forms the basis of the Cambridge Crowding Cards and the Sonksen–Silver acuity system (*Figure 9.2(a)*). The former consists of a central letter surrounded by four letters, one above and below together with one either side. The child identifies the central letter by pointing to the matching letter on an array. The test is designed to be presented at 3 m and is well within the cognitive capabilities of children over 3 years of age. In the Sonksen–Silver system the child has to identify letters from a linear array of five, and is given a keycard with letters arranged on an arc. A number of alternative tests are available which are described in Chapter 8.

In measuring the acuity of children in this age group the practitioner needs to observe the child closely. Difficulty in seeing the letters may be indicated if the child begins to peer, attempts to guess them, or easily becomes distracted. Equality of vision between the eyes as well as overall visual performance should be assessed.

The distance cover test may be performed using the spot light as fixation target, since this easily attracts the attention of young children. For older children a single letter may be a more appropriate target. The cover test should also be performed at near. As mentioned earlier it might be easier to use the thumb as the occluder. The effects on vision of the spectacle lenses can be assessed either by a parent holding lenses in front of one eye and occluding the other with the hand, or Halberg clips can be fixed onto a child's unglazed spectacle frame. Sometimes it has to be accepted that vision will need to be re-evaluated after spectacles have been made up for the child. *Table 9.1* describes the way in which visual acuity develops with age.

A number of useful tests are available for investigating the stereoscopic vision of children within this age group. The Lang Stereotest works on the principle of

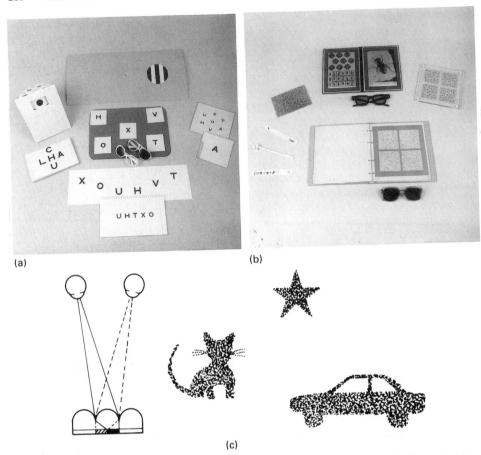

(a)   (b)

(c)

Figure 9.2. (a) Infant acuity assessment tests. The Keeler Acuity Cards (top) which may be used with a folding 'puppet screen'. Part of the five letter Sheridan–Gardiner Test is shown (centre) with spectacle frames adapted for occlusion. The flip-chart of the seven letter version together with the keycard to which the child points is shown (right). Other letter matching tests include the Sonksen–Silver Acuity System (bottom) and the Cambridge Crowding Cards (left), above which is the Catford drum. (b) Stereoscopic tests. The Titmus–Wirt test (top) with polaroid spectacles, the Frisby test (right) and the TNO test (bottom) are shown. Various fixation bars are shown (left) above which is the Lang Stereotest. (c) The detailed images of the Lang Stereotest (produced by Clement Clarke International Ltd).

cylindrical screens and does not require the use of a visor. It is placed 40 cm from the child, who will normally see three images (*Figure 9.2(c)*). The image of the cat, having a disparity of 1200 sec arc, is seen to be the closest – with little difference between the proximity of the star and car (600 sec arc and 550 sec arc respectively). The test plate needs to be positioned exactly on the fronto-parallel plane. The child may have to move their head to obtain the best viewing position or, alternatively, the practitioner may hold the plate and adjust it slightly. The child can be asked which object appears the closest or they may reach out in an attempt to pick it up. Gross stereopsis can be demonstrated by the greatly magnified, three-dimensional appearance of a housefly in the Titmus–Wirt test (*Figure 9.2(b)*). This is probably one of the most commonly used tests, comprising a series of plates consisting of vectographs with right and left pictures polarized at 45° and 135°, which are viewed

TABLE 9.1. Development of visual acuity with age

Age	PL	OKN	VEP	Recognition targets
2 Weeks	2/60	3/60		
1 Month	4/60		360	
2 Months	5/60	4/60	6/60	
3 Months	6/60		6/24	
4 Months	6/60	5/60	6/18	
5 Months		6/60	6/12	
6 Months	6/48	6/36	6/9	
1 Year	6/36			
2 Years	6/18			6/18
3 Years	6/9			6/12
4 Years	6/6			6/9
5 Years	6/5			6/9

The above table shows the development of visual acuity with age converted to Snellen notation. The results for preferential looking (PL) are those drawn from a number of studies (Mayer and Dobson, 1982; Allen, 1979; Gwiazda et al., 1978) whose exact psychophysical procedures vary slightly. Results show some similarity with those obtained for optico-kinetic nystagmus (OKN) by Fantz et al. (1962). Generally, visually evoked potentials (VEP) indicate acuity levels which are higher than those obtained by other methods, e.g. Sokol and Dobson (1976). Clearly the nature of the task is important, studies which involve recognition targets indicating lower acuity levels. The results are those derived from studies by Lippmann (1971), Woodruff (1972) and Roberts and Ludford (1977).

through a suitably polarized spectacle visor. To quantify stereopsis young children can be asked to look at three rows of animals, one of which stands out in each row, demonstrating stereoacuities of 400, 200 and 100 sec arc.

Ophthalmoscopy is best performed towards the end of the examination, by which time the child's confidence in the practitioner should have increased. With some children it is possible to get a very good ophthalmoscopic examination. Other children are less confident and only a brief view of the fundus may be obtained. Although the hydraulic chair may provide sufficient elevation, it is sometimes easier to examine the child with the practitioner seated and the child standing (*Figure 9.1(d)*).

At the end of the examination the practitioner should take care to explain his findings to the parents, indicating the state of health of the child's eyes, their level of vision, and whether or not a spectacle prescription is necessary.

It is generally unnecessary to prescribe spectacles for children with hypermetropia of less than 2.00 D or myopia of less than 1.00 D. Obviously, if a parent describes an occasional convergent squint then a cycloplegic examination should be performed and any significant hypermetropia corrected. Astigmatism of 1.00 D or less need not be corrected, provided it is in the vertical or horizontal meridian. Oblique astigmatism of less than 0.75 D similarly need not be corrected. It is advisable to correct anisometropia of 1.00 D and above.

The indications for a cycloplegic refraction are as follows:

(1) Any fluctuation of accommodation during the examination, seen by variation in the pupil size.
(2) An inability of the child to maintain fixation upon a distance target. It is sometimes easier to perform a cycloplegic refraction and ask the child to look at the retinoscopic light.
(3) Any history of squint.
(4) If a moderate degree of hypermetropia is revealed without a cycloplegic.

The details of cycloplegic refraction are considered in Chapter 10.

It is important then to decide on follow-up visits. If the child is presenting simply for a routine refraction then follow-up visits every 12 months should be satisfactory. If there is any question concerning the child's prescription, or visual acuity, then follow-up visits at 6- or even 3-month intervals should be considered. If spectacles are prescribed it is very important to give explicit instructions to the parents as to when the spectacles should be worn. In the case of a young child it is also important to notify the patient's medical practitioner.

Routine examination of babies or young toddlers

It is relatively unusual for a practitioner to be asked to examine the eyes of a very young baby or toddler. Parents may be concerned about the possibility of eye problems running in the family. Alternatively, they may be concerned that the child appears not to see well, or that the child squints. It is worth remembering that only 50% of squints are readily noticeable (Ingram, 1977). Invariably the child has to be held by a parent and consulting room lights have to be fully on. A young child might tend to hide behind a parent and literally peep at the examiner. The examiner should observe the child, deciding whether the eyes appear straight and normal. It should be remembered that broad epicanthal folds can give the appearance of a convergent squint. Conversely, their presence is no guarantee that a squint is not present. If broad epicanthal folds are present the apparent squint will disappear if the bridge of the nose is pinched slightly. Possibly the only value of the Hirshberg/Krimsky test, in which the location of the first Purkinje image is noted (Hirshberg) and aligned with prisms (Krimsky), is to investigate an apparent squint in a child with epicanthus. The test is otherwise a little coarse, a displacement of 1 mm in the reflected image indicating 20 Δ of squint, by which time it is readily noticeable.

As with older children the practitioner should take careful note of relevant history and signs. Parents can generally tell if the child appears to be seeing well and developing normally (see Chapter 2). With respect to the latter, the practitioner may ask if the infant's height and weight are normal for their age.

It is difficult to be specific about what a baby can see. It is generally held that infants of about 3 months of age have a resolution acuity of around 10 minutes of arc. The limiting factor appears to be the level of neural maturation rather than any optical consideration. It is generally possible to demonstrate fixation as early as 1 month, but some babies refuse to lock on to anything at this early stage. The ability to fix an interesting object is something which tends to develop between 1 and 3 months of age, as does accommodation.

There are a couple of simple tests of vision which can be performed on an infant. The examiner may cover each eye of the child in turn with his hand. As well as checking for the possibility of a squint, the child's response should be observed. If the child's vision is similar in each eye his response will remain unchanged as each eye is covered in turn. If the child's dominant eye is covered and vision in the other eye is poor then the child's response will be immediate. He may move the head, try to remove the cover or just cry. The examiner needs to use some sort of near-fixation target such as a toy, fixation bar or pen torch light.

Another quick test of infant vision is to hold a base-down prism (6 Δ) in front of one eye. If the eye moves upward, the child is clearly using the eye before which the prism has been placed. The examiner should elicit a comparable response from each eye.

A crude test of vision is provided by sprinkling a few candy strands ('hundreds and thousands') onto a clean tissue placed on a flat surface or parent's hand. One of the baby's fingers is moistened and touched onto a single sweet (*Figure 9.3(a)*). The finger is then guided to the child's mouth after which they usually repeat the procedure unaided. Each eye can then be covered in turn to see how the child performs in the monocular site. It should be remembered that the test depends on the child having attained a certain level of manual dexterity, necessitating hand–eye coordination which tends to appear at around 9 months (Sheridan, 1975). Young infants also have a very short attention span. The Catford drum has an oscillating spot which elicits opto-kinetic nystagmus and, thereby,

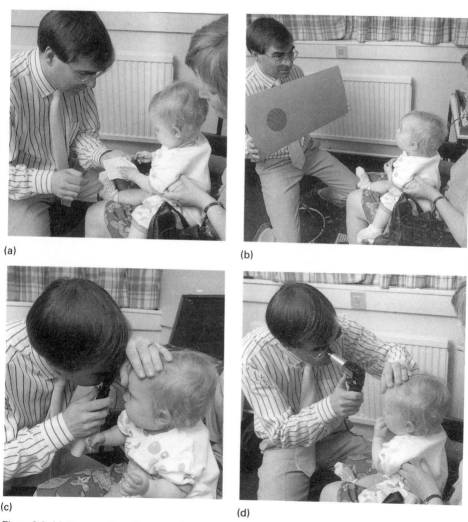

(a)   (b)

(c)   (d)

Figure 9.3. (a) The use of candy strands ('hundreds and thousands') as a crude estimate of infant vision. (b) The Keeler acuity cards provide a good estimate of infant acuity even without the use of the folding 'puppet screen'. (c) An infant may allow the practitioner to get close enough to perform direct ophthalmoscopy. (d) The AO indirect ophthalmoscope can be useful if the infant is dilated.

provides an assessment of acuity. Acuity is estimated from the smallest spot which continues to give OKN. Standardization, however, is poor with a tendency to markedly overestimate acuities in emmetropes and myopes.

As before, detailed discussion of methods of assessing acuity are contained in Chapter 8. The procedure most suitable for babies is preferential looking. Fantz (1958) described that an infant, of 6 months of age or younger, presented with two simultaneous objects in a distraction-free environment will tend to look at the most interesting of the two. The child is confronted with two objects, one a plain grey field and the other a grating pattern of equivalent mean luminance, for a brief period – early studies used 30-second exposure. The observer notes which object the child prefers to look at and the spatial frequency of the grating is increased until no preference is indicated by the baby (*Figure 9.3(b)*). This indicates that the baby no longer resolves the fine spatial detail of the grating since the lines are too thin to be differentiated from the plain grey field. Fantz defined acuity as the narrowest stripe (highest spatial frequency) that attracted the attention of 75% or more of the infants of that age. The Keeler acuity cards are a standard test based on these principles (*Figure 9.2(a)*). A more simple approach suitable for the consulting room is that of the Teller Cards which are simply held by the practitioner in front of the child (Teller, 1979). Preferential looking is most useful for babies between 1 and 6 months of age, since older infants become bored and too active (Atkinson *et al.*, 1982). Under 1 year of age satisfactory results can be obtained in around 97% of infants, but care must be taken with the ambient lighting. It may require a fair degree of practice to judge which card a rather active infant is fixing.

A version of preferential looking can be used in older non-verbal or neurologically impaired children where the child points or runs to the target to gain a reward. This is termed alley running.

Another useful test for young children is the Lang stereo test picture, described earlier. A positive result is indicated when the child attempts to reach out and grasp one of the objects. The eye movements of a child should also be observed. Stereoscopic clues disappear when the test card is held vertically. Hence a preferential looking technique can be used by positioning one test card horizontally and the other vertically. If the test indicates that a reasonably good level of stereopsis is present there is a fair likelihood of good vision in each eye, although infants with moderate amblyopia may be able to judge depth.

Objective assessment of refractive error

Some estimates of the refractive error present in babies may be obtained from the Bruckner Test. The ophthalmoscope light is directed at the child from a distance of 30 cm so that the light falls on both eyes. The practitioner should note an immediate pupil reflex, the position of the corneal reflex, together with the colour of the reflected light. The reflected light should be equal in colour and brightness in both eyes, any inequality indicating anisometropia.

Retinoscopy can be rather difficult to perform on young children and babies. Accommodation can fluctuate markedly and it is difficult for a child to maintain fixation for any length of time. In addition, relatively large pupil sizes tend to give distorted reflexes. The technique advocated by Mohindra (1975), and described earlier, may prove useful if performed in subdued light. Young babies were found to be most cooperative if retinoscopy was performed whilst they were being fed or given a pacifier. The young child fixes the retinoscope light almost automatically. It may be possible only for the practitioner to hold one pair of lenses in front of the baby's eyes to make a swift assessment of the refractive error. It should be borne in mind that some refractive errors in children may abate with time. It has been observed that most infants, of less than 1 year, exhibit considerable hypermetropia and astigmatism (see Chapter 7). It is generally found that over the following years there is a loss of astigmatism and emmetropinization of ametropia. Undoubtedly, skilled retinoscopy is the most sensitive and accurate objective method of assessing the refractive state of the eye. In this age group, if no reliable method of assessing acuity is possible and the eyes appear straight, the assessment of refractive error is the major indicator of normality. Objective methods of assessing acuity are described in Chapter 8.

Another useful objective method of assessing refractive error is that of isotropic photorefraction, a technique designed for rapid screening of a large number of children by unqualified staff. It involves a simple attachment to a wide aperture lens (F/1.2, 50 mm) of a standard 35 mm single lens reflex camera. This incorporates a fibreoptic light guide directing the electronic flash along the optic axis of the camera toward the patient's eyes. Light reflected from the fundus makes the pupils appear brightly illuminated on the subsequent photographs. Initially the camera is focused on the eyes of the baby who sits 75 cm away. This enables the pupil size to be measured, since it influences blur circle size, and the position of the corneal reflexes can be judged. The baby's eyes must be aligned with the camera axis, so the photographer has to stand behind the camera and attract the child's attention. Two additional photographs are then taken with the camera focused at 150 cm and 50 cm (i.e. 0.67 D in front and behind the child). If the eyes are hypermetropic relative to the working distance a smaller blur circle is obtained in the second photograph (focused at 150 cm) compared to the third (set at 50 cm) since the eyes are then focused behind the camera. In myopia the reverse is true. An elliptical blur circle indicates astigmatism. The technique can be used with or without a cycloplegic. The technique is said to compare well with retinoscopy, although the photorefractive estimates of hypermetropia tend to be lower than the retinoscopic values, necessitating a correction factor.

The large pupil size of children tends to permit a reasonable ophthalmoscopic view of the fundus, although the working distance may have to be somewhat long. Indirect ophthalmoscopy has been described as being useful for examining children because it is relatively unaffected by eye movements.

As always, findings should be discussed with the child's parents, who may need to be reassured. Obviously it is important that significant refractive errors are identified early to avoid poor preschool visual problems due to strabismus and amblyopia. Even a partial refractive correction worn during the early years reduces the incidence of strabismus and amblyopia. Nevertheless, the difficulty in getting a young child to wear any form of optical correction cannot be minimized and, unless absolutely necessary, is best avoided. Frequent review may be necessary to investigate whether the refractive error is stable. It is advisable to make several assessments of the refractive error on separate occasions before deciding on a refractive correction.

Routine examination of the school age child (over 5 years of age)

As the child becomes older the routine has a fairly similar pattern to that of an adult, but its extent will depend upon the child's span of concentration. This, together with the child's need to build up confidence in the practitioner, suggests that ophthalmoscopy is best performed towards the end of the examination. As with younger children the practitioner needs to assess how much ground can be covered in a single consultation. If further investigation of a particular aspect is indicated during the examination it may be useful to arrange a further consultation at a later date.

Children are often better behaved when they enter the consulting room on their own, thus deprived of an audience. It is preferable to move to this situation as quickly as possible. Practitioners need to be flexible about this because some children, whatever their age, are more comfortable when accompanied by an adult and their wishes should be respected.

The practitioner should engage the child in conversation early in the examination, putting them at ease and not discussing them as though they were not present. In this way history and symptoms should be established, as before, by speaking to both parent and child. The examiner should strive to establish a rapport with the child as well as their parent.

Initially the vision of each eye should be established, together with the cover test at distance and near. If the child is big enough a trial frame, preferably a lightweight one, can be used. Even so, this should be worn for as short a time as possible. As with younger children, an interesting fixation target reduces the natural tendency for the child to gaze around the room.

Attempts at a subjective refraction depend on the age of the patient. With young children the examiner needs to assess the quality of their subjective responses in order to decide what degree of reliance may be placed upon them. A young child often responds quite well to the cross-cylinder technique, but needs to be presented with clear, simple choices. The spherical element should, therefore, be varied in 0.50 DS steps and a 1.00 D interval cross-cylinder used. Older children whose visual acuity has attained optimal levels, and whose level of concentration is rather greater, can give very accurate subjective responses particularly if they are familiar with the routine.

The visual acuity of the majority of children within this age group can be determined in the usual way. The acquisition of reading skills is very variable. Many children will know the letters of the alphabet, particularly in lower case, before entering school. Some children continue to identify upper case (capital) letters phonetically for some time after starting school. If a child hesitates over a letter, the practitioner should ask if they can identify an equivalent larger letter. If the child continues to hesitate they should be asked if they can remember the name of the letter or the sound it makes. Some practitioners give children a key-card to hold displaying a circular arrangement of letters identical to those contained on the 6/6 or 6/9 Snellen lines. The key-card can be made from large print 'Letraset'. As with the Sheridan–Gardiner test the child simply matches the letters of the Snellen line with those on the key-card.

In addition to observing the usual binocular responses with a cover test, an attempt should be made at quantifying the degree of stereopsis which is present. A number of useful tests are available for children in this age group although, with care and depending upon the child, those designed for adults may be used successfully. After demonstrating the stereoscopic view of the housefly and observing the three rows of animals in the Titmus–Wirt test, stereoacuity can be measured. The test uses a series of nine pictures each having four rings, one of which appears to stand out, requiring stereopsis of between 800 and 40 sec arc. The Randot stereo test works in a similar fashion and can measure levels of stereopsis of between 400 and 20 sec arc. The TNO stereo test uses anaglyphic separation in which separate monocular images are printed in red and green ink on a white background. The child wears a red and green filter before each eye so that stereopsis of between 480 and 15 sec arc can be tested. The Frisby stereotest is useful for young children in that it does not require a visor to be worn. Stereo separation is achieved by printing the peripheral and central portions of a random pattern on the front and back surfaces of a perspex sheet. Different levels of stereopsis may be measured by varying the thickness of the perspex sheet. Stereoacuity can be tested at 340, 170 and 55 sec arc when used at 40 cm (*Figure 9.2(b)*).

Colour plays an increasingly important role in teaching and there is some value in establishing the normality, or otherwise, of children's colour vision. This is particularly important in boys, because of their greater frequency of colour vision defects. This is dealt with in detail in Chapter 12.

Children in this age group are generally fairly cooperative when performing ophthalmoscopy. The practitioner should explain that a bright light is to be shone into the eyes and that this is the last part of the examination. An interesting fixation target will help the child to look straight ahead rather than at the ophthalmoscope light. The pupil reactions may be tested at this point whilst the external eye is being examined. The pathological conditions which may be encountered in children are dealt with in Chapter 4 and mention is also made of those associated with chronic disorders of childhood in Chapter 3.

Older children, for a variety of reasons, can sometimes claim to have poor vision for which there is no basis in fact. There are a number of ways of assessing whether the acuity levels are the best that the child can achieve. It is possible to test at different distances, place two lenses in the trial frame which combine to give plano, or place a blurring lens before one eye whilst testing the acuity of the other. These serve to indicate the inconsistencies of the patient's responses.

At the conclusion of the consultation the findings need to be summarized for both parent and child. It is important that the child should not be ignored in this procedure and if spectacles are necessary it must be made clear when they should be worn. It may be preferable to explain findings to the child who is then free to leave the consulting room, after which the practitioner may freely talk to the parent. This is especially so when discussing the prognosis which may be, in both the child's and parent's view, rather depressing. It should be remembered that it can be very uncomfortable for a child to be the object of a conversation without being able to participate.

Obviously there are many clinical factors which have to be borne in mind when deciding whether to prescribe spectacles. Provided there is no amblyopia to be overcome, or squint, it is useful for spectacle wear to be introduced gradually. This allows the child, and their school friends, to adapt to the change in appearance which the spectacles bring. It also allows the child to determine for themselves the situations in which the spectacles are most useful.

As with young children, it is difficult to be specific about degrees of ametropia which should be corrected. With older children this can be more readily related to their symptoms. It should be borne in mind that the school work undertaken by older children is visually more demanding. The impact of a particular refractive error, however, undoubtedly depends upon a number of physiological factors specific to individuals. It is also useful to bear in mind the likely development of refractive errors considered in Chapter 7. Unilateral refractive errors should be corrected to avoid amblyopia, as should astigmatism, particularly when oblique, in excess of 0.50 D. Slightly more latitude is possible with regular astigmatism. Myopia of 0.50 D and above can cause problems with school work if viewing work on a chalkboard.

Young children can overcome a fair degree of hypermetropia and it may only be necessary to prescribe for errors in excess of + 1.50 D. The conditions under which a cycloplegic refraction should be performed have been discussed earlier.

Normally children should be examined every 12 months. Six-month intervals may be advisable for children for whom spectacles have been prescribed, or those whose results are in some way questionable. When spectacles are prescribed for the first time it is advisable to notify the child's medical practitioner and their teacher. In the case of the latter it is useful to specify under what conditions the spectacles should be worn.

References

ALLEN, J. (1979). Visual acuity development in human infants up to 6 months of age. Doctoral dissertation, University of Washington. University of Michigan Microfilms, Ann Arbor, Michigan.

ATKINSON, J., BRADDICK, O., DURDEN, K., WATSON, P.G. and ATKINSON, S. (1984). Screening for refractive errors in 6–9 month old infants by photorefraction. *British Journal of Ophthalmology*, **68**, 105–112.

ATKINSON, J., BRADDICK, O. and PIMM SMITH, E. (1982). Preferential looking for monocular and binocular acuity testing of infants. *British Journal of Ophthalmology*, **66**, 264–268.

FANTZ, R.L. (1958). Pattern vision in young infants. *Psychological Review*, **8**, 43–47.

FANTZ, R., ORDY, J. and UDELF, M. (1962). Maturation of pattern vision in infants during the first six months of life. *Journal of Comparative Physiology and Psychology*, **55**, 907–917.

GRAHAM, P.A. (1974). Epidemiology of strabismus. *British Journal of Ophthalmology*, **58**, 224–231.

GWIAZDA, J., BRILL, S., MOHINDRA, I. and HELD, R. (1978). Infant visual acuity and its meridional variation. *Vision Research*, **18**, 1557–1564.

INGRAM, R.M. (1977). The problem of screening children for visual defects. *British Journal of Ophthalmology*, **61**, 4–7.

INGRAM, R.M., WALKER, C., WILSON, J.M., ARNOLD, P.E. and DALLY, S. (1986) Prediction of amblyopia and squint by means of refraction at age 1 year. *British Journal of Ophthalmology*, **70**, 12–15.

LIPPMANN, O. (1971). Vision screening of young children. *American Journal of Public Health*, **61**, 1586–1601.

MARG, E. *et al.* (1976). Visual acuity development in human infants. *Investigative Ophthalmology*, **15**, 150–153.

MAYER, D.L. and DOBSON, V. (1982). Visual acuity development in infants and young children, as assessed by operant preferential looking. *Vision Research*, **22**, 1141–1151.

MOHINDRA, I. (1975). A technique for infant vision examination. *American Journal of Optometry and Physiological Optics*, **52**, 867–870.

MOHINDRA, I. (1977). Comparison of near retinoscopy and subjective refraction in adults. *American Journal of Optometry and Physiological Optics*, **54**, 319–322.

ROBERTS, J. and LUDFORD, J. (1977). Monocular visual acuity of persons 4–74 years. Vital Health Stats. Series 11 (No. 201). pp. 1–31.

SCHWARTING, B.H. (1954). Testing infants' vision: an apparatus for estimating the visual acuity of infants and young children. *American Journal of Ophthalmology*, **38**, 714.

SHERIDAN, M. (1975). *Children's Development Progress*, 3rd edn. NFER Publishing Company, Windsor, pp. 30–37.

SOKOL, S. and DOBSON, V. (1976). Pattern reversal visually evoked potential in infants. *Investigative Ophthalmology*, **15**, 58–62.

TELLER, D.Y. (1979). The forced-choice preferential looking procedure: a psychophysical technique for use with human infants. *Infant Behaviour and Development*, **2**, 135–153.

WOODRUFF, M.E. (1972). Observations on the visual acuity of children during the first five years of life. *American Journal of Optometry and Archives of the American Academy of Optometry*, **49**, 205–215.

10

Cycloplegic refraction

A.R. Shakespeare

Selection of cases

Cycloplegic agents are of inestimable value in the examination of children, particularly when binocular vision is at risk from incorrect assessment of refractive error. It follows, therefore, that any practitioner who feels unable or unwilling to use drugs should not undertake the examination of all children. Where initial screening suggests that the full refractive error must be established the child should be referred to another practitioner for cycloplegic refraction.

Not every child presenting for examination will require the use of a cycloplegic drug. If, for example, examination is requested on the grounds of a family history of myopia, the absence of this condition is usually easily established by retinoscopy even in the young child. Should unaided vision prove to be equal in each eye and appropriate to the age of the patient, the eyes appear healthy externally and internally and binocular vision seems to be present and stable, there is little point in instilling drugs. It is important that this initial examination may be remembered by the child as a pleasant experience during which interest has been maintained in a series of 'games' by a non-threatening clinician. Should a cycloplegic examination become necessary at a later date, the rapport already established is of great value.

The decision to use drugs will depend on a number of factors which may need to be weighed individually and in concert:

Family history

Ametropia particularly hypermetropia, squint or treatment for binocular problems, amblyopia, squint surgery or the onset of any visual problem especially at school or preschool age should be noted in close blood relatives. Relevant history in parents and siblings is of great import.

Patient history

In the case of the very young child a lot will depend on the observation of parents or others who spend time with the child, and of necessity much will be anecdotal. Health visitors and clinic nurses have their part of play and, at school age, the observation of teachers is usually accurate and objective. Learning difficulties and behavioural problems may well be related to visual difficulty and the teacher is well placed and properly trained to monitor progress in the classroom.

Difficulty with, or rejection of close work; poor hand–eye coordination during craft work or play; or slow reading ability in the young child, may suggest hypermetropia and possible binocular instability.

With increasing age, the risk of incipient myopia increases and the teacher is frequently the first to notice difficulty when the child is copying from the chalkboard.

Pre-cycloplegic examination

The nature and extent of the initial examination will, of course, depend on the age, attention span and cooperation of the child. History will usually be presented by a parent or guardian and the factors mentioned above should be taken into account. Where history or examination gives evidence of squint the possibility of injury during delivery should be borne in mind and it should be established whether the pregnancy and birth were normal.

Examination of the external eye and anterior segment can usually be achieved without difficulty even in the young child, and at the same time, pupil reactions which will normally be active except in the neonate or very young infant, may be noted for direct and consensual response. Eliciting a near reflex may be a little more difficult in the babe in arms although this is possible with a little ingenuity. For example, a favourite toy may be brought in to view from behind the patient. In the same way devices to attract and maintain distance fixation for short periods are required in order to undertake a satisfactory cover test. Comprehensive examination of the fundus may not be possible in the uncooperative child but it is usually possible to see discs and maculae. Given the right approach, most toddlers will permit ophthalmoscopy and, at school age, little difficulty should be experienced with these checks.

A whole battery of tests is available for estimation of visual acuity and every effort should be made to establish whether the acuity is normal for the age. It is especially important to know if there is a difference between the two eyes.

Retinoscopy should be attempted however young the child may be. Surprisingly accurate results can be obtained at this stage and the technique is a particularly useful indicator of the need for cycloplegic help. Examination should not be protracted, the aim being to make a rapid estimation of refractive error and to note the presence and degree of fluctuation in accommodation. If, on balance, it seems that cycloplegic examination will not be required, the retinoscopy result may be refined prior to any subjective tests.

The precycloplegic examination should, where possible, include a careful cover test, amplitude of accommodation, muscle balances or any other measurement which may be required to establish binocular status. Some of these tests may be repeated under cycloplegia to establish any change caused by the reduced amplitude of accommodation.

Cycloplegic drugs

Pharmacology

All cycloplegic drugs are antagonistic to the effects of acetylcholine, the neural mediator of the parasympathetic branch of the autonomic nervous system.

Parasympathetic innervation supplies the ciliary muscle and the sphincter pupillae muscle via the ciliary ganglion. Postganglionic nerve impulses cause a release of acetylcholine at the effector cell thereby causing contraction of the related muscle fibre. This muscle contraction produces accommodation via the ciliary muscle and miosis via the sphincter. It is true of the parasympathetic system generally that the ratio of postganglionic to preganglionic fibres is much lower than that found in the sympathetic system and this tends to give very precise control. Precision is enhanced by the fact that free acetylcholine is rapidly inactivated by the enzyme acetylcholinesterase.

Receptors in the parasympathetic system are classified according to their response to nicotine or muscarine and both ciliary and sphincter muscles are muscarinic in action. For this reason cycloplegic drugs are usually given the more precise definition 'antimuscarinic' rather than the more general description 'anticholinergic'.

Drugs which act on receptors to enhance the effect of acetylcholine are known as agonists and those which inhibit this action are known as antagonists. By virtue of a molecular structure which is similar to that of acetylcholine, antagonists occupy receptor sites without producing any pharmacological action. It should also be understood that the bond between acetylcholine and receptor is of very short duration whereas that between antagonist and receptor is much stronger and therefore of much greater duration. Variation in this bond strength seems to account for the variability in effect which is observable in different cycloplegics.

Choice of cycloplegic agent

Although a large range of drugs is available for cycloplegic examination a sensible approach would suggest that three agents will meet the needs of the optometrist and that one of these, cyclopentolate hydrochloride, will be used on most occasions since this drug will produce predictable and adequate cycloplegia even in relatively young children and, using weaker strengths, it may be used safely throughout the cycloplegic age range.

For children under the age of six or in other cases demanding potent cycloplegia, for example heavily pigmented eyes, atropine sulphate is the drug of choice.

At the other end of the scale tropicamide hydrochloride is a useful agent when modest cycloplegic effect will suffice.

Atropine sulphate

Availability and presentation

- Atropine Eye Drops 1% 10 ml.
- Atropine Eye Ointment 1% 3 g.
- Isopto Atropine (Alcon), eye drops 1%, hypromellose 0.5% 5 ml.
- Minims Atropine Sulphate (Smith & Nephew) 1% 20 × 0.5 ml.
- Opulets Atropine Sulphate (Alcon) 1% 20 × 0.5 ml.

Atropine is the most potent drug used by the optometrist and the most toxic. Since atropine is usually used for the examination of very young children ointment is preferred to watery drops. It is normally instilled, by the parent rather than the practitioner, two times per day for 3 days prior to the examination. Watery drops may drain via the puncti into the nasal mucosa. Significant systemic absorption can then take place which may lead to poisoning. Greasy ointments block the puncti thereby eliminating this risk.

Atropine is a Prescription only Medicine (PoM) and is obtained by issuing a signed order to the parent for presentation to the pharmacist. The signed order should contain the following information:

- Name and address of practitioner (use headed notepaper).
- Date.
- Name and address of patient.
- Age of patient.
- Purpose for which the drug is to be used ('for cycloplegic refraction').
- The quantity and strength to be supplied ('please supply Atropine Eye Ointment BP, 1% 3 g').
- Label: To be instilled morning and evening into both right and left eyes, on the days prior to the day of the eye examination, as directed.
- Signature of optometrist ....

Since a 3-g tube of ointment is fairly small, labelling instructions may be modified to 'to be used as directed', in which case a demonstration of instillation technique for the benefit of the parent may be accompanied by full written instructions.

The written instructions should, in addition to indicating the dosage, stress the poisonous nature of the ointment and the effect that even a trace of the ointment transferred to the eye of an adult may have in dilating the pupil. Supplementary advice may therefore be given along the following lines:

(1) The hands should be washed before and after each instillation.
(2) Any excess ointment should be removed from the lids with a clean tissue which should be destroyed.
(3) Any unused ointment should be destroyed.
(4) Between instillations, the tube should be kept in a secure place out of the reach of children.
(5) No ointment should be instilled on the morning of the examination (it produces a greasy retinoscopy reflex).
(6) Apart from widely dilated pupils and difficulty with close work, any unusual change in the child's appearance or manner should be reported at once and the use of the ointment discontinued.

This system of obtaining the drug and of instruction to the parent apply only to atropine. All other agents used by the optometrist are for office use and the system of supply is simpler (see later notes).

Complications

Although complications in the use of atropine sulphate are rare, two possibilities must be considered. First, and most likely, atropine, in common with any other drug, may produce an allergic response. The patient may suffer conjunctival injection, puffiness or swelling of the lids and a general histaminic response of the facial skin, which may show 'track marks' where tears have run down the cheek. This condition will clear after cessation of treatment but if the effect is severe, treatment with antihistamines, preferably systemic, may be required.

The second possibility is, of course, that of atropine poisoning which could only happen as a result of accidental ingestion of the ointment. Havener (1974) states that the fatal dose of atropine is about 100 mg for adults and 10 mg for children. It should therefore be remembered that a 3-g tube of 1% ointment contains 30 mg of atropine sulphate. Profound systemic reactions may be produced by ingestion of a very modest quantity of ointment.

The symptoms of atropine poisoning include:

- Dry mouth and throat, difficulty in swallowing.
- Severe thirst.
- Dry, hot and flushed skin. Fever and possibly a rash over the face, neck and upper trunk.
- Tachycardia, irritability or delirium.
- Rapid breathing. Possibly nausea and vomiting.

Where atropine poisoning is suspected transfer the child, as an emergency, to medical supervision at once. Telephone the hospital and advise the casualty officer that the child is en route and advise him or her of your suspicions.

- Do not delay matters by attempting to give an antidote.
- Do not give any emetic or make any other attempt to induce vomiting.

Instillation technique

Atropine ointment may be instilled directly into the lower fornix from the tube, or may be transferred to the eye with the aid of an ointment rod. The latter method is recommended as being safer and more predictable.

A short glass rod, the end of which has been fully smoothed in a flame, is first sterilized then rinsed and dried on a clean tissue. Milton (normal strength) or other hypochlorite solution, diluted in the ratio 1 : 10, is very suitable for this purpose.

As an alternative to the glass rod, disposable applicators individually packaged in a sealed, sterile envelope are now available from: Henleys Medical Supplies Ltd, Brownfields, Welwyn Garden City, Herts AL7 1AN. Telephone: 0707 333164.

A small quantity of the ointment, about the size of a grape pip, is squeezed onto the end of the rod. With the child looking upward, the lower lid is drawn away from the eye and the rod is gently placed in the lower fornix (*Figure 10.1(a)*). With the eye still directed upwards, the lower lid is released and, with a slow twisting action, the rod is removed (*Figure 10.1(b)*). The patient is then asked to close the eyes and the lids are gently massaged to spread the ointment evenly around the fornices. Little, if any, ointment should be lost but after repeating this procedure in the other eye the lids should be wiped with a tissue.

If a rod is not available, a short string of the ointment may be squeezed into the lower fornix and the flow broken against the lid margin. The eye should again be directed in an upward gaze. Prior to instillation a few millimetres of ointment should be discarded onto a tissue in case the neck of the tube has become contaminated. It is a wise precaution to thoroughly wipe the neck of the tube with a clean tissue immediately after use.

The suggestion has been made that instillation should be carried out when the child is sleeping, presumably in an effort to minimize distress. Although this may be possible with some children, there must be an element of risk attached to this method since the child may be disturbed and make a sudden, rapid and unforeseen movement, thereby increasing the chance of trauma. Instillation, with a little cooperation from the patient, is not a particularly stressful exercise and, following a demonstration by the practitioner, most parents can accomplish this task easily.

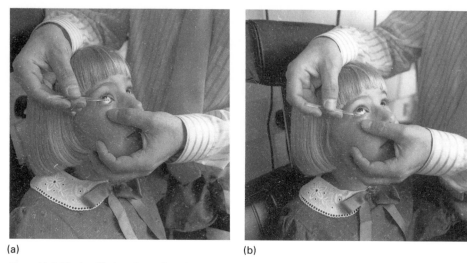

(a)   (b)

Figure 10.1. The instillation of atropine ointment. With the child looking upward, the rod containing the ointment is placed in the lower fornix (a). The lower lid is released and the rod removed with a slow twisting action (b). The lids are gently massaged to spread the ointment.

Refractive technique

Prior to refraction a brief external examination should be carried out. The atropinized patient should have a bright, clear, corneal reflex, thereby indicating that no ointment has been instilled in the last few hours. The pupils should be widely dilated and may even appear to be slightly decentred. No pupil reflex of any kind should be elicited. If pupil movement, however slight, can be detected, instillation has been far from adequate and it is virtually certain that cycloplegia is incomplete. The parent should be given further instruction and an appointment arranged for a later date.

Since atropine is normally only used for young children, objective assessment of refractive error assumes paramount importance. The precise method of examination will depend on the age of the patient and the likelihood of securing cooperation. A very young child should be seated on the mother's lap and no attempt should be made to use a trial frame. It is vital that the patient should retain a feeling of security in what may seem to be a hostile environment and the close proximity of the mother, who may help by supporting and steadying the child's head, is important.

Retinoscopy is then carried out by simply holding lenses in front of the eye under examination. The spherical component of the prescription is usually quickly established and this, now combined with trial cylinders, is used to determine astigmatism. With very little practice, axes can be estimated accurately and, if difficulty is experienced, the lens combination can be carried down to the desk and compared to the trial frame protractor. Care should be taken not to change the orientation of the lenses during this transfer.

Aberrations may in some patients be obtrusive. Because the pupils are so large, the peripheral zone may indicate an error which differs from that seen at the centre of the pupil. The effect, seen with a streak retinoscope, is of the streak bending or flexing at the periphery due to the differential speed or direction of movement.

Paradoxically, a peripheral movement 'with' the main one indicates a negative aberration and one that moves 'against' the central trend is a positive aberration. The entire area available should therefore be used only to assess the axis of astigmatism and the central zone of 3–4 mm only should be observed when assessing power.

Although the above instructions may sound fraught with difficulty, the ease with which most cycloplegic refractions on very young children can be carried out usually comes as a pleasant surprise. The patient may be encouraged to look at the retinoscope mirror and refraction is therefore carried out along the visual axes. Accommodation should be entirely absent, there are no pupil reflexes and the image from the dilated pupil is bright and clear. The procedure is therefore normally completed very quickly and well within the attention span of the patient.

Should there appear to be any variation in the refractive error during retinoscopy, some accommodational activity must be suspected and the parent again questioned about instillation technique.

In the case of the slightly older child, perhaps 4 to 6 years old, a lightweight trial frame may be used. An alternative may be created by using an ordinary children's frame to which Halberg clips have been attached.

Prescribing

TONUS ALLOWANCE

The ciliary muscle has both dependent and independent tone; since the latter is small it can be discounted for clinical purposes. However, the dependent tone which exists so long as the nerve supply is intact, is affected by the antimuscarinic effect of atropine and the prescription evolved therefore gives rise to an overprescription in the hypermetrope. *Table 10.1* may be used as a guide in order to adjust the final prescription.

It must be stressed that only the sphere should be modified on this basis and that, in any event, the final prescription remains a clinical decision. An accommodative squint in a very young child may respond better to the full atropine findings since the world of the very young is largely restricted to interest in near objects and maximal relaxation of accommodation is vital.

ASTIGMATISM

Astigmatism should, in the opinion of the writer, be corrected in full. The main object of undertaking a cycloplegic refraction is to deliver to each retina an image which is as clear as possible. Young patients do not usually suffer the problems of

TABLE 10.1. Tonus allowance when using atropine

Retinoscopy result	Modification to sphere	Resultant sphere
+6.00	−1.00	+5.00
+3.00	−1.00	+2.00
+1.00	−1.00	Plano
−1.00	−1.00	−2.00
−2.00	−0.50	−2.50
−3.00	0.00	−3.00
−4.00	0.00	−4.00

adaptation which may affect the adult who is suddenly presented with a dramatic change in retinal image size or form.

HYPERMETROPIA

Where a squint is associated with accommodative effort there is little doubt that a full correction should be prescribed independently of the age of the patient. If adaptive problems seem possible, particularly when high levels of previously uncorrected hypermetropia must be taken into account, spectacles should be made up as quickly as possible so that the patient may start wearing them before the effects of atropinization have worn off (see later). However a full correction is not always required. Prescribing should be directed towards the stabilization of binocular vision and the elimination of the presenting symptoms. If, with a reduced prescription, the cover test shows modest movement with rapid recovery or, better still, no movement at distance or near, a reduction of 0.75 D or 1.00 D is entirely justified. Adaptation and patient compliance are likely to be improved by this allowance.

MYOPIA

In recent years a number of workers have suggested that myopia may be controlled by undercorrection, particularly for reading. Since these theories have not gained total acceptance it seems appropriate in this section to suggest that although great care should be exercised in order to avoid overcorrection of the myopic child, the primary duty of the prescriber is to give the patient an acceptably high acuity. Lacking clear distance vision the child will be seriously disadvantaged at school and in playing many games. This seems to many clinicians to be an unacceptable penalty to impose during formative years. However, an increasing number of practitioners may be prepared to consider the provision of a bifocal correction for the young myope. Interested readers may wish to consider the evidence put forward by Kelly *et al.* (1975), Oakley and Young (1975) and others.

If conventional wisdom is to be followed a full correction must be consistent with attainment of binocularity and should not produce high levels of esotropia, particularly where this may give rise to decompensation.

Postcycloplegic examination

In some circumstances it may be advisable to conduct a postcycloplegic examination to establish the probable effect of the prescription on acuity or binocular stability. Should this be necessary 7–10 days will elapse before accommodation returns to normal and mydriasis may be present for 14 days or more. Parents should be warned of this duration and the possibility of photophobia.

Older children

Over the age of six, more information is usually available from the precycloplegic examination and full cycloplegia is rarely required. Weaker cycloplegics having a shorter duration of action may therefore be used. It is important in children of school age that the period of inhibition of close work should be kept as short as possible consistent with obtaining accurate results. Two cycloplegic agents are commonly used for this purpose and are described below.

Cyclopentolate hydrochloride

This synthetic drug first marketed in the 1950s is, by far, the most widely used agent for cycloplegia. Priestley and Medine (1951) suggested criteria for the ideal cycloplegic which include: (1) rapid effect; (2) extensive action; (3) prompt recovery; (4) complete dissociation of cycloplegic and mydriatic effects; and (5) no adverse local or systemic effects. They considered that cyclopentolate (then known as Compound 75 G.T.) more closely approached their ideal criteria than any other drug discovered up to that time. O'Connor Davies (1981) supports this conclusion and no drug has been marketed since then which provides the almost universal usefulness of cyclopentolate.

It should be stated that although it is possible to produce mydriasis with little or no cycloplegia, no available drug will produce cycloplegia without mydriasis and given the pharmacology of action it is difficult to imagine any drug which could do so.

Adverse local or systemic effects are possible with any drug and cyclopentolate hydrochloride which is normally buffered to around pH 5 in order to maintain stability in storage, will give rise to a mild burning or stinging sensation on instillation. Various writers have also reported temporary behavioural problems or personality changes following the use of cyclopentolate. Apt and Gaffney (1976) suggest that visual and tactile hallucinations are more common with cyclopentolate than atropine and psychotic reactions have been reported by Beswick (1962), Simcoe (1962) and Havener (1974). Lest the British reader should feel alarmed by these reports it must be stressed that all originate in the USA where greater strengths and higher doses of the drug are used than are common in the UK.

Availability and presentation

UK:

- Minims Cyclopentolate Hydrochloride (Smith & Nephew) 0.5% and 1% 20 × 0.5 ml.
- Mydrilate (Boehringer Ingleheim) 0.5% and 1% 5 ml.
- Opulets Cyclopentolate Hydrochloride (Alcon) 1% 20 × 0.5 ml. *Legal category:* PoM.

USA:

- Cyclogyl (Alcon).
- Ak-Pentolate (Akorn, Inc.).

Mydrilate is a multidose presentation, 5 ml being contained in a useful squeeze bottle which makes instillation convenient and easy. Care should be taken that the tip of the pipette does not touch the lid in order to avoid contamination and the risk of cross-infection between one patient and another. In any event, in clinic use, the eyedrops should be discarded 7 days after being opened. The expiry date given on the pack refers only to the shelf-life of the unopened dispenser. In a busy office where cycloplegic examination is undertaken frequently this presentation is useful and cost-effective.

Minims and Opulets are each single-dose applicators which are presented in packs of 20 and are convenient for the practitioner who uses drugs infrequently. The shelf-life is excellent but it should be stressed that each applicator is intended for use on one patient only and, since they contain no antimicrobial preservatives, they should be discarded immediately after use.

Instillation technique

Proper delivery of the drug to the eye is important in order to minimize the amount required, to secure a balanced dose to each eye thereby facilitating accurate comparison between the two. Careful instillation also avoids the risk of causing toxic systemic effects.

Good instillation using the right hand for the dropper can be achieved by standing on the left of the patient. The delivery hand may then be rested on the forehead of the patient to securely position the pipette immediately above the eye to be instilled and as near to the eye as possible without touching the lids or fornices (*Figure 10.2*). With the head tilted backwards the patient should be directed to look upward and the practitioner's left thumb or forefinger used to gently draw the lower lid away from the eye. The drop should then be squeezed into the lower fornix. The pipette should avoid the sweep of the lashes and, after drop delivery, the patient should be asked to look down. The cornea is thus bathed in the pool of solution contained by the lower fornix. The lower lid should then be released slowly and in a controlled manner thereby retaining most or all of the drop. Some lachrymation may be produced by cyclopentolate and a clean tissue should be at hand to blot the lids if necessary. In order to retain as much of the drop as possible and to reduce the risk of systemic effects, a nasolacrimal block should be applied by squeezing the nose between finger and thumb in the region of the canaliculi and exerting a slight pressure back towards the inner canthi. This block should be held for 1–2 minutes.

Dosage and strength

Cyclopentolate, although having a relatively short duration, is a powerful antimuscarinic and, in a Caucasian patient, will produce deep cycloplegia on

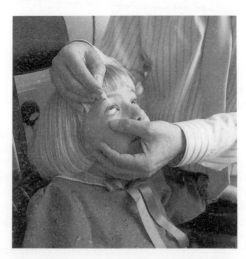

Figure 10.2. The installation of cycloplegic eyedrops. Standing to the left of the patient, the right hand can be rested on the forehead. The lower lid is drawn away from the eye with the other hand.

instillation of a single drop. In general the 1% strength should be used up to the age of 13 years, and 0.5% above this age. The degree of pigmentation in the eye is however of great relevance and will affect decisions about dosage and strength.

All drugs capable of penetrating the cornea to affect intrinsic structures may, in varying degrees, become 'bound' to melanin thereby reducing or slowing the supply to the neuroeffector sites. It may therefore be observed clinically that the same dose applied to eyes of differing pigmentation produces a differential effect. In the lightly pigmented eye the effect is quicker and, usually, more profound. The age range given above may therefore be shaded so that an 11-year-old patient with pale blue eyes may respond sufficiently to the 0.5% strength whereas at 17, a patient with very heavy pigmentation may need 1% for adequate cycloplegia. By the same token, the 8-year-old, Asian child may require two drops of the 1% solution. If in doubt the lower strength or dose should be given to be followed by a second drop if necessary. It is a sound general principle to use the minimum quantity of any drug consistent with producing the required effect.

Refractive procedure

Following instillation the eyes should be inspected after about 15 minutes. Some pupil dilation should be evident and the patient will probably report difficulty with reading. Accommodation is falling rapidly at this stage and maximal cycloplegia will normally be attained in 25–35 minutes. Note that maximal does not mean total. Unlike atropine, cyclopentolate does not destroy all muscle tone and a degree of residual accommodation may be measured. Various workers, Priestley and Medine (1951), Stolzar (1953) and O'Connor Davies (1972), have suggested figures slightly over 1 D and clinical observation by the writer confirms this figure. Depth of cycloplegia is therefore sufficient for most purposes and increasingly cyclopentolate is being used on pre-school age children in place of atropine. In very young children the dose may be increased to 2 or 3 drops at 5-minute intervals. It follows from the above that no allowance for tonus need be made in assessing the final prescription.

As with atropine, retinoscopy is usually straightforward and quickly accomplished. Pupil diameter will be large (around 8 mm) and aberrations should be taken into account. Distance fixation is advisable for final assessment, although initial estimates of refractive error may be made with the patient fixing the practitioner's forehead or retinoscope mirror until, working from in front of the patient, each eye has been largely corrected.

With the older child or young person, subjective confirmation of result and measurement of visual acuity can be recorded. Snellen acuity may be adversely affected by aberrations and a modest reduction at this stage is acceptable. If the visual acuity is substantially lower than expected from precycloplegic examination it may be necessary to delay the final prescription until a postcycloplegic check has been made.

Prescribing remains a clinical decision and should be directed towards the elimination of symptoms and the stabilization of binocular vision. Although knowledge of the full refractive error is always useful it does not follow that it must be prescribed in each case. For example, a previously uncorrected teenage student who has developed symptoms in the last 6 months is found to have a refractive error of Right + 4.00 and Left + 3.50. Since the hypermetropia has been present since early childhood, although largely latent and symptoms are recent, a much reduced Rx should remove the symptoms. At a later stage it will, in the normal course of events, be necessary to increase the level of correction but for several years the patient can more easily use the spectacle correction selectively, on a task-dependent basis.

A postcycloplegic examination may be required in order to make final decisions about the prescription and future management of the case. This step is frequently not required since the evidence gathered initially and under cycloplegia are usually enough to make firm decisions.

The cycloplegia induced by cyclopentolate usually lasts some 8–12 hours but the associated mydriasis is more likely to be in the region of 24–36 hours. Longer times are possible in heavily pigmented eyes. Although most youngsters adapt well to this situation, the possibility of temporary photophobia must be considered and, in bright weather, sunspecs may be helpful. In any event, the patient and/or parent should be warned in advance of the duration of action since the temporary ability to undertake close work may affect the scheduling of homework.

Tropicamide (bistropamide)

Availability and presentation

UK:

- Minims Tropicamide (Smith & Nephew) 0.5% and 1% 20 × 5 ml.
- Mydriacyl (Alcon) 0.5% and 1% 5 ml.

Legal category: PoM.

USA:

- Mydramide (BioProducts) 0.5% and 1%.
- Mydriacyl (Alcon).

This rapid-acting antimuscarinic agent is available in single and in multidose presentation in both 0.5% and 1% strengths. For cycloplegic use only 1% should be considered, 0.5% being reserved for mydriatic purposes.

Of all the available antimuscarinics tropicamide has the greatest separation of mydriatic and cycloplegic function which makes it the mydriatic of choice for many purposes (see later).

At least two drops of 1% should be instilled at 5-minute intervals. Shortly after the second instillation the pupils will begin to dilate and almost simultaneously a measurable drop in accommodation occurs. Full mydriasis is usual in about 15 minutes and maximal cycloplegia in 20 minutes. Residual accommodation of less than 2.00 D is typical, although the cycloplegia obtained with tropicamide is less predictable than with other agents and of much shorter duration. Unless the examination can be timed to complete all relevant tests in a period between 20 and 35 minutes from instillation, a third drop may be required to retain adequate cycloplegia. Gettes and Belmont (1961) found that a third drop was required in a significant number of cases and several workers (Milder, 1961; Hiatt and Jenkins, 1983) have compared tropicamide unfavourably with other cycloplegics.

Despite these apparent disadvantages tropicamide is a very useful and under-used drug. For the older child, cycloplegia is adequate for many purposes and recovery times are proportionately short. Full recovery of accommodation is likely within 6 hours and reading accommodation may be recovered in 1–4 hours. The pupils return to normal in 8–10 hours.

When the constraints of school work or other studies have to be considered the short recovery times make tropicamide attractive. In prescribing all of the foregoing advice should be considered. The mydriasis obtained with these dosages of tropicamide is profound and the possibility of aberrations affecting the result must be taken into account.

Summary of cycloplegic agents

For the practitioner who examines a large number of children and is therefore likely to undertake cycloplegic examination frequently the drug cabinet should contain a good selection of agents. Atropine is used rarely and, in any event, is always obtained for individual patients. Cyclopentolate in 0.5% and 1% strengths together with 1% tropicamide cover most eventualities. Minims or Opulets containing these drugs have a shelf-life of several years and are therefore convenient and, without doubt, the safest presentation when the risk of cross-contamination has to be considered. If, however, drugs are to be used frequently, multidose presentation should be considered on the grounds of cost.

If only one cycloplegic drug is to be kept for intermittent use, cyclopentolate 0.5% must be recommended. Predictable cycloplegia over a wide age range is available since, in the younger child, two drops may be instilled at 5-minute intervals instead of one drop of 1%.

Mydriatic agents

Profound mydriasis normally accompanies the cycloplegia obtained with any of the drugs discussed above. Fundus examination is therefore easy, the only limiting factor being the age and cooperation of the child. In certain circumstances careful examination of the fundus may be of paramount importance although cycloplegia is not required. Where diabetes is suspected or confirmed, the presence of retinal signs must not be overlooked and the progress of any retinopathy must be carefully monitored. Even allowing for the fact that children have relatively large pupils, early retinal signs may be missed, particularly near the posterior pole as a result of the active pupil contraction. Where facilities exist for retinal photography, mydriasis may be essential. Even the use of a non-mydriatic fundus camera may be enhanced and the procedure made quicker by the use of mydriatics.

Two types of agent will produce adequate mydriasis. Antimuscarinics usually produce wide pupil dilation even in weak strengths and the pupil is fixed. Tropicamide in 0.5% strength is the drug of choice for this purpose. One drop is usually adequate although a further drop may be instilled if, for example, heavy pigmentation inhibits the action of the drug. The writer's experience of taking several thousand fundus photographs, where the absence of a pupil reflex is a major advantage, suggests that the second drop is rarely required. Instillation may produce some reflex tearing but discomfort is minimal. Pupil dilation may begin at about 5 minutes and is usually maximal in 10–15 minutes. Recovery is variable and is between 6 and 10 hours.

Sympathomimetic drugs which stimulate the alpha receptors in the dilator muscle of the iris produce mydriasis with little or no cycloplegia, and may be used when fundus photography is not a consideration. Pupil dilation is less profound, although still adequate and pupil reactions remain intact. It may be argued that the presence of pupil activity makes this drug more confortable for the patient by reducing the risk of photophobia. Phenylephrine hydrochloride which is available in Minims in strengths of 2.5% and 10% is a direct-acting alpha stimulator and is the drug of choice for sympathomimetic mydriasis. Unless the eyes are heavily pigmented one drop of 2.5% will usually produce sufficient dilation.

Availability and presentation

UK:

- Minims Tropicamide 0.5% (Smith & Nephew) 20 × 0.5 ml.
- Mydriacyl (Alcon) 0.5% 5 ml.
- Phenylephrine Eye-drops 10% 10 ml.
- Minims Phenylephrine Hydrochloride (Smith & Nephew) 2.5% and 10% 20 × 0.5 ml.

USA:

Tropicamide
- Mydramide (BioProducts) 0.5%.
- Mydriacyl (Alcon; 0.5%.

Phenylephrine
- Ark-Dilate (Akorn) 2.5% and 10%.
- Cyclomydril (Alcon) 1% with 0.2% cyclopentolate.
- Efricel (BioProducts) 0.125%, 2.5% and 10%.
- Murocoll (Muro) 10% with 0.3% scopalamine.
- Mydfrin (Alcon) 2.5%.
- Neo-synephrine (Winthrop) 2.5% and 10%.
- Neo-synephrine viscous solution (Winthrop) 2.5% and 10%.

Miotic agents

The risk of inducing an angle closure glaucoma is statistically very slight and, in a child, is virtually non-existent. However if photophobia presents a problem the action of either drug may be reversed by the instillation of a miotic.

The mydriasis induced by tropicamide may be reversed by instilling pilocarpine 1% or 2% which will restore the pupil to normal although this will still take some hours. The net gain is therefore relatively slight. It should also be remembered that pilocarpine is a direct-acting parasympathomimetic drug which will act on the ciliary muscle and may well cause uncomfortable spasm of accommodation.

Following the instillation of phenylephrine the drug of choice for reversal is thymoxamine hydrochloride which is available in Minims in 0.5% strength. This drug is an alpha blocking agent which again acts directly on the alpha receptors of the dilator. This combination acts quickly and the pupil should return to normal size in 1–2 hours. One drop is usually sufficient to overcome the mydriasis induced by 2.5% phenylephrine. One disadvantage of using thymoxamine is that this drug has poor thermal stability and it should therefore be stored in a refrigerator set to 5° C.

It is, of course, possible to reverse the effects of phenylephrine with pilocarpine but this is not recommended. The simultaneous stimulation of two opposed muscles may well cause discomfort and since the iris is pulled taught against the lens this pupil block may cause an abrupt rise in intraocular pressure.

Availability and presentation

- Pilocarpine Eye-drops, pilocarpine hydrochloride 0.5%, 1% and 2% 10 ml.
- Isopto Carpine Eye-drops with hypromellose, pilocarpine hydrochloride 0.5%, 1% and 2%.
- Opulets Pilocarpine (Alcon) eye-drops pilocarpine hydrochloride 1%, 2% and 4% 20 × 5 ml.
- Minims Pilocarpine Nitrate (Smith & Nephew) 1%, 2% and 4% 20 × 5 ml.
- Minims Thymoxamine Hydrochloride 0.5%.

Legal category: PoM.
Note: At the time of writing Thymoxamine has been withdrawn from the market. It is probable that this situation is temporary but the reader is advised to establish availability before considering the use of phenylephrine as a mydriatic.

Legal aspects

In the UK the sale and supply of medicinal products is controlled by various Acts of Parliament. Those agents used by the optometrist are covered by the Medicines Act 1968, Part III of which divides products into three groups:

- General Sale List (GSL).
- Pharmacy Medicines (P).
- Prescription Only Medicines (PoM).

The latter group may normally be supplied only on the prescription of a doctor, dentist or veterinary surgeon. However, as a result of various Statutory Instruments and Amendment Orders all the drugs normally used by the UK optometrist are made available. With the exception of phenylephrine, which is category P, all the drugs mentioned in this chapter are Prescription Only Medicines and are incorporated in SI 1980/1923.

The normal method of obtaining these drugs is to issue to the pharmacist a signed order which should be on headed notepaper and should contain the following information:

- Date.
- Quantity, strength, form and type of drug.
- An indication that the drugs are to be used in professional practice.

Provided that the sale is under the supervision of a registered pharmacist, category P drugs are available to the general public and a verbal order for phenylephrine will suffice, although it is more usual for this to be included with other drugs in the signed order.

References

APT, L. and GAFFNEY, W.L. (1976). Toxicity of topical eye medication used in childhood strabismus. *Symposium on Ocular Therapy*, **8**, 1–9.

BESWICK, J.A. (1962). Psychosis from cyclopentolate (letter). *American Journal of Ophthalmology*, **53(5)**, 879–880.

GETTES, B.C. and BELMONT, O. (1961). Tropicamide. Comparative cycloplegic effects. *Archives of Ophthalmology*, **66**, 336.

HAVENER, W.H. (1974). Autonomic drugs. In *Ocular Pharmacology*, 3rd edn. Mosby, St Louis, pp. 214–323.

HIATT, R.L. and JENKINS, G. (1983). Comparison of atropine and tropicamide in esotropia. *Annals of Ophthalmology*, **15**, 341–343.

KELLY, T. STUART-BLACK, CHATFIELD, C. and TUSTIN, G. (1975). Clinical assessment of the arrest of myopia. *British Journal of Ophthalmology*, **59**, 529–538.

MILDER, B. (1961). Tropicamide as a cycloplegic agent. *Archives of Ophthalmology*, **66**, 70.

OAKLEY, K.H. and YOUNG, L.A. (1975). Bifocal control of myopia. *American Journal of Optometry and Physiological Optics*, **52**, 758–764.

O'CONNOR DAVIES, P.H. (1981). Other cycloplegics. In *The Actions and Uses of Ophthalmic Drugs*, 2nd edn. Butterworths, London, pp. 122–123.

PRIESTLEY, B.S. and MEDINE, M.M. (1951). A new mydriatic and cycloplegic drug. *American Journal of Ophthalmology*, **34**, 572.

SIMCOE, C.W. (1962). Cyclopentolate (Cyclogyl) toxicity. *Archives of Ophthalmology*, **67(4)**, 406–408.

STOLZAR, I.H. (1953). A new group of cycloplegic drugs. *American Journal of Ophthalmology*, **36**, 110.

11

Binocular vision

David Pickwell

The advice of an optometrist is often sought by parents who feel that their child appears to have a problem with binocular vision, either because this has been reported by teachers or during school health checks or because they themselves have noticed that the child apparently squints.

The duty of the optometrist is three-fold:

(1) *Examination:* to establish if a problem is present.
(2) *Evaluation:* to decide if the anomaly will respond to optometric treatment or requires referral.
(3) *Management:* to give any appropriate optometric treatment or to refer.

Examination

The routine method for the examination of children depends on the age of the child and is considered more fully in Chapter 9. For children under the age of 6 years the normal routine optometric examination has to be modified as the understanding, cooperation and the reliability of the patient will be less than older children and adults. As a guide, the procedures likely to be possible and appropriate at each age are shown in *Table 11.1*. There is a close relationship between amblyopia and binocular vision problems in children. Therefore it is necessary to emphasize acuity measurements as well as the investigation of the other sensory and the motor aspects of binocular vision. In all examination routines there must be an element of screening which involves selecting the procedures most likely to detect anomalies in a reasonable time. With young children this screening element must be greater because of the reduced cooperation and the shorter time for which the attention of the child can be maintained.

As with all optometric examination, the possibility of active pathology must be investigated (*Figure 11.1*). Although a fairly rare condition, retinoblastoma can present as a squint, and therefore the possibility of this serious condition needs to be investigated in patients under the age of 4 years. The signs are opaque white patches on the fundus. It is not unusual for a squint to occur as the lesion prevents fusion, and this squint can be the first sign noticed by the parents.

Other signs of pathological or congenital binocular anomalies in children are abnormalities in lid apertures and lid movements, and non-comitancy of the deviation. The lid openings in children are of more rounded proportions than in

TABLE 11.1. Routine for examination of young children with binocular vision anomalies at different ages. The arrows show that the procedure is appropriate also to the age group in the next column on the right

Under 3 months	*3–12 months*	*1–2½ years*	*2½–4½ years*
Parent's observation	→	→	→
Family history	→	→	→
Screen for pathological signs:			
Comitancy / Lid signs	→	→	→
Fundus colour	→	→	→
Bruckner test	→ Attempt ophthalmoscopy / Pupil 'swinging flashlight test'	→	→
Fixation check	→ Look for nystagmus	→	→
Cover test:			
For amblyopia / Deviations	→ Infantile esotropia / Dissociated vertical deviation	→	→ and acquire deviations
		Stereo-tests	→
Prism test	→	→	→
Acuity:			
(cover test)	→ (OKN or PL)	→ Ffooks test (sometimes possible)	→ Sheridan–Gardner STYCAR E test
Refraction			
Screening for high error / astigmatism / anisometropia	→		
Consider cycloplegic	→	→ Attempt refraction	Refraction
			4Δ prism test for microtropia →

Note: over the age of five years, a normal routine eye examination can be attempted.

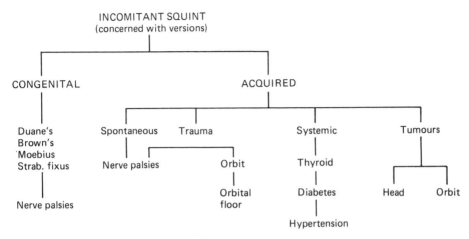

Figure 11.1. Incomitant deviations: summary of deviations. The congenital deviations are likely in children. The acquired deviations may be possible

adults, but the vertical dimensions should be equal in the two eyes to within 3 mm. They should remain equal as the eyes track horizontally across the motor field during the motility test. An obvious sign of Duane's retraction syndrome is unsymmetrical lid openings which vary with different positions of the eyes. When the patient is looking to the left, the left lids are more widely opened than the right, and the right lid opening is greater when the patient looks to the right. Restrictions in ocular movements will be noted in the affected eye. These restrictions vary depending on the type of the anomaly, but there is always restriction of eye movement.

Other common congenital ocular-motor restrictions include Brown's syndrome in which elevation of one eye is restricted when the eye is adducted. A VIth nerve palsy is not uncommon and results in a convergent squint of early onset.

It is obvious that these deviations are non-comitant in nature and that the motility test is vital in their investigation. This should be carried out by asking the patient to keep the head still whilst following with the eyes a pen-torch light moved in the motor field. From the primary position, the light is moved upwards and downwards whilst the practitioner watches to ensure that both eyes follow the light equally, and the lid movements are coordinated with those of the eyes. The light is then moved horizontally across the motor field from the primary position to check that the lateral and medial rectus muscles are functioning normally and the lid openings are constant. The horizontal movement is then repeated across the top of the motor field. Any restrictions in the elevation of either eye is noted as the eyes track across the upper part of the motor field. When the eye is turned inwards (toward the nose) its elevation is normally maintained by the inferior oblique muscle. In inferior oblique palsy, there will be a restriction of movement of the affected eye in the upper nasal part of the motor field. A squint may be seen, and diplopia may be experienced by the patient. This is also the appearance in Brown's syndrome (see above). A superior rectus palsy is less likely to occur as an isolated muscle palsy. Moving the pen-torch horizontally across the lower part of the field may indicate a restriction of movement of one eye due to a palsy of the depressor muscles. This is particularly important in superior oblique or IVth nerve palsies when there is a restriction of one eye when looking down and inwards.

Acquired muscle palsies occur infrequently in children, but they are usually accompanied by incomitant diplopia. This can be analysed with the motility test which should be carried out on all patients as described above (Boylan and Clement, 1987).

Most of the procedures in *Table 11.1* are dealt with in other chapters of this book. However the Bruckner test (Griffin and Cotter, 1986) is worth particular description with reference to binocular vision because anisometropia is often associated with squint. An ophthalmoscope is directed at the child's face from a distance of about 30 cm so that the light patch falls on both eyes, and by looking through the sight-hole the following can be noted:

- The immediate pupil reflex.
- The position of the corneal reflection and therefore any obvious squint or departure from central fixation.
- The colour of the reflection of light from the fundus. This should have the same appearance and light distribution in both eyes. Any difference may be accounted for in terms of anisometropia. This is the main benefit of the Bruckner test: it gives a very quick indication of the state of the refractive error.
- Any white patches indicating retinoblastoma may also be apparent, but the test does not by itself constitute a full search (see above).

The cover test is a very important part of the routine investigation in binocular vision cases. It is the only objective method of detecting smaller angle squint which is available in normal optometric practice. The cover test will distinguish an apparent squint caused by a nasal epicanthal fold and an actual deviation. Ideally it should be carried out with the patient fixing a target which provides precise accommodation so that an assessment of a deviation relative to the accommodation can be carried out. This is not always possible with very young patients when a more gross target in the form of a small toy may have to be used. The test should be carried out for near and for distance fixation if possible. With very young patients, fixation for the distance cover test may be more difficult. By covering and uncovering each eye in turn, deviations present in the patient's habitual vision may be detected. This is the only method of distinguishing between a squint and heterophoria: alternating the cover between the two eyes often increasing the angle of a squint making it easier to see. When only one eye is covered for a short time, there is little dissociation. As the cover is kept in place for a longer time the dissociation will be more. In the alternating cover test the dissociation is complete. If the angle increases with the degree of dissociation, anomalous single vision is present showing that sensory adaptations to the squint have occurred and these allow the angle to be reduced by peripheral fusion.

Binocular sensory adpatations occur in most squints. This means that in spite of a foveal image in one eye and a peripheral image in the squinting eye, there is no diplopia. This anomalous type of binocular vision in squints is traditionally known as abnormal retinal correspondence (ARC).

Evaluation and management

The motility test will indicate that the deviation is non-comitant (see above). These cases usually require medical investigation. Many of them are congenital anomalies of the ocular motor system and will not respond to optometric treatment.

When trying to evaluate a case of comitant squint, the nature of squint must be kept in mind. The deviation is partly the result of the motor factors that determine the eyes' position and partly due to the anomalous correspondence that develops between the two eyes and causes fusion when one eye is in the deviated position. The macular region of the squinting eye is suppressed. The peripheral retinal input is adapted so that the motor system has a false sense of the squinting eye's position and fusion takes place at the angle of the squint. This anomalous fusion develops very readily in infants and if it is allowed to persist can become impossible to break down.

The examination should allow classification of the deviation (*Figure 11.2*). In the case of squint, it will be seen that the age of onset of the squint is critical.

Onset under the age of 1 year

Where the squint first appears before the age of 1 year, 'infantile esotropia syndrome', it is unlikely that the deviation will respond to optometric treatment. The role of the optometrist in such cases is one of recognition as early as possible and referral for a surgeon's opinion if this has not already been taken. In cases where surgery has been attempted or rejected as inappropriate, the optometrist's role is one of providing spectacles or any other form of optometric treatment required.

It is not always easy to determine the age of onset of the squint in older patients. Sometimes early photographs will help. Although the infant may show epicanthus in photographs, infantile esotropia usually has a large angle, about 40 Δ. This type of deviation also shows a moderate to high degree of hyperopia. There may also be crossed fixation – the right eye is used to fix objects in the left of the motor field and the left eye used for the right half of the field. The change of fixation can be seen as

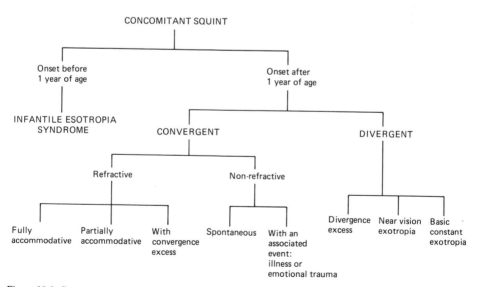

Figure 11.2. Convergent squint: summary chart of main types of concomitant deviations likely to be seen in optometric practice

TABLE 11.2. Convergent squint with an onset over the age of 1 year, summarizing the main diagnostic features and management

A. Fully accommodative	B. Partially accommodative	C. Convergence excess
Diagnosis		
*Hyperopic correction fully relieves the deviation	Characteristics from A and C	Refractive correction does not change the angle
Deviation for near and distance vision are the same	Sensory adaptations are very likely	*Marked increase in deviation for near vision
Low base-in prism vergences		Normal base-in prism vergences
Normal AC/A ratio		High AC/A ratio
Sensory adaptations in long-standing cases		Sensory adaptations in long-standing cases
Management		
Full prescription	Full prescription	Full prescription with bifocal addition to relieve the deviation for near vision (seg. set high)
Check in 1 month	Check in 1 month	
Treat sensory adaptations by physiological diplopia	Treat sensory adaptations and develop base-in prism vergences	Treat amblyopia by occlusion
Develop base-in prism vergence	Consider referral to surgeon if no early restoration of binocular vision	

* Principal features.

the patient follows an object moving horizontally across the field: a sudden flick of the eyes is observed as the object is moved slightly beyond the midline. This jump of the eyes when following a target moved horizontally across the field is a very useful diagnostic sign for infantile esotropia. There may also be nystagmus or latent nystagmus which only shows when one eye is covered. Dissociated vertical deviation (DVD) may also be present: whichever eye is covered, it moves slowly upward and slowly returns when the cover is removed. The exact characteristics of infantile esotropia depends on its cause and nature.

It must be emphasized that there is no effective optometric treatment for infantile esotropia. Surgical management can sometimes be successful in restoring binocular vision in some types of infantile esotropia if undertaken early enough. It is therefore important that optometrists refer as soon as the condition is detected. When the patient presents at an older age but the squint is obviously of very early onset, it is very unlikely that binocular vision will be restored by any means. In these cases a cosmetic operation may be considered. Indeed a cosmetic improvement is the usual outcome of surgery for infantile squints.

Onset over the age of 1 year

When it can be established that the age of onset of the squint is over the age of 1 year, we should consider convergent and divergent deviations separately (*Table 11.2*).

Convergent squint

It is important in convergent squint to distinguish between refractive and non-refractive deviations. In general, refractive squint responds more easily to optometric treatment than many non-refractive cases. There are three broad divisions of refractive squint, detailed below.

REFRACTIVE SQUINT

Accommodative

As can be seen from *Table 11.2*, the main characteristic of accommodative squint is that the deviation is completely relieved by the correction for hyperopia. A full cycloplegic refractive correction is prescribed for constant wear. It should be demonstrated to the patient and parent that the spectacles straighten the squint and that they are not prescribed to improve the acuity. After 4 weeks, a check must be carried out to see if the correction has established binocular vision or if there is still any marked amblyopia or suppression. If binocular vision has been established, the acuity in the previously squinting eye will normally have improved a little and should continue to improve to a level close to that of the other eye. Where no improvement in acuity is found, a short period of occlusion with appropriate exercises requiring the patient to work at the limit of the acuity is usually the quickest method with younger children. Some treatment for suppression may also be required. In older children it is often more satisfactory to proceed with the suppression treatment and avoid all the problems of trying to persuade them to wear a patch. The rationale behind this is to bring the previously squinting eye into use with the other eye so that the acuity will improve by use of both eyes together. If required, orthoptic exercises for suppression should be given. These may include stereoscope exercises with cards that assist overcoming suppression such as the 'Simultaneous Macular Vision' cards (F series) in the Bradford Stereoscope Training Cards set (Pickwell, 1978). Bar reading or other physiological diplopia-type exercises might also be useful (see later under 'Partially accommodative esotropia').

When the prescription has been worn for 3 months and binocular vision established, base-out prism vergence exercises may be useful in strengthening the motor fusion to prevent any subsequent breakdown of binocular vision.

It should be noted that the management of fully accommodative squint is entirely optometric and they seldom require other treatment. Referral is seldom needed.

Convergence excess esotropia

The main characteristic of convergence excess is a significant increase in the angle of the deviation for near vision. There may be either a very small angle or no squint for distance fixation and where there is no squint, the acuity in the squinting eye may be good. These patients have a high AC/A ratio: a small change in accommodation brings about a larger than average change in convergence. This means that the angle of the squint for near vision can be relieved by prescribing a reading addition to the distance correction which relieves the accommodation and therefore the overconvergence. The amount required is found by trying spherical binocular additions in steps of 0.50 DS and checking with the cover-test to find the lowest addition that shows no movement. The spectacles are made in the form of 'Executive' or straight-top bifocals with the segment top in line with the centre of the pupil when the eyes are in the primary position. This high segment top ensures that the patient looks through the segment for near vision. A trial period can be made with a pair of segments cut from a Fresnel lens, but in most cases this is not satisfactory for the long-term use required.

Sometimes simple suppression exercises are required, but once it has been established that the bifocals consolidate binocular vision, the patient should be seen at 6-monthly intervals. Each time a change of spectacles is required, the near addition may be reduced slightly. In most cases, phasing out the addition is a long process and may take several years. Many of these patients have significant hyperopia and may therefore require spectacles in the long term anyway.

Partially accommodative esotropia

In partially accommodative squints, there are characteristics present of both the fully accommodative and convergence excess types of squint. The angle of the deviation is reduced by the spectacle correction to a smaller residual angle. However there is often some increase in the angle for near vision and this may remain when the spectacles for distance have been prescribed. There is usually amblyopia in the deviated eye.

Optometric treatment of these patients is very much a matter of clinical judgement of the individual case. The general principles apply that the more longstanding the squint and the older the patient, the more intractable the condition is to treatment. Where the residual angle is small and the deviation has been present for only a few years, the deviation may respond to optometric management. Spectacles are prescribed to reduce the angle as much as possible and also to present each eye with a sharp image. This reduction in angle and a clearer image in the squinting eye will also help to break down the anomalous correspondence and suppression. Occassionally it may even create diplopia. Clearly this is undesirable if it leaves an angle too large to be overcome by the patient. The treatment of squinting should be discontinued in these cases. In other patients, the spectacle correction eliminates the squint for distance vision and the case can then be treated as convergence excess.

Where there is marked amblyopia, this must receive attention. In patients under the age of 7 years, this is best done by a period of occlusion. In older patients, where the acuity is 6/12 or better, treatment by physiological diplopia methods may establish binocular vision and assist in improving the acuity.

In a lot of cases it may be possible to find a fixation distance for near vision where there is no cover-test movement. This provides a starting point for treatment by physiological diplopia methods. A small object for fixation is placed where the visual axes appear to cross and the cover-test applied. If a squint is shown, it is explained to the patient that the eyes are 'turning in too much' and that they are looking 'too close'. By 'mental effort' (imagining a more distant object) it may be possible to obtain bifoveal fixation of the small fixation object. This can be checked by observing the lack of movement on the cover test. In some cases, it is possible to move the object nearer to obtain fixation with both eyes. Sometimes a reading addition will assist in inhibiting the excessive convergence. However, in some cases the sensory adaptations to the motor deviation are so firmly established that fusion with anomalous correspondence always occurs and more rigorous methods are required to break this down. Prescribing a prismatic overcorrection for the squint in the form of about 5 more than the prism-bar measurement of the deviation will sometimes be effective (Hugonnier and Clayette-Hugonnier, 1969). Care must be taken to ensure that this does not produce intractable diplopia: frequent checks are required to demonstrate that binocular fixation is possible as soon as normal correspondence has been established.

When a position where binocular fixation at one distance is established, the patient is taught to appreciate physiological diplopia by the introduction of a second object at a different distance from the eyes and on the median line (Pickwell, 1989). It may be necessary to occlude the dominant eye briefly to demonstrate both diplopic images of the second object. Home exercises may then be appropriate. These will take the form of moving the second object slowly towards the fixation object until the patient reports that physiological diplopia of the second object is lost or that single vision of the fixation object is no longer possible. The second object is then moved back to a position where normal fixation with physiological diplopia of the second object is restored. The movement of this second object closer to fixation is repeated until physiological diplopia can still be appreciated when the two objects are only 2–3 cm apart.

If the fixation point is for near vision, that is there is still a squint for distance fixation, the second object may be placed either closer to the eyes than fixation and therefore seen in crossed physiological diplopia, or it can be further away giving uncrossed diplopia. Crossed physiological diplopia is easier for some patients to appreciate, but in patients with a strong convergence excess element the nearer object stimulates the convergence and the squint returns. When the second object lies further from the eyes than the fixation, its image falls on the nasal retina which is an area where the sensory adaptations are firmly established. Therefore if uncrossed physiological diplopia can be appreciated, it may be taken as a good sign of likely success by this method.

The objective of physiological diplopia methods is to employ the physiological appreciation of diplopia to correct the anomalous correspondence and to overcome the suppression. It is not a good method of reducing the angle of the squint, therefore the emphasis should be on moving the second object whilst retaining the physiological diplopia. The fixation object should not be moved from the position where bifoveal fixation is established. If the method is used for small residual angles, less than 10°, the intention is that when the sensory adaptations have been overcome it will be within the ability of the motor system to straighten the eyes. Large residual angles may need surgery and early referral is appropriate in these cases. It is not helpful to anyone to retain a patient beyond the time when it is obvious that treatment by optometric methods is not likely to be successful.

NON-REFRACTIVE CONVERGENT SQUINT

In many squints, the angle of the deviation is not affected by correcting the refractive error. Spectacles may be required to relieve the symptoms of hyperopia if these are present, or they may correct any anisometropia. In the latter case, the spectacles may also overcome the sensory adaptations to the squint and the patient could experience diplopia. This is most likely in patients of 7–12 years of age. Before prescribing spectacles in such cases it is important to consider whether the angle of the deviation is small enough to allow single binocular vision once the anomalous correspondence and suppression have been broken down. Consolidation of single binocular vision may be assisted by developing the base-in prism vergences.

In some non-refractive esotropia the onset of the squint can be associated with a particular event. The most usual is a squint which follows a marked deterioration in general health. In cases where there has been binocular vision prior to some illness it is usually possible to restore it once the patient has recovered good general health. Spectacles should be prescribed for any significant refractive error and the base-in prism vergences developed.

When the event associated with the onset of the squint is traumatic, more caution needs to be exercised. In cases of physical trauma, medical examination is advised.

Cases where the child's squint comes on following psychological trauma are not easy to treat. The effects of the trauma can be very lasting.

Divergent squint

There are three broad types of comitant divergent squint (*Table 11.3*), each requiring a different approach.

DIVERGENCE EXCESS

The essential diagnostic feature of divergence excess is that the deviation is larger for distance vision than for near. In most cases there is an intermittent divergent squint for distance which is more obvious when the patient is not concentrating on vision or day-dreaming. There is often single binocular vision for near fixation. Usually the child does not complain of symptoms, although sometimes diplopia may be reported in response to questions. The angle of the deviation sometimes increases when the patient looks up – V syndrome. There is usually little or no refractive error and the condition is more prevalent in females (Pickwell, 1979). It is sometimes classified as either 'true' or 'simulated' divergence excess depending on whether the lack of a squint for near vision is due to inherent anomalies in the motor system or due to very high tonic convergence in young children (von Noorden, 1984). This distinction seems to be more relevant to surgical management than to optometric treatment.

In its typical form, the condition is usually met in optometric practices in young teenage patients when they come complaining that other people notice the eyes sometimes adopt an odd position. If it is intermittent for distance with binocular vision for close work, some simple orthoptic exercises can often help. The patient is shown how to appreciate crossed physiological diplopia whilst fixing an object at about 40 cm, and also uncrossed physiological diplopia of a nearer object whilst

TABLE 11.3. Primary divergent squint: summary of main diagnostic features and the management

A. *Divergence excess* *(a) true, or (b) simulated*	B. *Near-vision exotropia* *(convergence insuf. type)*	C. *Basic constant exotropia*
Diagnosis		
Squint for distance vision	Squint for near vision	Constant squint for distance
Usually intermittent	Binocular at distance	and near
Binocular vision at near	Late onset (over 16)	Often alternating with nearly
Squint obvious during:	Symptoms	equal acuities
Inattention	Often myopia	Early onset likely
Poor health	Equal acuities	No symptoms
Sunny climates		
No symptoms		
Low refractive error		
Mainly in females		
V syndrome		
Management		
Orthoptic for:	Correct refractive error	Correct refractive error
Suppression	Orthoptics	Try negative additions and
Base-out vergences	Base-out vergences	orthoptics
Physiological diplopia	Relieving prisms	Refer for cosmetic reasons
	Refer in angles over 20°	

fixing a distant one. A home exercise consists of alternating between the two conditions. A continuous display of physiological diplopia can also be demonstrated by asking the patient to fix a bead (or small hexagonal nut) threaded on a string stretched from a point between the patient's eyes and a point about 3 m away. The bead should be seen singly and the string as two lines crossing through the bead in the form of a diagonal cross. Suppression is indicated by an inability to see one limb of the cross. An exercise consists in moving the bead along the string and away from the eyes whilst maintaining the cross appearance (Pickwell, 1989).

It usually helps to exercise the base-out prism vergences concurrently with the physiological diplopia exercise. This can be done with a stereoscope and cards such as the Bradford F series, or the Wells cards in which decreasing the separation exercises convergence.

NEAR-VISION EXOTROPIA

Sometimes patients with convergence insufficiency become decompensated in the mid or late teenage years and a divergent squint occurs for near vision only. There are usually symptoms associated with reading which may consist of headaches and intermittant diplopia. The acuities are usually good and equal, and there is often myopia.

The management consists of correcting any refractive error by spectacles for constant wear in order to establish a proper accommodation/convergence relationship. Orthoptic exercises will usually help. These can take the form of improving the convergence by pencil-to-nose exercises, or improving the positive fusional reserve by base-out prism vergence exercises. Relieving prisms incorporated in the spectacles are sometimes required. The amount is determined by finding the smallest prism which will give a good recovery on the cover test.

Where the angle of the deviation is over 15–20°, the case is likely to require surgical relief.

BASIC CONSTANT EXOTROPIA

Constant exotropia for distance and for near vision is likely to have been present from a very early age. There are unlikely to be any symptoms as full adaptation will have occurred. In most cases it is an alternating deviation. Sometimes the patient can change fixation from one eye to the other at will, and sometimes one eye is used for distance fixation and the other for near. In other cases fixation can be changed by covering the fixing eye and the patient does not immediately change back.

In patients under the age of 7 years, binocular vision may be restored by prescribing negative additions to the distance correction. Obviously this works better if there is a high AC/A ratio. Pairs of negative spheres are added to the prescription in steps of − 0.50 DS until binocular vision is demonstrated with the cover test. Of course this puts an added stress on the accommodative system and the case needs to be checked frequently to ensure that binocular single vision is present. Once it has been firmly established, base-out prism vergences may be developed to give sufficient fusional reserve. The negative additions are reduced with each new pair of spectacles so that when the patient's amplitude of accommodation begins to reduce a normal distance correction can be prescribed.

Where this line of treatment is inappropriate due to the patient's age or no satisfactory negative addition being found, a surgeon's opinion should be sought.

This account does not constitute a comprehensive list of all types of squint. It does however offer sufficient for the practitioner to get a broad understanding of the nature and the management of squint. A particularly important aim is to recognize that some squints have an optometric method of treatment. Those that do not should be identified and referred as early as possible. Early recognition is often the key to the successful management of squint.

Heterophoria

Most children have heterophoria and in the majority it is esophoria that is fully compensated and requires no attention. There is a significant number of children in whom the heterophoria becomes decompensated, either due to innate anatomical and physiological factors or to stress, and in many cases to a combination of both. When this occurs before the age of about 6 years, sensory adaptation readily takes place so that children seldom report symptoms and the first sign may be intermittent squint. The parent may report that the squint has been noticed when the child is tired. The practitioner should look for any signs of squint or that binocular vision easily breaks down. There may be a slow hesitant recovery on applying the cover-test. If the alternating cover-test is applied, the angle of the deviation may increase markedly and in some cases there may be no immediate recovery when the cover is removed, that is, the heterophoria is converted into a tempory squint by the alternating cover. Often some sensory adaptions or amblyopia may be already manifest by the time the patient is brought from examination. The cause of this may be apparent in the form of significant refractive error; hyperopia, anisometropia or high astigmatism. Obviously a pair of spectacles for constant wear in the first place is required and may prevent the establishment of constant squint. In other cases the type of squint likely to ensue may be apparent and can be considered as described above. Again the importance of early action as preventative measures must be emphasized.

Patients over the age of 6 years usually have established good binocular reflexes so that sensory adaptations are less likely to occur. Therefore, symptoms are present when the stress combines with any inherent abnormal factors and the heterophoria becomes decompensated. It is important with this age group to appreciate that heterophoria problems are usually attributable to some change that has occurred. This may be a deterioration in the patient's general health or some other disturbance in the well-being of the child such as a high level of anxiety or emotional stress. It may also be due to more direct stress on the ocular motor system. Uncorrected refractive error becomes more of a problem as the patient gets older. Close work is increased and at some point the amplitude of accommodation reduces. The patient may need to acquire new visual habits such as increasing the near working distance, or working in improved illumination (Pickwell, Yekta and Jenkins, 1987). It is important that care be taken when the patient's history and symptoms are recorded to identify any changes in the general well-being or in the visual circumstances which will contribute to the decompensation of the binocular vision. The general principle of management in heterophoria problems is to diagnose the factors likely to cause decompensation and then to give attention to removing as many of these as possible. Sometimes improving the visual habits by insisting on a proper working distance and conditions will remove the symptoms without any other measures. The cooperation of parents and teachers, to keep reminding the child, is usually required to ensure that this is done. In very many cases the correction of the refractive error goes a long way to restoring symptom-free binocular vision. Simple orthoptic exercises often help, and prism relief is occasionally required.

With children there are several particular conditions that occur more frequently.

Convergence excess

In young patients the convergence impulses are often very high and this means that esophoria can become a problem for close work. This is exacerbated if there is uncorrected hyperopia which causes an unusually high degree of accommodation for near vision. The problem may be further heightened if the patient reads at very close distance. The symptoms are frontal headache, intermittant blurred near vision and a failure of accommodation to relax when looking up after reading, accommodative inertia. These symptoms usually follow long periods of close work. With some children a spasm of accommodation may be present which may even lead to psuedo-myopia. Large esophoric movements will be noted with the cover-test. The remedy is to prescribe the full cycloplegic findings of refractive error, less any allowance for tonus. This may blur distance vision at first but this will become clear quite quickly if the spectacles are worn constantly for the first few weeks. Obviously attention must be given to a proper working distance of not less than 35 cm. Sometimes it is necessary to develop the base-in prism vergences if the symptoms persist.

Convergence insufficiency

It is interesting that although the convergence impulses can be very high in many children, convergence insufficiency can be a problem with others. These patients find difficulty in maintaining sufficient convergence for long periods of close work. This causes intermittant diplopia and headaches associated with reading. The near point of convergence is measured on a near-point rule. The 'jump convergence test' is carried out by asking the patient to look at a distance object whilst a second fixation target is placed at about 15 cm from the eyes. The patient is instructed to look at the nearer object on the command 'now'. When the command is given, the eyes of a normal person can be seen to execute a smooth convergent movement. In convergence insufficiency, the near point of convergence may be greater than 10–15 cm. Jump convergence may be hesitant and slow, and sometimes a versional movement occurs before the convergence. In these cases, both eyes move in the same direction so that one fixes the near target. Then the second eye convergences to take up fixation also (Pickwell and Hampshire, 1981). The management is described above under near-vision exotropia.

The condition may be accompanied by accommodative insufficiency so that a teenage patient has a low amplitude of accommodation as well as poor convergence. Rarely this may be caused by trauma in which case the onset will be sudden and marked by an inability to obtain either clear or single vision. In other cases when convergence and accommodative insufficiency are present together, orthoptic exercises seldom produce any improvement. A small reading addition and base-in prism relief should be considered. The exact amounts can be decided by subjective responses and should be checked by noting their effect on convergence and the total accommodation available with the reading addition. The condition is usually temporary and the reading addition with the prismatic correction can be abandoned when recovery occurs. Some cases have a recent history of infectious illness, glandular fever, mumps, etc. Recovery of good health assists the visual problem.

A variant of accommodative insufficiency is fatigue of accommodation in which the patient cannot sustain clear near vision for long periods of close work, although the amplitude appears normal for the age in the clinic at the time of measurement. There is often a history of recent illness. In most cases correction of the hyperopia with spectacles helps. If there is also convergence insufficiency, convergence exercises will help. These may take the form of pencil-to-nose exercises. Sometimes an exercise specifically for the accommodative problem will also assist. The patient is loaned a pair of negative spheres (1.00 or 1.50 DS) and is asked to practise changing the accommodation to see clearly as the lenses are placed before the eyes for a few seconds and then removed. This is repeated for several minutes several times a day.

Nystagmus

Examination of nystagmus should include noting any symptoms. In nystagmus caused by active pathology there is usually a nauseating oscillation of the visual field with the eye movement. The longstanding or congenital types of nystagmus seen in some children do not show this symptom. The examination should record if the oscillation is slow in one direction and quick in the other (jerky nystagmus), or is the same slow speed in both directions (pendular). It should be classified according to degree. First-degree nystagmus is present in peripheral gaze only; second-degree is present in the primary position, and third-degree is present in all parts of the motor field. It should be noted whether the movement is horizontal, vertical, diagonal or rotary. The amplitude of the movement in degrees is estimated and recorded, and a judgement made as to whether the oscillation is fast, medium or slow.

Nystagmus in children can be part of the infantile esotropia syndrome as described above. However it can also occur without a squint as a primary condition. These other congenital forms are usually classified under several headings, detailed below.

Ocular (or sensory) nystagmus

This is due to some disturbance in establishing the fixation reflex. It is common in albinism and also in some congenital cataract. Similarly foveal fixation may be prevented by lesions in the central retina or by optic atrophy in very early life. The signs of the primary condition will be apparent. In these cases optometric help in the form of a spectacle correction with tinted lenses may be useful.

Hereditary nystagmus

Hereditary nystagmus has a variable pattern of signs. Sometimes the hereditary nature of the condition is obvious because other members of the family have a history of nystagmus. An important feature in distinguishing this congenital nystagmus from that which is acquired due to pathology of the nervous system, is that there is no oscillopsia in congenital nystagmus; apparent movement of the visual field as the eyes move. The child does not complain of symptoms, and there is no history of inner ear troubles which can be associated with some nystagmus in children. However the acuity may be reduced due to the eye movements. When fixing in the primary position, the nystagmus is usually pendular but it may be jerky in peripheral gaze or if it is associated with a squint. It may also be reduced in amplitude or eliminated in one position of peripheral gaze; often about 10–15° from the primary position. This is sometimes called the 'nul position'. It may cause an abnormal head position which is particularly noticeable when measuring the acuity, as the child turns the head to obtain the clearest vision. The nystagmus is often accentuated by occluding one eye. It may be less or absent as the patient converges in near vision. Neurological examination usually includes a critical observation of the optokinetic movements (OKN) which are abnormal. Hereditary nystagmus tends to lessen as the patient gets older and in some cases may disappear after adolescence.

During refractive examination of these patients, a fogging sphere rather than an occluder should be used, and a trial frame allows the patient to hold the head in the nul position which a refractor head does not. Both reduce the magnitude of the nystagmus. It is sometimes possible to reduce the nystagmus significantly by prescribing base-out prism so that the eyes are in a convergent position. A further reduction may be possible by prisms which turn the eyes towards the nul position. The weight of the lenses can put a restriction on the extent of this help. In some cases it may be appropriate to consider treatment for any amblyopia, but a fogging method should be used rather than occlusion.

It is often helpful to assure the patient and the parents that hereditary nystagmus tends to improve and is very unlikely to get worse.

Latent nystagmus

Latent nystagmus has the clinical appearance of a milder form of hereditary nystagmus. Oscillations of one or both eyes are brought on only by occluding or dimming the image of one eye. It may be associated with dissociated vertical deviation (DVD). It is usually jerky in nature, but it causes the patient no problems, and requires no treatment. A fogging sphere should be used in refractive examination rather than an occluder.

References

BOYLAN, C. and CLEMENT, R.A. (1987). Excursion tests of ocular motility. *Ophthalmic and Physiological Optics*, 7, 31–35.

GRIFFIN, J.R. and COTTER, S.A. (1986). Evaluation of the clinical usefulness of the Bruckner Test. *American Journal of Optometry*, 63, 957–961.

HUGONNIER, R. and CLAYETTE-HUGONNIER, S. (1969). *Strabismus, Heterophoria and Ocular Motor Palsy*, translated and edited by S. Verroneau-Troutmen. Mosby, St Louis.

NOORDEN, G.K. VON (1984) *Burian-von Noorden's Binocular Vision and Ocular Motility*, 3rd edn. Mosby, St Louis, p. 305.

PICKWELL, D. (1989). *Binocular Vision Anomalies: Investigation and Treatment*, 2nd edn. Butterworths, London.

PICKWELL, L.D. (1978). The use of stereoscope cards in orthoptics. *Ophthalmic Optician*, 18(5), 167–168.

PICKWELL, L.D. (1979). Prevalence and treatment of divergence excess. *American Journal of Optometry*, 56, 78–81.

PICKWELL, L.D. and HAMPSHIRE, R. (1981) The significance of inadequate convergence. *Ophthalmic and Physiological Optics*, 1, 13–18.

PICKWELL, L.D., YEKTA, A.A. and JENKINS, T.C.A. (1987). The effect of reading in low illumination on fixation disparity. *American Journal of Optometry*, 64, 513–518.

12

Colour vision assessment in children

Suman C. Patel and Terry Buckingham

Introduction

As Newton demonstrated that white light could be fragmented into its spectral components, so their recombination provides a basis for the understanding of human colour perception. *Figure 12.1* is the typical diagrammatic representation of the rules governing the addition of spectral colours. The primary colours, red, green and blue, are located at the apices of an equilateral triangle and the secondary colours, obtained by the addition of the primaries, along the sides of the triangle. The trichromatic generalization is that almost all colours can be matched with an additive mixture of three fixed primary colours whose radiant powers have been adjusted. When colour pigments or dyes are combined subtractive colour mixing occurs. Cyan (a greenish-blue), magenta (a bluish-crimson) and yellow may then be regarded as primaries, with cyan and yellow being mixed to give green. The relationship between the subtractive primaries, cyan, magenta and yellow, and the additive primaries is most readily revealed if they are referred to as negative-red, negative-green and negative-blue respectively.

The additive laws of colour mixing formed the basis of the trichromatic theory of human colour vision proposed by Thomas Young in 1801, and developed about half a century later by Herman von Helmholtz. It suggested that signals generated by each of three cone types were transmitted directly to the brain via three separate colour channels. There were, however, a number of colour phenomena, such as complementary colours and afterimages, that defied explanation in terms of the trichromatic theory. Two spectral colours are said to be complementary, or nearly so, if they can be combined to form white light. Such colours would lie on the axis through the white point of the centre of the triangle in *Figure 12.1*. Hence, blue (580 nm) and yellow (480 nm) are complementary and can be mixed to produce white light. Complementary colours are often seen as afterimages from prolonged viewing of spectral lights. The opponent theory of colour vision was developed by Ewald Hering in about 1870 to account for these phenomena. Essentially this suggested that colour information was encoded by means of two chromatic channels (red-green and blue-yellow), together with an achromatic (black-white) luminance channel. An opponent theory would account for the empirical observation that some intermediate hues, such as reddish-greens or yellowish-blues, are never perceived.

Only a combination of both trichromatic and opponent theories could account for the results of colour matching, discrimination and appearance, as well as chromatic adaptation. Muller (1930) is generally credited as being the first to introduce the

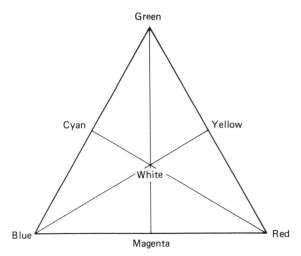

Figure 12.1. A diagrammatic representation of the rules governing spectral colour addition. Colours which are on the opposite ends of an axis passing through white are complementary. Colours along the sides of the triangles are termed analogous colours

zone-theory concept. Zone-theories of colour vision combine both classical approaches by postulating that each is applicable to separate sequential zones in the visual pathway. The Young–Helmholtz theory accounts for the experimental data of colour matching operating at receptor levels, whilst the two chromatic and single achromatic signals generated within the neural network mirror the Hering paradigm. A diagrammatic representation of the way in which colour information is processed in the visual pathway as far as the lateral geniculate body is given in *Figure 12.2*.

At cortical levels an area designated V4, containing a high concentration of colour-coded and colour-sensitive cells, would appear to play a major role in colour perception. Colour information seems to be held separate from that relating to other visual information about form and movement (Zeki, 1990).

Colour vision defects

The ability to match or discriminate between colours, forms the basis of most colour vision tests. Colour matching is based on the phenomenon of metamerism, in which stimuli appear identical despite having different spectral compositions. Such metameric colour matches achieved under particular incident lighting conditions may not hold if the conditions are changed. Markedly defective colour vision – typically as a result of a failure in the red or green signalling mechanism – results in a dichromat who requires only two primaries to match a particular wavelength. Their colour discrimination threshold is raised and hue discrimination so poor (*Figure 12.3*) that only two families of colours are seen either side of a neutral or white point – a specific wavelength on the boundary of the triangle in *Figure 12.1*, which appears grey or achromatic. This point is located at about 492 nm in those who are red defective (protanopes) and at about 498 nm in those who are green defective (deuteranopes). About 2.6% of males and 0.05% of females are dichromats. A very

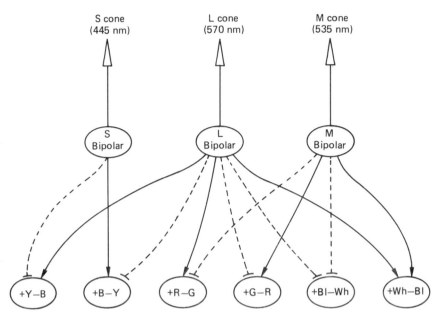

Figure 12.2. A schematic diagram of the processing of colour information as far as the LGN, showing excitatory (→) and inhibitory (---|) inputs. L cones, having a maximum absorption at 570 nm, input into all pathways.

small proportion of the population (0.005%) are monochromats, matching any colour with a single primary. Monochromats have no colour discrimination and make judgements based solely on brightness.

A small proportion of trichromats, about 5.5% males and 0.4% females, make abnormal colour matches, the degree of which may be slight or marked. This would suggest that all three colour mechanisms are present but that one is abnormal. Such subjects are referred to as anomalous trichromats. It can be difficult to distinguish between a markedly affected anomalous trichromat and a dichromat.

The distribution of genetically inherited colour vision defects is given in *Table 12.1*. Although congenitally inherited colour defects produce colour deficits for specific colours, no other visual function is affected. The common red-green colour defects (protan or deutan) are inherited in a sex-linked manner, the mode of inheritance is described in *Figure 12.4*. Their incidence is not equal, deuteranomaly being the most common. The incidence of deuteranomaly is about 4.5% in men compared to around 1% in each of protanomaly and protanopia with a slightly higher incidence of deuteranopia (about 1.5%). Obviously where the genetic pool is confined, as a result of geographical or cultural isolation, the incidence of colour vision defects may increase. Unlike other colour vision anomalies, tritan defects are found to follow an autosomal dominant trait. Monochromatism is rather rare, occurring in about 5 cases per 100 000 (0.005%) in males. Its occurrence in females is extremely rare. Rod monochromats generally display reduced visual acuity of about 6/60 or less. Rarely, visual acuity may remain relatively unaffected at around 6/18 to 6/24.

Acquired colour defects arise as a result of ocular or systemic pathology and are associated with losses in visual acuity and visual fields. Indeed, these latter features

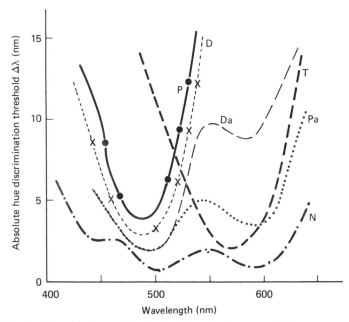

Figure 12.3. Hue discrimination in normal and colour defective observers. The just noticeable difference in wavelength is plotted as a function of wavelength. N, normal trichomat; P, protanope; Pa, protanomalous; D, deuteranope; Da, deuteranomalous; T, tritanomalous

may be more readily detectable than the associated acquired colour vision defects. An observant patient may report the onset of changes in their colour perception, or notice a difference between each eye. Typically the colour defect appears irregular and changes with the progress of the condition, so that interocular difference in colour perception are frequently reported. Although red-green defects are sometimes reported, it is often blue perception which is first affected by pathology.

TABLE 12.1. The distribution of genetically inherited colour vision defects. Such a distribution may be regarded as approximate since a number of factors, such as cultural and geographical, are likely to affect the genetic pool

Colour vision category	Inheritance	Male incidence (%)	Female incidence (%)
Normal trichromatic		92.0	99.5
Anomalous trichromatism			
Protanomalous	X–R	0.90	0.02
Deuteranomalous	X–R	4.60	0.38
Tritanomalous	A–D	Rare	Rare
Dichromatism			
Protanopic	X–R	1.21	0.02
Deuteranopic	X–R	1.43	0.01
Tritanopic	A–D	0.001	0.001
Monochromatism			
Cone	?	Rarest	Rarest
Rod	A–R or X–R	0.005	Insignificant

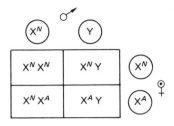

Case 1: Father normal
Mother, a carrier
Half of the female children are
likely to be normal, the other half carriers
Half of the male offspring normal
the other half colour defective

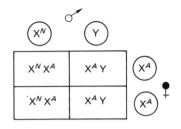

Case 2: Father normal
Mother colour defective
All female children carriers
All male children defective

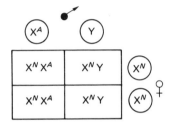

Case 3: Father colour defective
Mother normal
All female children carriers
All male children normal

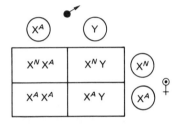

Case 4: Father colour defective
Mother colour carrier
Half the female children carriers,
the remainder colour defective
Half the male offspring normal,
the other half colour defective

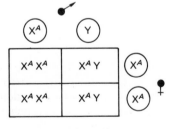

Case 5: Father and mother both
colour defective
All female children defective
All male children defective

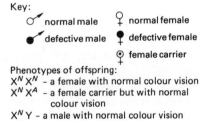

Key:
○ normal male   ♀ normal female
● defective male   ● defective female
⊙ female carrier

Phenotypes of offspring:
$X^N X^N$ – a female with normal colour vision
$X^N X^A$ – a female carrier but with normal
colour vision
$X^N Y$ – a male with normal colour vision
$X^A Y$ – a male with defective colour vision
$X^A X^A$ – a female with defective colour vision
X and Y are chromosomes
N normal, A defective genes

Figure 12.4. Genetic inheritance of colour defects.

Importance of investigating colour vision in children

Many systems for teaching both reading (e.g. Gattegno, 1964) and arithmetic (e.g. Cuisenaire and Gattegno, 1957) utilize colour. Whilst colour cueing can facilitate the acquisition of vocabulary and visual sequencing (Hallahan and Kauffman, 1975), confusion over colour can impair learning at a critical age of educational development. Mistakes made over colours can destabilize associations between vision and language for some children. It has been suggested that defective colour vision may be a factor in some cases of specific learning disability. A greater incidence of defective colour vision has been observed in the educationally handicapped (Espinda, 1973; Litton, 1979) and those having a poorer primary school reading performance (Grosvenor, 1977). Deficiencies in colour vision have also been directly implicated in intelligence test performance (Mitchell and Pollack, 1974). Some have argued that dichromatism can be responsible for a non-achieving attitude in school (Synder, 1973; Heath, 1974). Others, however, have failed to observe any association between defective colour vision and academic performance (Mandola, 1969; Lampe, Doster and Beal, 1973). Dwyer (1991) suggests that such children are incorrectly diagnosed as colour defective because they cannot respond appropriately to the tests as a result of language or other difficulties, for example, labelling confusion. Those testing such children must adopt a level of language appropriate for the child's stage of development. Obviously some children's capacity for digit reconstruction (as with the Ishihara test) and familiarity with pictorial material (such as found with the Matsubara test) is limited, together with their ability at labelling. Some apparent reversals of sequence (such as 23 for 32) and 'labelling confusions' (such as 28 for 23 and 78 for 73) may not be due to colour vision deficiency. When placed under stress children with learning difficulties are more likely to make inappropriate or guessed responses. The production of false positives in any pseudoisochromatic plate test can be argued to represent a mismatch between the intellectual capacity of the subject and the cognitive demands of the test. It would appear that, by virtue of its multifactorial basis, there is no unambiguous evidence of significantly greater levels of colour vision anomalies amongst those exhibiting a poor educational performance. Yet when defective colour vision is demonstrated, the effect of the disability on learning progress should be considered and appropriate allowances made.

Those who are congenitally colour defective may be unaware of their own deficiencies and early diagnosis is valuable, not only in this respect, but also in planning vocational or career choices (Taylor, 1971; Thuline, 1972). A colour vision defect may prevent entry into a particular career principally for reasons of safety (e.g. the armed services, the merchant navy, transport services, police and fire services) or because critical colour judgements have to be made (e.g. chemical engineering, pharmacy, the textile and printing trades). In some careers a colour vision defect does not debar entry, but can be a handicap (e.g. cartography, decorating and design work) depending on the type and severity of the defect. In general, protans are potentially more likely to experience difficulties in such matters as identifying red traffic signals under reduced visibility at night or in fog.

Appropriate colour vision tests

Although older children may perform colour vision tests as accurately as adults, many tests have limited application for young children. These are considered in more detail.

Pseudoisochromatic plates

These are designed for use under a standard illuminant such as a MacBeth easel lamp or at a north-facing window where the variations in incident daylight are less marked. Generally about 4 seconds is allowed for adults to distinguish each plate, but rather longer may have to be allowed for children depending on their age.

American Optical Company (Hardy, Rand and Rittler) plates

Gallagher and Gallagher (1964) used a simple screening method based on a selected number of the AO H-R-R plates. These utilize the geometric patterns of a circle, triangle and cross. They observed significant degrees of colour vision deficiency to be present in about 3% of preschool or first-grade children, which could constitute a practical handicap in correctly discriminating colours. Their approach was to present the demonstration plate first followed by the high chroma plates which would enable all but the severely colour defective to have a degree of success. This allows children to become better acquainted with the test procedure. In certain circumstances it may be necessary to include more than one test plate to identify those unable to understand the test instructions – or those malingering. The child is asked, 'Tell me what you see in this picture'. They are then instructed to 'Show me with your brush where the symbol is'. Finally, the child is asked to name the symbol. Supplementary tests are performed on those who fail on significant plates to estimate the severity of the defect in which they point to a symbol with a soft camel-hair brush. This screening procedure can be completed in 3 minutes in most cases – those with colour defects who are slightly more hesitant may take up to 5 minutes. Testing time should be kept to a minimum to avoid fatigue, straying attention or confusion. This test, which is no longer available commercially, can distinguish mild to severe colour vision defects and contains both tritan and 'tetartan' plates. The latter plates were included when the possibility of a fourth colour defect in yellow discrimination was postulated, most now regarding these as additional tritan plates.

The Ishihara test

Although the most commonly used test for detecting red-green colour defects in adults, its use is inappropriate for children who have not reached the age of about 7 years. To a child of limited experience the coloured dot numbers lack clarity and have configurations which differ from those numbers commonly shown to children in that age-group. It should be remembered that most young children are only familiar with numbers between 1 and 10. None the less some children, usually males, may produce a pattern of inaccurate perceptual and labelling responses including reversals, confusion with similar digits, difficulty or hesitation in reading plates with twin numbers. It should be remembered that such guesswork and lack of response may reflect difficulty with language or procedural understanding. Justen and Harth (1976) suggested that young children with learning difficulties experienced greater problems with figure-ground discrimination, which is required by all pseudoiso-chromatic plate tests. Those children who give responses indicative of colour vision defects may be investigated further by 'trails' tests, Guy's and Matsubara tests. A simple matching procedure may also be used on the anomaloscope by the children capable of understanding and performing the procedure. Adams (1974) found that about half of those who fail pseudoisochromatic plate tests, and are subsequently tested by the D-15 test, do not have a colour vision defect of such severity to warrant consideration as an educational handicap.

The Guy's colour vision test

Whilst open to criticism, the Guy's test has clear potential for use with children having delayed language development or poor manual dexterity. It is valuable for use with those having an educational handicap. The child is required to pick up one of six plastic letters matching that seen on the pseudoisochromatic plate. Two or more matching errors tend to suggest that a colour defect is present.

The Matsubara test

This test makes use of pictographs requiring verbal responses which children having limited language development might be able to produce. A normal trichromat would produce no errors, but a single error should not be regarded as abnormal in this group.

Farnsworth–Munsell tests

These comprise the Farnsworth–Munsell 100-hue test and the Farnsworth D-15 panel.

The Farnworth D-15 test is used under MacBeth illuminant 'C'. A specific colour cap is given to the child who is asked to select another which matches the cap best of all. The child is then asked to match successive caps until all 15 have been arranged, normally as a sequence of gradually changing hues. The caps are then scored and charted. This allows classification of deutan, protan or tritan colour defects, the number of errors indicating whether the defect is moderate or severe. The test, however, is relatively insensitive to mild colour vision defects.

A more sensitive test is provided by the 100-hue test, paradigmatically similar to the D-15 test, in which 85 colour caps are arranged in gradually changing hues. The sum of the numerical difference between adjacent colour caps is calculated and the score for each plotted on a polar diagram. Errors in the arrangement of hues generate confusion axes which are diagnostic of the type of colour defect. The severity of the defect is derived from the total error score. A 'practice effect' may be observed and the total error score may fall at a second attempt. Obviously there are more subtle hue changes between caps and its complexity makes it suitable only for those children who could perform the D-15 test with ease. The test is useful for monitoring acquired colour vision defects.

Lantern tests

The lantern tests rely on a rapid linguistic response to the colour shown. As such they have limited application for use with young children who may not be able to respond quickly and accurately.

The anomaloscope

This may be regarded as the definitive and ultimate means of specifying colour vision defects. The Pickford–Nicholson anomaloscope can be used on children as young as 4 years of age in the manner recommended for adults, except that it is transformed into a matching game (Pickford and Lakowski, 1960). Hill *et al.* (1982) used the red-green equation as a criterion for evaluating colour vision tests in children, the results

TABLE 12.2. The pass–fail error rate for colour vision normals and defectives obtained from a sample of 439 children aged 4–11 years (Hill *et al.*, 1982a). The validating criterion was that of the Pickford–Nicholson anomaloscope

	Pass	*Fail*
Ishihara 1966 (wavy lines)		
Defective	6	22
Normal	350	61
HRR (matching cut-out symbols)		
Defective	6	22
Normal	351	60
Guy's (matching letters)		
Defective	2	26
Normal	231	180
Matsubara (object naming)		
Defective	7	21
Normal	261	150

of which are shown in *Table 12.2*. A pass-fail criterion was set for all tests which were received binocularly under illuminant C at 600 lux. A sample of 440 boys aged between 3 and 11 years was used. A total of 28 were indicated to be colour defective, suggesting an incidence of 6.3%, agreeing well with the previously published findings for the west of Scotland when demographic variations are taken into account. They consider that it is possible to obtain sensible and reliable results from young children using an anomaloscope. They noted a very high proportion of false positives (i.e. colour normal children who failed the test) which on average exceeded comparable values for adults by a factor of 10. Such error rates might be regarded as quite unacceptable clinically and were greatest for the younger age groups. Surprisingly those tests which provided the poorest performance were the Guy's and the Matsubara tests, both of which were designed specifically for children. It appears that for all four tests in the study if a child fails a single test there is a much greater likelihood that he is normal than colour defective. The lower incidence of colour defects amongst females would indicate that there is no value in screening females for colour vision defects. Only a test capable of producing a positive error rate of the order of 2 in 10 000 would be acceptable. Only with the Ishihara test would it be possible to approach the false-positive error rate by males simply by altering the fail criteria of the test (Hill and Aspinall, 1982a).

When to screen colour vision

Arguably there are two critical ages at which colour vision should be tested. These are the preschool ages of 4–5 years and at 10–11 years. Verriest (1981) argued that preschool age children were too young to provide a satisfactory and meaningful performance because they were likely to experience conceptual and perceptual difficulty with a particular testing regimen. There are grounds for believing that colour vision develops as the fovea matures. Limited hue discrimination is found in infants between 2 and 3 months of age (Peeples and Teller, 1975; Bornstein, 1976),

TABLE 12.3. A comparison between children and adults of the Baysian probabilities associated with colour normals passing, or colour defectives failing, four colour vision tests (from Hill and Aspinall, 1980)

Test	Children*		Adults†	
	P(N/Pass)	P(D/Fail)	P(N, Pass)	P(D, Fail)
Ishihara 1966 (wavy lines)	0.97	0.32	0.99	0.82
HRR (matching symbols)	0.97	0.32	0.98	0.94
Guys (matching letters)	0.99	0.12	—	—
Matsubara (object naming)	0.97	0.15	0.97	0.73

* Aged 4–11 years; $n = 439$.
† Aged 15–28 years; $n = 100$.

which is likely to improve markedly as the fovea develops. Effective screening for colour defects depends on both the cognitive skills demanded of the test as well as the attributes of test sensitivity and specificity with respect to the rationale of the screening programme. Children of any age after 4 years can respond appropriately to a given test, such as pseudoisochromatic plates, when cognitive and digit identification demands are reduced. Hill *et al.* (1982) compared the results from four colour vision tests with those from the Pickford–Nicholson anomaloscope used on 439 colour normal and defective children aged 4–11 years. The pass-fail error rates are listed in *Table 12.2*. In addition a comparison between the performance of children and adults on four colour vision tests is given in *Table 12.3*. This lists the probabilities of colour normals passing and colour defectives failing the tests. Clearly some tests appear more successful than others in accurately detecting colour defective children. This would tend to suggest that in an ideal screening procedure, a battery of at least two supplementary tests should be included. The child's composite performance can then be assessed rather than basing this on a single test result. In view of the marked trade-off between false positives and false negatives, it is valuable to decide whether the screening programme is aimed at detecting colour vision deficiency or normality. The important rationale is to distinguish between those who would benefit from further examination and those who would not (Aspinall and Hill, 1984). It tends to be the case that poor performance on a colour vision test is usually due to design limitations rather than the child's restricted perceptual development. Indeed, it has been demonstrated that, given appropriate test material and instructions, children as young as 4 years of age can satisfactorily perform tests of identification and interpretation (Donaldson, 1978).

Conclusions

The anomaloscope represents the most accurate way of establishing the normality, or otherwise, of a child's colour vision. Those clinical colour vision tests commonly available are only valuable if used as part of a battery of tests. General screening for colour vision defects is particularly difficult at an early age. However, in the early teenage years it may become statistically acceptable to screen the colour vision of males. Other groups of children, such as females who report having difficulty over colour and those children whose educational progress is questioned, would require rather fuller investigation.

References and further reading

ADAMS, A.J. (1974). Colour vision testing in optometric practice. *Journal of the American Optometric Association*, **45**, 35–42.

ASPINALL, P.A. and HILL, A.R. (1980). An application of decision theory to colour vision testing. In *Colour Vision Deficiencies V*, edited by G. Verriest. Hilgar, Bristol, pp. 164–171.

ASPINALL, P.A. and HILL, A.R. (1984). Is screening worthwhile? In *Progress in Child Health*, edited by A. MacFarlane. Churchill Livingstone, Edinburgh, pp. 243–259.

BORNSTEIN, M. (1976). Infants are trichromate. *Journal of Experimental Child Psychology*, **21**, 873–890.

CUISENAIRE, G. and GATTEGNO, C. (1957). *Numbers in Colours, A New Method of Teaching Arithmetic in Primary Schools*, 3rd edn. Cuisenaire, New York.

DONALDSON, M. (1978). *Children's minds*. Fontana, London.

DWYER, J.I. (1991). Colour vision defects in children with learning difficulties. *Clinical and Experimental Optometry*, **74**, 30–38.

ESPINDA, S.D. (1973). Color vision deficiency: a learning disability? *Journal of Learning Disabilities*, **6**, 163–166.

GALLAGHER, J.R. and GALLAGHER, C.D. (1964). Colour vision screening of Pre-school and First grade children. *Archives of Ophthalmology*, **72**, 200–211.

GARDINER, P.A. (1973). Colour vision test for young children and the handicapped. *Developmental Medical Child Neurology*, **15**, 437–440.

GATTEGNO, C. (1964). *Words in Colour*. Encyclopedia Brittanica, Chicago.

GROSVENOR, T. (1977). Are visual anomalies related to reading ability? *Journal of the American Optometric Association*, **48**, 510–517.

HALLAHAN, D.P. and KAUFFMAN, J.M. (1975). Research on the education of distractible and hyperactive children. In *Perceptual and Learning Difficulty in Children*, vol. 2, *Research and Theory*, edited by W.D. Cruickshank and D.P. Hallahan. University Press, Syracuse.

HEATH, G.G. (1974). The handicap of colour blindness. *Journal of the Optometric Association*, **45**, 62–69.

HILL, A.R. and ASPINALL, P.A. (1980). An application of decision analysis to colour vision testing. In *Colour Vision Deficiencies V*, edited by G. Verriest. Hilgar, Bristol, pp. 164–171.

HILL, A.R. and ASPINALL, P.A. (1982a). Pass/fail criteria in colour vision tests and their effect on decision confidence. *Documenta Ophthalmologica Proceedings Series*, **33**, 157–162.

HILL, A.R. and ASPINALL, P.A. (1982b). Tetartanomaly in a mixed heterozygote. *Documenta Ophthalmologica Proceedings Series*, **33**, 333–336.

HILL, A.R., HERON, H., LLOYD, M. and LOWTHER, P. (1982). An evaluation of some colour vision tests for children. *Documenta Ophthalmologica Proceedings Series*, **33**, 183–187.

JUSTEN, J.E. and HARTH, R. (1976). The relationship between figure-ground discrimination and colour blindness in learning-disabled children. *Journal of Learning Disabilities*, **9**, 96–99.

LAMPE, J.M., DOSTER, M.E. and BEAL, B.B. (1973). Summary of a 3-year study of academic and school achievement between color-deficient and normal primary age pupils. (Phase 2). *Journal of School Health*, **43**, 309–411.

LITTON, F.W. (1979). Colour vision deficiency in L.D. children. *Academic Therapy*, **14**, 437–443.

MANDOLA, J. (1969). The role of color vision anomalies in elementary school achievement. *Journal of School Health*, **39**, 633–636.

MITCHELL, N.B. and POLLACK, R.H. (1974). Block design performance as a function of hue and race. *Journal of Experimental Psychology*, **17**, 377–382.

MULLER, G.E. (1930). Uber die Farbenempfindungen. *Z. Psychol., Erganzungsb.*, **17**, 18.

PEEPLES, D. and TELLER, D.Y. (1975). Color vision and brightness discrimination in two-month old human infants. *Science*, **189**, 1102–1103.

PICKFORD, R.W. and LAKOWSKI, R. (1960). The Pickford–Nicholson anomaloscope. *British Journal of Physiological Optics*, **17**, 131–150.

SYNDER, C.R. (1973). The psychological implications of being color blind. *Journal of Special Education*, **7**, 51–54.

TAYLOR, W.O.G. (1971). Effects on employment of defects in colour vision. *British Journal of Ophthalmology*, **55**, 753–760.

TELLER, D.Y., PEEPLES, D. and SEKEL, M. (1978). Discrimination of chromatic from white light by two-month old human infants. *Vision Research*, **18**, 41–48.

THULINE, H.C. (1972). Colour blindness in children. *Clinical Pediatrics*, **11**, 295–299.

VERRIEST, G. (1981). Colour vision test in children. *Atti. Fon. G. Ronchi*, **36**, 83–119.

VERRIEST, G., VAN LAETHAM, J. and UVIJLA, A. (1982). A new assessment of the normal ranges of the Farnsworth 100-hue test scores. *American Journal of Ophthalmology*, **93**, 635–642.

VERRIEST, G., UVIJLS, A., GANDIBLEU, M.F., MALFROIDT, A. and DECO, M.R. (1982). Colour vision tests in children. *Documenta Ophthalmologica Proceedings Series*, **33**, 175–178.

VERRIEST, G. and UVIJLA, A. (1977). Special increment thresholds on a white background in different age groups of normal subjects and in acquired ocular diseases. *Documenta Ophthalmologica*, **43**, 217–248.

ZEKI, S. (1990). Colour vision and functional specialisation in the visual cortex. *Discussion in Neuroscience, Disner*, **VI**, No. 2, 1–64.

13

Dispensing for the child patient

W.S. Topliss

Introduction

The skill in obtaining a prescription for a child patient is completely nullified if the lenses are not correctly centred and positioned before the eyes. The fit of the spectacles on the nose and ears is crucial for comfort and absolutely vital if the lens prescription is a high one. When dealing with children the practitioner may have to rely simply on visual clues, and personal experience, to tell whether a frame is fitting correctly since the child may be unable or unwilling to say how the frame feels. Children who are wearing spectacles for the first time find this an unusual experience and tend to remove their spectacles. They have to be encouraged to wear them, but this is extremely difficult if the frame tends to irritate and is uncomfortable. Very soon it becomes a battle for parents to get their child to wear their spectacles – one which parents invariably lose. In addition to being uncomfortable, ill-positioned spectacles alter back vertex distance and, if not level, generate unwanted relative prismatic effects. It is worth bearing in mind that, when a child has to wear spectacles for the first time, there is often considerable impact upon parents who see their child's appearance dramatically changed. Quite simply, if the spectacles appear unsightly it is less likely that they will be worn.

General considerations in frame fitting

Children's spectacle frames take a fair degree of punishment during wear and play. Good quality metal frames tend to withstand this more easily than plastic ones. Since metal bends under stress, frames which have been grossly deformed can be straightened to restore them close to their original appearance. This may have to be done on a number of occasions and if the frame breaks a solder repair may be possible. Plastic frames, which have less 'give' in them, have a tendency to break when stressed. A repair is not easily effected within the practice and although a new component may be obtained there is always the risk that the frame design may be discontinued.

Children's frames suffer rather rough handling when they are removed and are frequently knocked when worn. Sprung joints are, therefore, very useful since they flex without damaging the sides. Curl sides may have to be used with very young children, particularly with those having a large refractive error. The sheer bulk of the

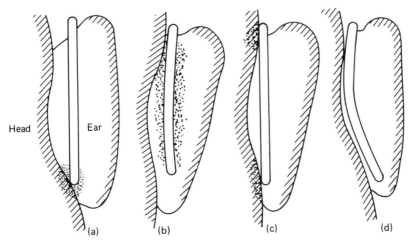

Figure 13.1. Sides must also be contoured to fit the head behind the ears, allowing for the depression of the mastoid bone; (a) side angled in too much, concentrating pressure on one point at the side of the head; (b) the other extreme, here all the weight is on the ear and will cause discomfort. The sides should be angled in more; (c) an improvement, the side makes contact only at the top of the ear and end of the side, but a gap is left over the mastoid dip; (d) side contoured to a perfect fit (From Topliss, 1975)

lenses, combined with the poorly developed bridge of the nose, causes the frame to be rather unstable. Curl sides can be rather uncomfortable if not carefully fitted and children tend to prefer hockey-end sides as soon as their facial features have developed sufficiently (*Figure 13.1*). It is wise to note the length and angle of the sides which will be required, since these are better altered at the workshop whilst the frame is being glazed (*Figure 13.2*). The total length of curl sides should be specified so that their ends are not visible below the ears.

Lenses constitute the major bulk of any pair of spectacles. Care should be taken that the overall size of the frame is not so large that lens weight becomes a problem. When selecting the size of frame for the child it should just clear the cheeks and

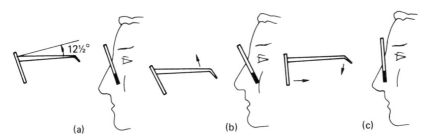

Figure 13.2. The side length or angle may need altering when the frame is in the workshop for lens glazing. The final angling, length to bend of the sides, the temple and head widths must be adjusted during the final fit. Ideally, the frame should just clear the cheeks and the eyebrows: (a) normal angle for a side – approximately 12.5°; (b) Bottom rim touching cheek, which will lead to discomfort and 'steaming up' of lens – the sides should be angled up to move the bottom of the rim out; (c) bottom of rim too far from cheek, leading to interference with vision when wearer looks down – the sides must be angled down to bring bottom of rim in (From Topliss, 1975)

eyebrows, with the normal downward angle between the side and the plane of the front in the region of 12½ degrees for a high joint frame. The prominent cheeks of some children may require this angle to be reduced, as would centrally fitted sides. If the child has prominent eyebrows and cheeks then a frame having a shallower depth should be chosen. Side angle and lens depth are important when considering the frame fit on the nose. Young children generally have a rather flat nose so that a frame that has adjustable pads might command the best fit.

Bridge types

There are three main bridge fittings which are encountered:

(1) The regular bridge. The shape and contour of this bridge corresponds to the nose itself, spreading the weight of the frame and lenses evenly over as large an area as possible.
(2) Plastics pad bridge. This type of bridge is unsuitable for children without a well-developed bridge. The weight of the frame and lenses is borne on the pads. The frontal angle and splay angle are the most important characteristics of this bridge (*Figure 13.3*).

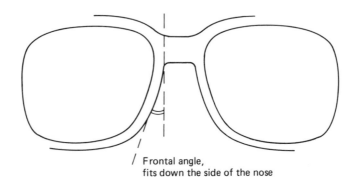

/ Frontal angle,
fits down the side of the nose

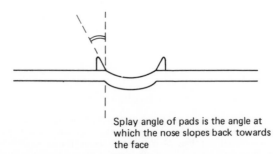

Splay angle of pads is the angle at which the nose slopes back towards the face

Figure 13.3. With both frontal angle and splay angle it is important to get the maximum amount of frame into contact with the nose in order to spread the weight of the spectacles and give maximum comfort to the patient (From Topliss, 1975)

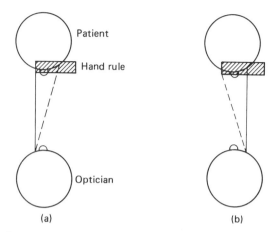

Figure 13.4. Stages in the measurement: (a) optometrist has left eye open and right eye closed; patient looks into optician's open eye; (b) patient looks into examiner's open right eye (from Topliss, 1975)

(3) Metal pad bridge. This form of bridge offers the most scope for young children since the pad arms can be manipulated allowing a good fit on almost any child's nose. It also allows the frame to clear cheeks and eyebrows. There are a couple of useful adjuncts to this range. Pad bridges, which are linked by a flexible plastic strap, can combine the advantages of pad and regular bridge fitting so that even support is obtained across the bridge of the nose. In addition, plastic comfort bridges are available with inset metal supports at the sides which can be manipulated to adjust the shape of bridge.

Pupillary distance

The conventional manner of measuring the pupillary distance is for the practitioner to measure from the temporal limbus of one eye to the nasal limbus of the other eye, whilst the patient fixates the examiner's right and left eye respectively (*Figure 13.4*). Children do not concentrate for any length of time, so that it may be useful for the practitioner to hold a small object in his hand just below his eye for the child to look at. Alternatively, a squeaky toy may prove very useful in getting the child to maintain

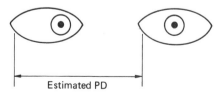

Figure 13.5. When the patient has a squint the reading can be taken using the inner canthus of one eye, and the outer canthus of the other eye as reference points. The reading should be near enough for normal purposes, as any small error of prismatic effect introduced will not be of great importance (From Topliss, 1975)

some degree of fixation. With young children a number of measurements may have to be made before ascertaining the interpupillary distance. This technique is perfectly adequate for most prescriptions, assuming that significant facial asymmetry is not present.

If the patient has a squint the above method of measurement is not suitable. The approximate pupillary distance can be measured with a rule from the inner canthus of one eye to the outer canthus of the other eye (*Figure 13.5*). Alternatively monocular pupillary distances may be measured with one eye occluded whilst the child looks at the examiner's eye.

If significant horizontal asymmetry is present then half pupillary distances should be measured, particularly if the lens powers of the right and left eyes are quite different.

The visual system is less tolerant of prismatic imbalance in the vertical plane than in the horizontal plane. If significant vertical asymmetry is present try to fit the frame to the patient so that it appears level with the eyebrows, and at the same time the distance between the lower eyelid and the bottom of the rim of the frame is equal for both eyes. If the frame fits correctly in relation to the two eyes, it may not look straight when the top rim is compared with the eyebrows. In this case you may have to explain the problem to the patient or to the child's parents. The frame should then be adjusted for the best possible compromise. The position of the optical centres should be measured with the frame in position. The height of the centres can be measured either in relation to the spectacle frame datum line or vertically from the bottom rim. Alternatively, a felt-tip pen can be used to mark the pupil centres on demonstration lenses contained within the spectacle frame. If the frame is not already glazed with plano demonstration lenses a piece of transparent sticky tape can be put across the rims to allow the pupil centre to be marked as before.

Spectacle lenses

People in all industrial countries are becoming increasingly aware of the need for safety. The dangers from industrial, chemical, mechanical and radiation injuries are at last being realized and protection sought. Consequently more thought is being given to protective lenses for children, particularly with the increasingly hazardous sports that they undertake – as if the dangers of the playground are not in themselves enough.

Glass is a highly brittle substance which upon impact shatters into innumerable sharp splinters. Any accident which causes an impact to the lenses may lead to a serious eye injury. Children are much more likely than adults to indulge in activities which lead to shattered spectacle lenses. There are a number of ways in which some degree of protection can be afforded, and these are detailed below.

Heat-toughened lenses

It can be shown that glass under tension breaks quite easily, yet under compression it is quite strong. To produce compression in a lens it must be heated to near melting point and then suddenly cooled. This is achieved by heating the otherwise completed lens in a small oven to a temperature of about 650° C for a specified time, depending upon the type, weight and size of the particular lens. At the end of this specified time the lens is removed from the oven and positioned between two nozzles which allow

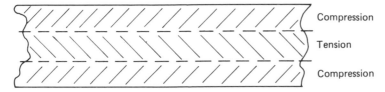

Figure 13.6. Section through heat-toughened glass. The outer layers are under compression while the intermediate mass is under tension (From Topliss, 1975)

compressed air to blow onto both surfaces of the glass simultaneously for a short period. The two outer surfaces of the lens cool quickly because of the air blown onto them, whilst its centre remains comparatively fluid for some little time. As the centre cools to the same temperature as the outer glass, it contracts and exerts a tension on the cool outer layers producing a 'skin' of compressed glass, the centre of the lens being under great tensile stress (*Figure 13.6*). Hence the sudden cooling process produces the compression and tension within the lens which gives it the required strength.

When a lens has been toughened in this manner, a certain amount of strain is produced in the glass which may be seen using a crossed polaroid strain viewer, the strain pattern in the lens being similar in appearance to a Maltese cross. The actual pattern, however, will vary with the power and thickness of the lens and the size of the cold air nozzle used to quench the lens.

Each lens is tested to British Standards quality and should withstand a steel ball of 32 mm diameter weighing 130 g, dropped from a height of 1.83 m onto it. This strength would give children most of the protection they need. Certain types of lenses may not be accepted for toughening: drilled or grooved lenses, minus lenses with a power over -10.00 D and large diameter lenses.

A toughened lens is not unbreakable, and should not be described as such. When a break does occur, the glass crumbles into pieces which may be rolled between finger and thumb without cutting.

Plastic lenses

CR-39

Allyl diglycol carbonate was developed by the Columbia Chemical Company division of the Pittsburgh Plate Glass Company at the end of the 1930s, hence the name Columbia Resin CR-39.

The liquid CR-39 monomer is heated with a catalyst to form a hard clear thermosetting substance which will not re-soften under heat. Glass moulds are used to cast the lenses or alternatively cast blanks may be surfaced in the same way as ordinary glass lenses.

CR-39 has a high impact resistance but when it does break it will break into a number of both large and small pieces, some of which may be sharp. However, it is still classed as a safety lens, and its optical properties are equal to those of glass lenses. The weight of a plastic lens is only half that of a similar glass lens so it is an ideal medium for high-powered prescriptions. CR-39 can be dyed to any number of colour combinations and can be antireflection coated and hard coated. The use of CR-39 lenses is rising every year, demonstrating their popularity.

Polycarbonate

Undoubtedly the best lens available for absolute safety. The author has seen a lens withstand repeated impact from 0.22 mm gun pellets fired at the lens from a distance of 45 cm. In fact, its strength to weight ratio is equal to that of aluminium and twice that of zinc. Compared to aluminium and zinc, its impact strength is four times greater. Polycarbonate can withstand five times the impact energy of CR-39. These lenses should be regarded as essential for children or adults who play games which could be dangerous, such as cricket or squash. The lenses can be both tinted and hard coated. Until the development of abrasive resistant coatings, polycarbonate was too soft to be an effective safety lens. Silicone-based polymer coatings can be applied to the lenses by either a dip or spin coating method and leave the lens with a hard surface.

Cosmetic dispensing

With a positive approach children can enjoy trying on different frame styles after the eye examination. These days children appear much more certain of how they wish to look and the range of frames available is extensive. Obviously the frame must be suitable for the child's prescription. From what has been said earlier the art of cosmetic dispensing is not inappropriate. Frame selection, combined with experience and a little thought, will help to achieve a balanced picture of the child's face.

Figure 13.7 shows the proportions of three crosses. If the child's face is imagined as a cross with the eyebrows forming the horizontal element, then is it an (a), (b) or (c) face? The object is to try to alter, or maintain, the balance of the face when wearing spectacles so that it more nearly resembles the proportions of (a). The way in which this might be achieved is to follow a technique called the 'box line and balance' method. The box (*Figure 13.8*) may be rectangular or square, depending upon eyebrow position and fullness of cheeks. The depth of the face will be either average, long or short. A spectacle frame having a shallow depth will make the face appear

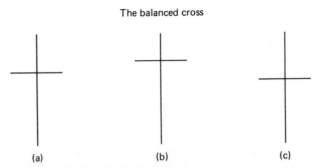

The balanced cross

(a)   (b)   (c)

Figure 13.7. Demonstration of placing essentially similar elements in different relationships to produce surprisingly different effects: (a) horizontal bar crossing at two-thirds the height of the vertical produces a figure of well-balanced appearance; (b) placing the crossbar higher up the vertical makes the figure look taller; (c) apparent shortening and stubbiness result from positioning the crossbar near the centre (From Topliss, 1975)

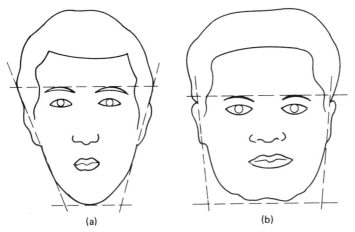

(a)   (b)

Figure 13.8. The face related to a 'box': (a) deep rectangular, calling for a deep eyeshape and solid-colour rim; (b) short, square type for which a shallow frame will be preferable, either two-tone or in supra style (From Topliss, 1975)

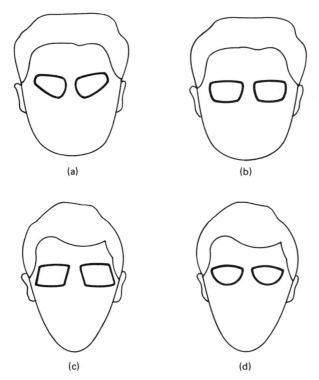

(a)   (b)

(c)   (d)

Figure 13.9. The 'line' approach: (a) the harlequin shape will make the cheeks look fatter and squarer; (b) a frame which follows the line of the cheek produces a more balanced effect; (c) square-shaped frames on a face with a pointed chin will make the chin look even more pointed; (d) choosing a frame shape which follows the line of the cheek will give the chin a wider appearance (From Topliss, 1975)

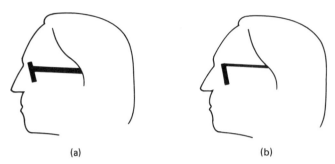

(a)   (b)

Figure 13.10. Identical profiles wearing (a) a frame with a thick side and centre joint; (b) frame with a thin side and a high joint. The thick side 'shortens' the face; the other has the reverse effect (From Topliss, 1975)

longer and vice versa. The line of the patient's chin and jaw gives an indication of the most suitable frame shape. Ideally the bottom rim of the frame should follow the line of the chin and jaw. This avoids emphasizing the lower part of the face, making the cheeks appear fatter or thinner (*Figure 13.9*). Spectacle frames having a dark-coloured bridge tend to emphasize a child's short stubby nose and give the appearance of the eyes being close together. A clear bridge tends to 'lengthen' the nose and give the appearance of the eyes being more widely spaced. A similar effect may be obtained from a metal frame with adjustable pads, which will probably also give a good fit. The cosmetic effect of high and centre joint sides, together with their thickness, is described in *Figure 13.10*.

Reference

TOPLISS, W.C. (1975). *Optical Dispensing and Workshop Practice*, Butterworth, London.

14

Paediatric contact lens practice

A.G. Sabell and A.J. Kempster

Introduction

Contact lenses are not commonly worn by younger children. Those with lower refractive errors are normally and quite adequately corrected by means of spectacles. For such refractive errors, the use of contact lenses should be actively discouraged. Having said that, there will remain a small proportion of child patients for whom a contact lens correction will appear to have distinct advantages over spectacles. For these cases of 'clinical necessity' the use of contact lenses will be justifiable and beneficial whatever degree of persistence may be needed to achieve success.

Indications for contact lenses during childhood

When considering adult contact lens patients it is often convenient to define several distinct age groups. Thus many of the 16 to 35 year-old patients will fall into the category of 'vanity' wearers whose motivation is dislike of their own appearance in spectacles. Others will find for certain occupations or hobbies that the wearing of spectacles is an impediment. These are strongly motivating factors often producing a great incentive to persevere and to overcome difficulties over adaptation to contact lenses when these problems occur. In contrast, the middle age range, perhaps from 40 to 60 years of age, may have slightly different reasons for wanting to wear contact lenses. Although the 'vanity' factor may still exist, other features begin to impinge, notably the onset of presbyopia and its implications. For instance, the incovenience of a second pair of spectacles or the dislike of bifocal or varifocal glasses may be solved by a distance correction by contact lenses and the use simply of reading spectacles. If the practitioner has sufficient stamina, he may even be prepared to recommend bifocal contact lenses in some cases! New contact lens wearers within this age group will be less common and most of the group will be composed of existing contact lens wearers who have 'graduated' from the earlier group and who have no definite reasons for abandoning the mode of vision correction to which they are accustomed. The third age group, often of 65 years upwards, will perhaps contain a somewhat increased group of first-time users of contact lenses. These however will be the cases of 'clinically indicated' lenses. These three age categories will be well recognized by the average practitioner.

The fourth group, consisting of child patients although having a much smaller spread of ages, does show a number of distinct subdivisions. These may be created by factors such as:

(1) Ease of determining the fit of a contact lens.
(2) How cooperative the child is likely to be.
(3) The ability of the child to insert and remove their own lenses and, if this is not possible, the ability of the parents to perform this task adequately.

With paediatric contact lens practice, these are the sort of factors which will govern the practitioner's choice of lens form. As with the adult groups, they will not constitute rigid divisions and great variations do occur. This is especially true of the factor of cooperation. Some young children will be found to have a very placid temperament and allow manipulation of the eyes with little or no protest. Others, sometimes much older children, seem totally unable to relax or to cooperate. This one suspects is often the outcome of the home environment and parental attitudes.

Management of the child patient

Older children can be regarded essentially as 'miniature adults' and as such the practitioner will require as many different communication skills as those used with adult patients. The term 'child' covers all ages from the infant to the teenager. It is fairly obvious that different skills will be required dependent upon the age of the patient. There are however a few general rules that apply from toddlers to the upper junior school age.

The type of personality encountered with these child patients will be as varied as with adults. It is important for the practitioner to approach the child with confidence. The great difference between adults and children is that the child has no fear until an event has been experienced, unless of course that fear has been instituted by the behaviour of a parent or another child. Provided each time the child patient is seen, a rapport is gradually built up between the practitioner and patient, it is possible to execute rather uncomfortable procedures with few problems. It is essential to explain in simple terms what the procedure entails. The whole examination should be approached with an element of fun and, whenever possible, games should be invented. The whole idea is to jolly the patient along, a technique occasionally necessary with some adult patients. The authors' experience has shown that it is of utmost importance to tell the child truthfully, if of suitable age, if something is going to be uncomfortable. As an example, when inserting an hydrogel lens, it is helpful to say 'this lens may tickle for a few moments but it will not hurt'. The word tickle is used because it can be understood by the child. It is a word often used by children to describe the sensation of a soft contact lens in an unadapted eye. It has been found that using children's own words to describe situations is very helpful. The authors also believe that in some situations, a reward such as a sweet or a badge can relieve a difficult situation. Such bribes should never be given unless adequately earned by the child by virtue of cooperating with the practitioner.

Fear can undoubtedly be transmitted from the parent or guardian. This may be very difficult for the practitioner to combat since the fear may be unspoken and in any case is usually unfounded. It is therefore important to spend time explaining to the parent in advance, exactly what will be involved in the fitting of the contact lenses. In some cases it may be worth inviting the parent, if particularly apprehensive, to have a contact lens put onto their eye in order to convince them that the procedure is innocuous. It has been suggested that in some cases, when teaching the parent to insert and remove lenses from their child's eyes, their confidence might be enhanced by allowing them first to insert and remove a lens using the practitioner as their patient. The remedy for a particular fear may have to vary from case to case, and will depend upon its cause. There will be occasions when persons other than the parent may be more helpful in overcoming such problems; elder brothers or sisters, aunts, uncles or even teachers may provide invaluable assistance. Children are usually very truthful and if asked, will tell the practitioner whom they would prefer to insert their contact lens. Beware, they will also announce with great clarity which practitioner they like best. Time spent explaining things to parents and to children is always time well spent, a fact that is all too easily forgotten in the middle of a busy clinic.

So what, loosely speaking, are the age groups into which the child patient is likely to fall? In the opinion of the authors they are as follows:

- Under 1 year.
- 1–3 years.
- 4–6 years.
- 6–10 years.
- 10 years and over.

The approach to be adopted with each group will vary. With the first two groups, although the child will not understand that what is happening to them is for their benefit and they will probably protest loudly, with the first group they have not yet developed arm and leg muscles of sufficient power to produce an inconvenient level of resistance. However, as age increases within this group, so do the problems of management.

As the child passes into the second age group their muscular development is such that physical resistance becomes an increasing problem and assistance beyond that of the parent may be necessary. Both volume of noise emmitted and physical resistance may present the practitioner with increasing problems. The most common need for contact lenses in these two groups will be aphakia, either unilateral or bilateral. It is essential, if visual development is to be maximized, for congenital cataracts to be removed at the earliest opportunity; if possible as early as 2–4 weeks old has been stated by some surgeons (Davies and Tarbuck, 1977). The aphakic correction is necessary as soon as possible following surgery, usually within a week or so. A slight overcorrection of 2 or 3 D is commonly used since the child's visual attention is usually directed at near objects. Some surgeons have been in the practice of inserting a soft extended wear lens immediately on completion of surgery (Davies and Tarbuck, 1977). Others prefer to apply the contact lens about a week later; often, in bilateral cataracts when the second eye is being treated (Willshaw, 1985, personal communication). This allows a second opportunity to assess the refractive error under anaesthesia. The first lenses will commonly be in the order of $+30+35\,D$. Such a lens will clearly have a substantial centre thickness and oxygen transmission will accordingly be somewhat limited. Fortunately the need for such a high plus steadily declines over the following months and the correction can be reorientated to distance vision requirements allowing further reduction in lens thickness. Just as the age group will often determine the form of lens used, so it will bring about the need to vary one's fitting procedures.

The usual type of lens to be fitted initially will probably be an extended-wear hydrogel. Very young children usually sit happily on the lap of one or other of the parents, preferably with their head cradled in the adult's arm on the side nearest to the practitioner. From this position it is usually relatively easy to place the contact lens into position. With some of the more difficult infants, this may be more readily accomplished while the child is asleep or in the process of waking or even on occasion when the child is feeding. Very young infants do not usually rub out their lenses as do the slightly older ones. Towards their first birthday, lens insertion and removal become increasingly difficult and an assistant will be found to be invaluable to restrain the 'flailing' arms and legs. It is usual to wrap the child tightly in a blanket or sheet whilst lying on an examination couch in order to make the procedure possible. The practitioner stands at the head of the couch to insert the lens while the assistant is positioned at the side to ensure that the arms and legs do not escape from the folds of the blanket (*Figure 14.1*). It is possible with very small infants to have the child lying along the thighs of the practitioner and the assistant, who sit on two chairs facing each other. This method has been described in several textbooks of ophthalmology over many years (Duke Elder, 1962). Tightly wrapping the child during such procedures is said to not only prevent injury to arms and legs lashing vigorously around but to make the child feel secure, it is worth noting that even when securely wrapped in a tight blanket the head can be vigorously moved from side to side, a considerable obstacle to the insertion of a soft contact lens. Thus in some cases an assistant to hold the head steady may be a considerable advantage.

Many of the above comments become even more important when the child passes to the second age group of 1–3 years. This is the most difficult age group to fit with contact lenses for the first time. The child fitted at the age of less than 6 months and having worn contact lenses from that point may be less troublesome through this 1–3-year phase than one introduced to contact lenses at this point. Again, the extended-wear soft lens is likely to be the best choice for an initial trial. As will be seen later, other lens forms may be required including the scleral lens. It may be found necessary, when a child is teething and more prone to rubbing their eyes, to dispense with contact lenses and to return to them when this phase is passed. In some

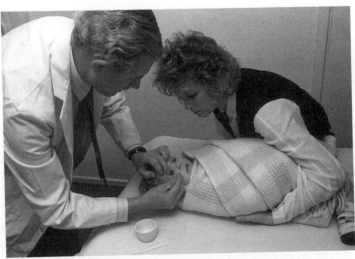

Figure 14.1. Blanket restraint used when inserting contact lenses into infant eyes

cases this is deemed to be clinically undesirable and it may be necessary to battle on using contact lenses. One of the authors recalls a case in which five soft lenses were inserted before the child finally succumbed and fell asleep with exhaustion from crying. This did not represent success however and the child was back again next morning for more of the same treatment, having displaced the lens during the night. Unless there is a bottomless pit of resources, it is better to admit defeat and abandon contact lenses until the teething period is over. Even in unilateral aphakia one can prescribe a spectacle correction for the aphakic eye with an occluding lens for the good eye to be worn for part of each day to prevent development of amblyopia. Such spectacles may need to be used for a period of about 6 months before further contact lens trials can resume. It is only fair to say that one occasionally encounters infants who steadfastly reject the wearing of spectacles, so this option may not always be a smooth alternative.

When this troublesome period is passing and the infant reaches his/her third birthday, it becomes increasingly possible to have a reasonable conversation with the patient. Gradually a relationship can be built up and once established satisfactorily, this is rarely broken. A problem can arise from this in that the child may then become reluctant to change from one practitioner to another. Whenever possible, it is advisable to accustom the child to more than one person. Adaptation to two practitioners may not be feasible but continuity can often be provided by the assistant member of staff such as a nurse or orthoptist. The value of such auxiliary staff is of the greatest importance and every opportunity should be taken to involve them in the clinical procedures. When children reach the age of 3 years, it may be possible to consider changing to daily-wear soft lenses. The success of such a venture may depend on the degree of involvement which has been achieved by the parents. Some parents may persistently resist all attempts to get them to undertake responsibility for removal and daily cleaning of the child's lenses. In these cases one must continue further with the extended-wear lens and hope that the future may bring about a change of attitude.

In the 3–6 year age group the child should be appreciably easier to deal with and may be fitted with a wider range of lens types. Even so, considerable differences will be encountered from one child to another. The average 6 year old, given supervision, will often be able to remove their own soft lenses and may even be able to replace them. The level of supervision needed will depend on the child's natural dexterity as well as the capability of the parent. Although children have small fingers they can find it difficult to manipulate small objects such as a contact lens. They are usually very capable of holding their own eyelids apart while an adult applies the contact lens. Such participation is helpful to the process of obtaining cooperation and is to be encouraged. Gradually, as their dexterity improves they become able to insert and remove their own lenses, possibly at first with an adult holding the eyelids for them. It should be possible around the age of 6 or 7, for them to undertake the whole procedure for themselves. It is still advisable that the lens cleaning and storage procedures be performed by an adult to ensure efficacy and to avoid unnecessary damage to the lenses.

By this time, it will be found that most children can be fascinated by fluorescein patterns in fitting rigid lenses. It is helpful to show them the appearance of their own eye by placing a handbag mirror behind the lens of the u.v. lamp. By introducing this 'game' into the fitting procedure their attention can often be diverted away from the initial sensations of the lenses. It is also possible that the judicious use of local anaesthetic at this stage in the fitting of hard lenses can ease the process. If time allows this 'fluorescein' game to be played fully, some older children can even be taught to distinguish between a flat fit and a steep one with corneal lenses.

The 6 to 10 year olds are moving into the 'miniature adult' category and often present no more difficulty in fitting than adults. Again there is considerable variability and attitudes will usually be the product of parental influence. Usually the more intelligent children become the most time consuming since they expect to be given adequate answers to a seemingly unending succession of questions. It is clearly of the greatest importance that the practitioner should answer these to the best of his ability. In this age group the children become very interested in instruments and can often be encouraged by being given the opportunity to look through such things as keratometers and slit-lamp microscopes, possibly using a favourite teddy-bear or doll as subject (*Figure 14.2*). It may be possible to allow the child to apply an old, scrap contact lens to the eye of such a teddy-bear. Encouraging such familiarity with the clinical instruments and with the handling of the lenses can give the child a sense of security within the practice environment. Indeed, one of the authors has gone so far as to accept a role reversal and allowed some children within this age group to place contact lenses on her own eye in the belief that the child is made to feel in command of the situation and thereby takes up the challenge of getting to wear the lenses successfully. The hypothesis being that if the practitioner can tolerate the contact lens, there is no reason why the child should fail to cope. With this age group it is most helpful when assistants who come into the consulting room while the fitting is proceeding, make suitable complementary remarks to the child regarding their good appearance in the lenses and/or their good behaviour during the fitting. Children usually respond very favourably to such encouragement. A mirror is an invaluable part of the equipment of the consulting room for the child to examine their own appearance when wearing the lenses. This is especially true when dealing with children with high refractive errors since they frequently are subjected to uncomple-

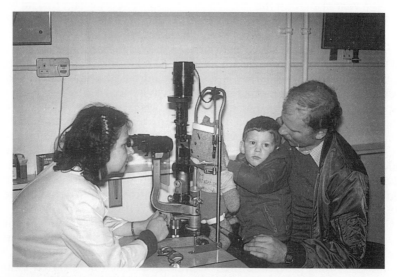

Figure 14.2. The use of a teddy bear to aid cooperation of a young child during introduction to keratometry or slit-lamp examination

mentary remarks at school with regard to the appearance of their spectacles. The use of such subtle devices can be very useful in boosting motivation to wear the contact lenses. Children usually do not want to be different from the others in their group and are generally happier to discover the normality of their appearance when wearing the contact lenses.

To all intents and purposes the over 10-year-old group are treated as adults. They may have certain limitation in vocabulary but this variability will be found also among some adult patients. They usually respond best when they are treated as adults. One should not underestimate the psychological impact of having to wear very high powered spectacle lenses, and it has been often quoted over the past 50 years in various textbooks on contact lenses that personality change has been observed in adults who have changed from long-term spectacle wear to the use of contact lenses (Obrig, 1942). Such changes are also observed in these highly ametropic older children and at times can be most dramatic. Children who cannot be persuaded to speak in reply to the practitioner's questions suddenly begin to respond and to communicate. Changes of this type are enormously encouraging to the practitioner who then begins to realize the great benefits which his skills can bring.

Fitting procedures

Keratometry

While fitting principles for children are no different to those adopted for adults, it becomes obvious to all who attempt this that certain modifications and compromises must be accepted. An immediate example springing to mind is that of keratometry. This requires cooperation of the patient in placement of the head, in retaining a stationary posture and in steadiness of fixation. With young children this is impossible, although great personal variations are to be found within each age group.

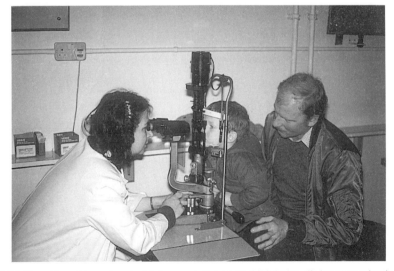

Figure 14.3. Parent's assistance is valuable in supporting small child during slit-lamp examination or keratometry

It is impossible therefore to specify an age at which successful keratometry can be expected. One just has to try and to be prepared to abandon the attempt if it proves impracticable. Assistance of a parent or other support staff is usually needed to support the child and to hold the head steady and in the correct position on the chinrest (*Figure 14.3*). Even so, one is still dependent on reasonable fixation to achieve a successful measurement. If the child is distressed, this is impossible and the attempt should be abandoned. Presentation of the procedure as a 'game' to be played between the patient and the practitioner is frequently useful at the early attempts. Once successful, such procedures can usually be repeated on future occasions with increasing ease.

Clearly with very young children keratometry will be impractical. Attempts have been made to perform keratometry under general anaesthesia (Absell *et al.*, 1990), either by having the instrument mounted on a special vertical stand as with the operating microscope, or even with some instruments to use it hand held. The Zeiss Jena keratometer head is suitable for this, being reasonably compact and readily removeable from its normal mounting (*Figure 14.4*). Even so, in the authors' experience, the results often leave much to be desired in terms of accuracy. The eye under general anaesthesia is often elevated and a speculum and/or the use of fixation forceps by an assistant may be needed (*Figure 14.5*).

Fitting without keratometry

It may therefore be more practical to select the first soft lens on an arbitrary basis and to modify one's decisions according to results. Such a system is recommended by Wilson and Millis (1988b) who suggest the use of back surface radii of 7.50 mm for infants up to about 1 year old. Thereafter they believe that 7.80 mm may be appropriate for the next year or two with possible further flattening later. These figures are quoted on the basis of a total diameter of 13.00 mm and may clearly need

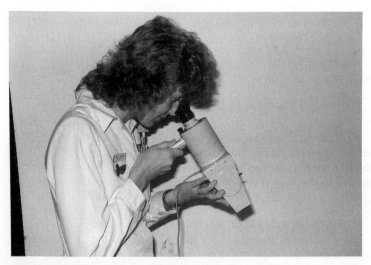

Figure 14.4. The Zeiss Jena keratometer head detached from its mounting for hand-held use on child under general anaesthesia

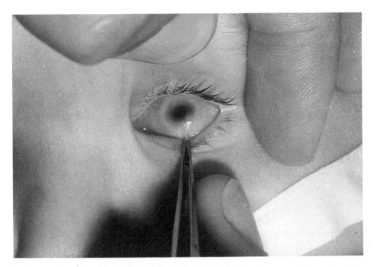

Figure 14.5. Infant eye held in suitable position for keratometry under general anaesthesia

modification if the TD needs to be varied. Such changes in diameter will depend on the size of the eye and, in buphthalmos for example, the TD may need to be as large as 16.00 mm and radii correspondingly flatter.

One of the main problems associated with extended-wear soft lenses in infancy will be ejection from the eye. This is usually the result of eye rubbing; not from discomfort so much as from reflex rubbing during the process of waking up after sleep or, as has been mentioned, during teething. Parents must be instructed to check that lenses are still in place each morning and at intervals throughout the day. Displaced lenses if found are returned to the practitioner in a vial provided containing preserved saline so that they can be inspected and, if in suitable condition, cleaned and re-sterilized for future use. The provision of preserved saline for these return vials is of vital importance since if the vial contains unpreserved saline it is often found that by the time the lens can be inspected it is already contaminated by a fungus mycelium which has encroached into the lens substance and which cannot be removed. Thus salvaging of the lens is unfortunately not always possible and the cost of keeping infants in extended-wear soft lenses is not inconsiderable. However when compared with cost of many other forms of medical and surgical treatment, these costs are well justified. Spare lenses are kept in a personal stock for each patient and where possible parents should be instructed in inserting a replacement lens and can thus hold some spare lenses at home. This may not always lie within the competence of parents and in this case they need to be able to contact the hospital and arrange a visit without undue delay for a new lens to be inserted. For this reason a good emergency cover service is needed and may often be provided by support staff.

In terms of reducing such loss rates, the authors find that moving to a larger TD is helpful in many cases. Wilson and Millis (1988a) suggest that high water content soft lenses should be ordered somewhat thicker than might be used for adult eyes. This, as well as helping to mask some corneal astigmatism, makes insertion of the lens easier. Again, the level of patient cooperation varies enormously and advice has been given elsewhere in this chapter on such procedures. Unfortunately, making the aphakic soft lens appreciably thicker, while being advantageous to insertion, renders removal more difficult particularly from very small eyes. One of the authors has produced a pair of 'soft-nosed forceps' to aïd removal of difficult lenses from the eyes of infants, these are in effect miniature fingers made of silicone rubber (*Figure 14.6*) and have proved useful in some cases. One of the greatest difficulties in the insertion of thin soft lenses into the eyes of uncooperative small children lies in the extraordinary power of the orbicularis muscle. Manual efforts to retract the lids tend to result in a spontaneous lid eversion which defeats the object of effective soft lens placement. Under these conditions, a rigid lens is much easier to insert. A further device constructed by the author to assist under such circumstances is a soft lens applicator made of PMMA (*Figure 14.7*). The soft lens is placed into the cup of the applicator which provides the stability and effectively converts the lens to a rigid one until it is flat against the surface of the eye. Care is needed in the removal of the applicator to ensure that the soft lens is not ejected also.

Thus one commences by inserting a selected lens of estimated specification determined by visual observation of the eye. From inspection of the centration and movement of this lens, the practitioner decides whether the fit is satisfactory or requires modification. This observation is more difficult with infants than with other children since the controlled versional movements of the eyes cannot be requested. Nor can the infant be asked to blink to order. Thus one can only watch for a while in the hope that the child will produce movements which allow some judgement to be reached. Some of the older infants react adversely to such close range observation and it is not uncommon to find that the eyes are held tightly shut, especially if a light is brought close to the child's face. This may in some cases be a photophobic response but in many instances it is a signal of disapproval of any form of interference. Many infants register such objection to the physical manipulation of the eyelids even though the procedure may create no discomfort. That this protest is a 'matter of principle' is demonstrated by the rapid cessation of noise as soon as the manipulation ceases. The practitioner must learn to attach little importance to such a response but

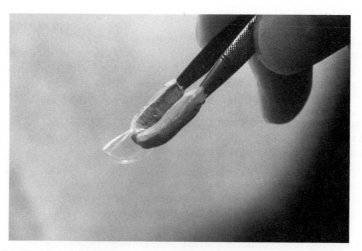

Figure 14.6. Sabell's soft-nosed forceps for removal of hydrogel contact lenses from infant eyes

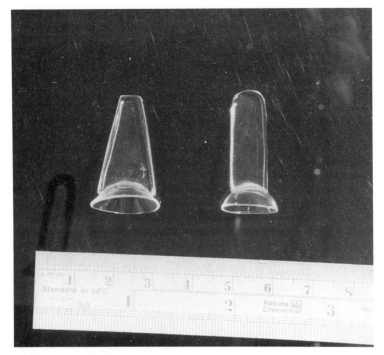

Figure 14.7. Sabell's applicator for insertion of extended-wear soft contact lenses to infant eyes

it is useful to reassure the parent(s) that what one is doing is not causing physical pain. Some parents, particularly when the infant is their first child, may become rather anxious over such a noisy response and may be worried that the procedure may be causing marked discomfort. In the case of one of the authors, the need to use a hearing aid has proved to be a boon since it can be switched off at such times (*Figure 14.8*).

Assuming one is satisfied that the lens does not appear abnormally steep nor obviously too mobile, an attempt at retinoscopy can be made. Since many children in this very early age group will be aphakics, the problems associated with varying accommodation will not arise. Despite this, other factors may render retinoscopy less than easy and one may need to wait until one of the routine examinations under anaesthesia (EUA) before coming to a firm conclusion about the accuracy of the refractive correction. An arbitrary selection of lens power will have been made in the first instance. In the case of the very young, say less than 6 months old, a + 35.00 D lens is the likely choice. The required optical power will decline quite rapidly as the eyes grow and successively weaker lenses can be employed.

Choice of lens form

Extended or daily-wear hydrogels

Since no great handling differences exist between extended wear (EW) and daily wear (DW) soft lenses, this choice will depend on other factors. The occurrence of

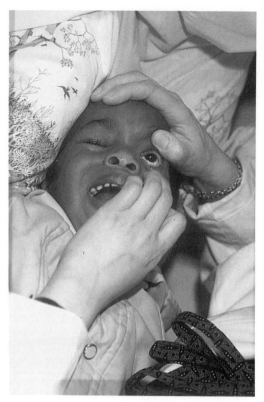

Figure 14.8. A noisy response from some young children to the insertion or removal of a contact lens

adverse reactions to EW soft lenses clearly forces the practitioner to seek less hazardous alternatives. These reactions are fortunately not very frequent provided that the risks are understood by all parties. Statistics have been frequently quoted, indicating a higher risk of corneal infection in wearers of EW soft lenses (Dart, 1988; Glynn *et al.*, 1991). There is clearly a need to have available a 24-hour emergency cover service. Parents must be made aware of the need to watch for signs and symptoms indicating a potentially adverse response. These have been frequently listed as pain, redness, eyelid or conjuctival swelling or discharge, and white spots or haziness of the cornea. Complaints from the patient of deterioration of vision are more applicable to older children than to infants. It is interesting to remember that these signs and symptoms are basically those of inflammation as recorded by Celsus around AD 30. The need to seek prompt advice should these signs be detected is impressed on the parents (and provided they are of the calibre to respond), then probably the risks attached to the use of EW lenses are justifiable where the need to wear contact lenses rather than spectacles is clinically indicated. The potential risks attached to EW contact lenses impose the need for more frequent review by the practitioner than would be the case with daily wear. This, naturally, creates an additional time burden on the practitioner. It has been frequently stated that patients supplied with EW lenses should be followed up at initially frequent intervals. Wilson and Millis (1988a) quote these as after 24 hours, 1–2 weeks, 1 month and thereafter every 2 months or sooner should the need arise. The reader can well imagine the load that such a programme imposes on a busy ophthalmic clinic dealing with considerable numbers of aphakic and other contact lens wearers. Of necessity certain modification to such a rigid schedule frequently has to be made and 'clinical judgement' exercised for each individual case. There will always be the need to have cover available commonly by staff other than the contact lens practitioner. This may well be where the independent optometrist working outside the hospital may find himself at some disadvantage, unless his working relationships with his local hospital are good and the facilities available in that hospital are such that suitable support services are possible.

Thus the employment of DW soft lenses, or indeed of rigid lenses, would appear to be desirable when and where this can be achieved. In the case of young children this choice may be limited by the ability, or indeed the willingness, of parents to undertake the necessary handling and maintenance routines. There may also be social factors which impose limitations on the parents: work commitments where both parents are forced to have employment; or in the case of some one-parent families regular daily attention to the child's contact lenses may impose an unwanted additional burden. Families involving abnormally large numbers of young children or in some cases of handicapped children may well make such extra tasks unacceptable. If doubt exists about the ability of parents to follow the maintenance tasks imposed by DW soft lenses, it could be argued that rigid lenses, particularly in PMMA may well reduce infection risks (Weissman and Stein, 1989). Thus, even when the child has reached an age when he or she could be switched from EW to DW lenses, circumstances may dictate that in some cases, the EW programme be continued. In all these instances there must be a sound clinical reason for contact lenses and not simply the vanity of parents not wishing to admit that their offspring is dependent on spectacles.

Other factors influence the choice between daily or extended wear, one of these may be the degree to which surface deposits are formed on the EW soft lenses. This is notoriously variable and while the average patient may be capable of retaining EW soft lenses for a 2 to 3-month period, some require much more frequent removal for cleaning. One lad of about 6 years of age needed to have his lenses exchanged every third day because of rapid build up of lipid and other deposits. If the lenses were retained for some 3 or 4 weeks, not only was vision seriously impaired, but the deposits became impossible to remove from his lenses. Luckily in this instance, his mother was very willing and able to perform the necessary maintenance. Even so, such problems do encourage the return to spectacles or to some radically different form of contact lens. At the more normal exchange periods, the cleaning may be performed by optometric support staff or the lenses may be sent to a contact lens laboratory for intensive cleaning. The alternative system is to retain the lenses in use until they are deemed to be expendable. This on the surface appears to be a financially wasteful exercise but when one considers the time and effort expended on lens cleaning or the expense of having this done commercially for large numbers of lenses, it may well be a justifiable option. Up to the present, the available systems of disposable soft lenses do not seem to cater for the high optical powers often required in paediatric practice. Certainly when the practitioner himself chooses to undertake the cleaning of EW soft lenses which are being worn for 3-month periods, he rapidly becomes aware of the limitations of the commercially available cleaning regimens. Luckily lens calculi or the so-called 'jelly bumps' are uncommon on the lenses of younger children. Stubborn central film of the type described as due to calcium phosphate is not infrequently encountered on high-powered aphakia lenses worn by very young children. It seems likely that the protective barrier of the contact lens impairs the necessity for frequent blinking, and central drying of the bulbous front surface of a $+30.00$ or $+35.00$ D soft lens allows this rapid deposition. At this very early age, the resultant reduction in vision is, in itself, not an adequate stimulation to the blink reflex. Unless such lenses are exchanged at frequent intervals they become quite impossible to clean satisfactorily resulting, at this very early age, in an undesirable impairment of vision.

While such factors as potential hazards and lens deposition may make the change to daily wear desirable, other aspects may prompt the delaying of such a change. As the infant approaches the age of 1 year they begin to reach a phase in which their resentment of physical interference can be expressed in terms other than the purely vocal. Physical resistance to the insertion or removal of a contact lens becomes an increasing problem. Techniques for dealing with this difficulty have been discussed earlier in this chapter. Such obstacles to peace and tranquility may tempt the practitioner to persist with the EW regimen although it is likely that the regular daily exchange of lenses, if the effort is made, would do much to encourage the child to accept the normality of such interference. It is with this 1 to 3-year-old group that the problem of frequent lens loss is most likely to occur. Even slight sensations of irritation will result in eye rubbing and it is impossible to convey to the child the need to restrain such an impulse. Often eye rubbing will occur during the process of waking and parents must check for the presence of the lenses and in their absence should search the bed or cot for the missing item. It may be useful for the practitioner to have available an old soft lens in a dehydrated state to be able to show the parents as an indication of the sort of thing which they will be looking for. This loss rate is not completely overcome by changing to DW soft or indeed to corneal lenses but may constitute a valid indication for the fitting of scleral lenses.

Damage to the lenses is not a great issue during the wearing of EW soft lenses but may occur during the cleaning process. Vigorous cleaning in order to remove stubborn deposits may result in the loss of edge sections or the creation of splits or holes in the lens. Occasionally such high water content lenses can become grossly flat and correspondingly large during the intensive cleaning programme. Such complications illustrate some of the inherent disadvantages of the hydrogel lens.

Older children tend to be introduced directly into DW lenses or even to rigid lenses if circumstances permit. With soft DW lenses, many children from the age of 5 or 6 can quite expertly remove these from their own eyes although they will probably need an adult to insert them for some time to come. Discolouration of soft lenses is a well-documented phenomenon and is most frequently encountered in the adult wearer (Kleist, 1979). One or two examples of repeated discolouration in lenses worn by older children have been observed by the authors. In one instance the lens colour was not constant but would vary from one visit to another and was regarded with extreme suspicion. Although the cause was never established in this case, on a previous occasion another small lad had admitted that his exotically coloured pink soft lenses was the result of touching each lens with a felt-tipped pen!

Corneal lenses for children

The corneal lens is perhaps the most obvious choice for older children except when very high refractive corrections are required. The teenager, having reached the stage of wishing to be without spectacles for whatever reason, will usually have adequate motivation to see them through the few days of adaptation. With adult patients the rigid lens and in particular the PMMA lens, provided it is well designed and well fitted, is likely to give many years of useful service, the likelihood of acquired intolerance being much less than with soft lenses. We now see healthy adult patients who are still happily wearing PMMA corneal lenses after periods of up to 30 years. In the opinion of the authors, the co-polymer RGP lenses should only be employed when good clinical reasons exist and not be regarded as automatically the lens of first choice.

Younger children may not take so readily to the initial sensation produced by a rigid corneal lens, especially if they have previously enjoyed the comfort of soft lenses. It may be difficult to convey to them the clinical reasons why one believes that the soft lens is no longer a safe or suitable form of correction. Corneal lenses do, of course, have their limitations where high powers are needed. Good edge profile and control of edge thickness is of vital importance and high minus corneal lenses can sometimes present difficulties in this respect. The high plus corneal lenses, especially in aphakia, often present centration problems despite ingenious compensatory features such as the negative carrier introduced some years ago (Mandell, 1968). In these aphakia lenses, centration can be improved by fitting larger lenses which in any case may prove initially more comfortable. An extreme example would be the APEX lens of the 1960s (Bagshaw, Gordon and Stanworth, 1966). However, such designs are at the expense of good oxygenation and even if one adopts a gas-permeable material, this may be of limited compensation when the optical power is in the order of $+20.00\,D$.

While the fitting of corneal lenses will be normal for the older child, several clinicians have recommended the use of rigid corneal lenses for very young aphakic infants, claiming that the loss rate is lower than with EW soft lenses (Rose *et al.*, 1985). The procedure for fitting the older child with corneal lenses is essentially that used for adults. Keratometry should not present difficulties unless nystagmus is present, although the authors occasionally encounter the so-called 'hyperactive child' who seems to have extreme difficulty in maintaining sufficient concentration to fixate the keratometer target long enough for the examiner to obtain a reading. Even in such cases, patience and persistence by the practitioner can usually achieve usable results. Keratometry can be followed by conventional fluorescein assessment and this may be the method of choice where keratometry has been unsuccessful. Where the provision of contact lenses is a matter of clinical necessity, there is no reason why the assessment of fit cannot be carried out using local anaesthesia which will aid relaxation and enhance cooperation of the patient with regard to eye movements. Thus a more reliable opinion on fit of the lens may be obtained. With this age group the assessment of refraction by objective and subjective means should give no difficulty. In some cases of mental impairment one may need to rely on objective refraction and in extreme cases even this may be difficult owing to poor fixation.

For the fitting of very young aphakics with corneal lenses the fluorescein assessment will need to be made under general anaesthesia. The difficulty of keratometry under general anaesthetics has been mentioned earlier and it may therefore be more efficient to proceed directly to fitting by fluorescein. Unlike the fitting of soft lenses, reasonable precision will be required and such observations, using fluorescein, are not usually possible with young children except under anaesthesia. Even so one will have limited information on lens riding characteristics and lens movement during normal wear. It is highly desirable that the fit assessment and more especially the refraction be performed using fitting lenses somewhere near the power required for the finished correction. Thus fitting sets of corneal lenses powered at say +/−10.00 D, and at +/−20.00 D may be required. Estimation of size of lens necessary to expect reasonable centration during wear is important. It may be possible to judge this by moving the lens on the cornea either with a finger or by manipulating the lids.

Rigid lenses have several clear advantages over soft lenses for these infants. The automatic correction of corneal astigmatism in most cases is an obvious example. The lower rate of deposit formation, especially with the PMMA lens, is a considerable advantage. It has been suggested that certain materials in the GP range allow extended wear, but even if one prefers a regimen of daily wear, the rigid corneal lens is easier to insert into the eyes of uncooperative infants. Their smaller size and lack of that annoying habit of bending uncontrollably are both most advantageous features. Provided that a good fit assessment has been made, corneal lenses should not suffer from the instant ejection sometimes encountered when trying to insert soft lenses. Removal on the other hand may not be so easy as with the soft lens, although the difficulties of achieving that have been mentioned earlier. The accidental displacement of a corneal lens onto the conjunctiva and especially into the upper fornix may provide parents with problems until they have acquired the necessary expertise. In that respect at least the well-fitting soft lens does not give difficulty.

Scleral lenses in paediatric practice

In the present-day world of contact lenses it is sometimes admitted that a place still exists for the scleral contact lens. Such observations are usually heard only from practitioners dealing with therapeutically indicated contact lenses. This is certainly true in the paediatric field as well as for adult patients. In the opinion of the authors, the usefulness of the scleral lens extends far beyond its use as a prosthetic appliance. For many clinically indicated conditions, scleral lenses offer a superior option to other forms of contact lens. The factors which these days are seen to limit the usage of scleral lenses for this group of patients are:

(1) The additional time to be spent over their fitting.
(2) The availability of the workshop equipment necessary for such work.
(3) The acquisition of the necessary skills and the experience needed to make adequate judgements.

While it is true that the time needed to assess the fit of a corneal lens or a soft lens may be slightly shorter, the time difference is more often the product of inexperience in dealing with scleral lenses. It is most noticeable at the present time how few students can say that they have had any clinical experience of handling scleral lenses during their undergraduate training. The number of eye hospitals or eye departments in general hospitals from which scleral lenses are available is today somewhat limited. The decline in usage of scleral lenses during the last half of the 1950s was in part due to the apparent simplicity with which toleration could be built up by patients using corneal lenses. In the same way the 1970s saw an upsurge in the fitting of soft lenses because, to many, this looked a less demanding and more rapidly executed procedure than the fitting of PMMA corneal lenses. Success with the scleral lens is the product of good design and careful determination of fit by the practitioner. The needs of the scleral lens, however, extend beyond the selection of a preformed fit as with corneal and soft lenses. With these, the practitioner needs to be personally involved in the physical creation of the fit relationship. He needs to be able to change the dimensions of the lenses on the spot. It is no use thinking that each alteration can be sent back for his manufacturer to perform. Not only would this extend the time taken up by the fitting but also grossly inflate the costs of the process. Even if this were not the case, it is increasingly difficult today to find laboratories which retain the equipment and the staff expertise to perform these tasks adequately. For success, therefore, the practitioner himself must accept responsibility for such lens or shell modification. The fitting of scleral lenses is very much an art process, and as such it retains a considerable appeal to a very small number of practitioners. It is quicker and more effective for the person who makes the observations of fit to carry out the modifications needed than to convey the needs to a second person and usually to supervise the way in which the adjustments are carried out. The toleration and functional efficacy of the scleral lens are the direct product of such observations, decisions and actions on the part of the contact lens practitioner. The pressures on time within the present-day optometry courses in universities rarely permit the luxury of practical experience of fitting this type of lens.

The scleral lens is therefore often regarded as an anachronism, as is all too often the PMMA corneal lens. For patients with clinical indications for contact lenses, nothing could be further from the truth. Where facilities exist for the supplying of well-fitted scleral lenses, they will be found to be of the greatest help for appropriate patients and will be employed on an increasing scale. Where such facilities are lacking, the staff will do the best they can with lens forms which are available, and will refer only those patients for whom nothing but scleral lenses will suffice. It would seem therefore that many of their patients will be making do with a second best form of correction. Referral of patients for scleral lenses may these days necessitate such patients travelling considerable distances.

For children the scleral lens proves to be a useful solution to a number of problems. Extreme refractive errors can be accommodated. The high loss rate experienced with some children using soft lenses is eliminated. The problems of lens cleaning and lens storage are very considerably simplified. Where insertion and removal has to be carried out by parents, this is found to be much more easily performed than with soft lenses or corneal lenses. One usually finds that the children can undertake lens insertion and removal at a much earlier age with scleral lenses than would be possible using either corneal or soft lenses. High corneal astigmatism which with corneal lenses would entail the fitting of more complex toroidal designs with all their associated problems is usually resolvable more simply by means of the scleral lens. Cases which require non-rotating lenses as a carrier for front surface cylindrical corrections are often better served by this form of lens.

The fitting of scleral lenses for children

Although the preformed scleral lens has a useful role in introducing a child to the feel of a scleral lens, the additional time required to try in and examine a multiplicity of fitting lenses is rarely justified. It is much quicker and usually more effective to fit scleral lenses from eye impressions. The indication for using scleral lenses rarely arises in the under 1-year-old group of children. In the next group of 1 to 3 year olds sclerals will be mainly for prosthetic appliances, often for unilateral microphthalmos. In these cases, when the cornea is clear and the iris appears bright and of similar colour to its fellow, it may be sufficient to fit a clear lens or shell to regulate the size of the palpebral aperture. A shell slightly thicker than normal may be all that is required. Should the discrepancy be marked and a shell thicker than about

2.50 mm be needed, the clear appliance becomes of limited value. This is because the separation of the lids from the globe becomes apparent and tends to create an appearance similar to ectropion. In these cases as well as those in which the cornea or iris is of abnormal appearance, a painted shell or lens will be needed.

The other main indication for scleral lenses within this age group will be because of excessive loss of hydrogel lenses. This is likely to be mainly in aphakic infants, with the occasional high myope.

While it would be theoretically possible to fit preformed scleral lenses to the 1 to 3 year olds under general anaesthesia, this would of necessity be a more prolonged procedure than impressions and therefore unjustified. A further disadvantage of preformed scleral lenses in the eyes of infants seems to be their tendency to rotate out of position in the case of some children. This is accentuated by an eye rubbing tendency and this may be prevalent during the adaptation stages of wear. An impression-fitted lens should eliminate this problem.

When taking impressions under general anaesthesia (*Figure 14.9*) one needs to be aware that the eyes frequently elevate and the impression tray needs to be

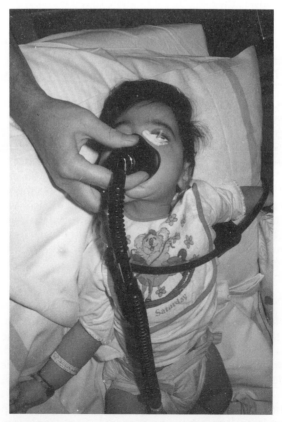

Figure 14.9. Left eye impression under general anaesthesia using Sabell's thin-handled infant impression tray

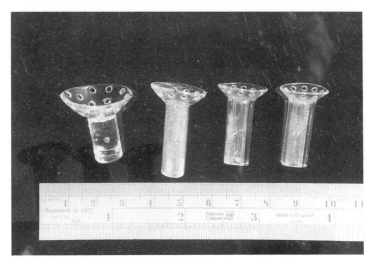

Figure 14.10. Standard adult impression trays edged down for use with small children, compared to a small sized adult impression tray on left. Note the unnecessary bulk of the handles

supported in a similar position to achieve a reasonable proportioned cast of the scleral zone. For impressions on young infants, and particularly those with congenital microphthalmos, a special range of tiny impression trays will be required. For older children, the smaller end of the set of adult trays is usually suitable. Adult impression trays can in some cases be cut down to infant size (*Figure 14.10*), but it is usually more effective to create one's own set to suit individual needs. The handles of adult shells are often inconveniently bulky when used on tiny eyes and, unless the injection technique is to be used, trays with much finer stems can be produced. If the practitioner has facilities for pressing his own trial shells, as should be the case, the making of such small impression trays will present no problem. A selection of infant trays made by the author are shown in (*Figure 14.11*). The smallest of this set was made for use with a microphthalmic eye in an infant aged 6 months.

In older children, scleral lenses may prove useful where excessive deposits are produced on soft lenses and where the refractive error may be inconveniently high for a corneal lens. In the case of one child fitted by one of the authors, a bilateral aphakic with the Hallermann–Strieff syndrome (Grattan, Liddle and Willshaw, 1989) and an abnormally high refractive error, the loss rate with soft lenses was such that it was decided to try sclerals. This little boy, now aged 7½, very happily wears scleral lenses of + 35.00 D in both eyes. Equally some older children, having lived for some time with the low physical stimulus of soft lenses, may be reluctant to tolerate the initial sensation of a corneal lens. Here also, the scleral lens may prove superior.

The need for cosmetic scleral lenses following injury is not uncommon among older children. Perforating injury to the cornea in this age group is often the result of games involving catapults, darts, bows and arrows, and air guns. While an approximate cosmetic match can sometimes be attained with a cosmetic soft lens, a more natural result can usually result from a hand-painted acrylic scleral lens or shell. Thus the scleral lens still constitutes an essential option for the paediatric contact lens practitioner.

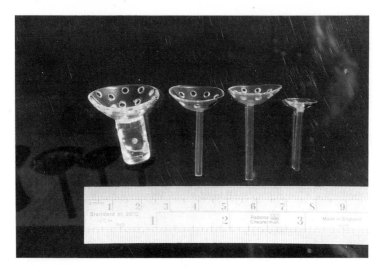

Figure 14.11. Sabell's infant impression trays with thinner handles compared to small size of adult tray. The far right hand tray is used for congenital microphthalmos in young infants

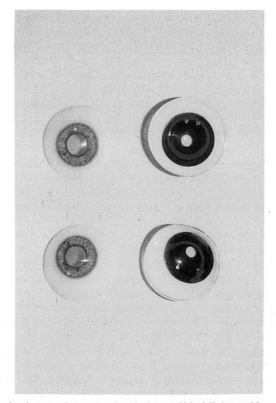

Figure 14.12. Albino scleral contact lenses showing the internal black lining and front view of painted iris

Albinism has been a condition for which scleral contact lenses have been employed for many years, incorporating a painted iris and sclera with opaque black lining (*Figure 14.12*). Given the availability of facilities for the fitting of acrylic lenses of this type, they are usually found to be superior to the present-day cosmetic soft lenses (Lewis, 1971; Kemmetmuller, 1981).

In older children, one will also begin to encounter the occasional young keratoconic. Whilst corneal lenses will suffice for the early stages, these young-onset patients are likely to progress to a level of ectasia which will call for the employment of scleral lenses.

Conclusion

In paediatric contact lens practice, the range of conditions encountered will be similar to those in adult patients seen within the hospital service. Typically, the largest groups will consist of aphakics, both unilateral and bilateral, and also high myopes. The aphakic group will contain those resulting from the removal of congenital cataracts as well as the rather less frequent consequence of traumatic cataract, usually unilateral. Within this last group one is likely to encounter corneal irregularity and opacification, and possibly traumatic or surgical iris coloboma or even aniridia. Another small group likely to be encountered are children with subluxated lenses. If the crystalline lens displacement is sufficient it may be found more effective to utilize the aphakic zone rather than deal with a sometimes high level of lenticular astigmatism from the phakic portion of the pupil.

Contact lenses in childhood may be desirable in refractive anisometropia in addition to that resulting from monocular aphakia. To a smaller extent, congenital corneal opacity or congenital iris coloboma may come within the contact lens practitioner's care. Occasionally a child with intractable diplopia will benefit from the use of an occlusive contact lens. Post-keratoplasty use of contact lenses is rather less common among children than adults but will nevertheless be occasionally required.

Among the conditions demanding the use of cosmetic lenses or shells will be albinism, microphthalmos and the occasional phthisical eye. There will also be found the post-enucleation cases, occasionally even bilateral enucleation. There is of course with these bilateral cosmetic applicances, the consolation to the practitioner that the problems of colour matching are eliminated!

Thus the use of the full range of lens types and materials as applied in adult contact lens practice will be required. The difference will lie in the lower levels of patient cooperation to be expected and the need to encourage the support and cooperation of additional persons, usually the parents. For the practitioner there is a necessity to be able to vary his or her approach according to the age and needs of the particular child. Since many of these young contact lens patients will be suffering from pathological or post-traumatic disorders, the contact lens practitioner is only a portion of a broader team involved in the care of the patient. This fact may call for some reorientation on the part of the independent optometrist who has for so long cherished the ideal of unilateral decision making. It also means that, within the UK at least, the bulk of paediatric contact lens work will be conducted within hospitals.

References

ABSELL, P.A., CHIANG, B., SOMERS, M.E. and MORGAN, K. (1990) 'Keratometry in children'. *Contact Lens Association for Optometry,* **16**, 99–102.

BAGSHAW, J., GORDON, S.P. and STANWORTH, A. (1966). A modified corneal contact lens: binocular single vision in unilateral aphakia. *British Orthoptic Journal,* **23**, 19–30.

DART, J. (1988). Predisposing factors in microbial keratitis: the significance of contact lens wear. *British Journal of Ophthalmology,* **72**, 926–930.

DAVIES, P.D. and TARBUCK, D.T.H. (1977). Management of cataracts in infancy and childhood. *Transactions of the Ophthalmological Society of the United Kingdom,* **97**, 148–152.

DUKE-ELDER, SIR, S. (ed.) (1962). *A system of Ophthalmology,* vol VII. Kimpton, London, pp. 235–236.

GLYNN, R.J., SCHEIN, O.D., SEDDON, J.M. *et al.* (1991). The incidence of ulcerative keratitis among aphakic contact lens wearers in New England. *Archives of Ophthalmology,* **109**, 104–107.

GRATTAN, C.E., LIDDLE, B.J. and WILLSHAW, H.E. (1989). Atrophic alopecia in the Hallermann–Strieff syndrome. *Clinical and Experimental Dermatology,* **14**, 250–252.

KEMMETMULLER, H. (1981). The optical aid in albinism. *The Contact Lens Journal,* **10**, 2–9.

KLEIST, F.D. (1979). Appearance and nature of hydrophilic contact lens deposits. *International Contact Lens Clinics,* **6**, 120–130.

LEWIS, E.M.T. (1971). Contact lenses for infants and children. *British Journal of Physiological Optics,* **26**, 61–68.

MANDELL, R.B. (1968). A method to determine the dimensions of a minus carrier contact lens. *Journal of the American Optometric Association,* **39**, 641–642.

OBRIG, T.E. (1942). *Contact Lenses,* 1st edn. Chilton Company, Philadelphia, pp. 87–92.

ROSE, L., PE'ER, J., COHEN, E. and BENEZRA, D. (1985). Fitting infants with hard contact lenses. In *Transactions of The British Contact Lens Association Annual Clinical Conference.* (Blackpool 1985).

WEISSMAN, B.A. and STEIN, J. (1989). Corneal infection and contact lens wear. *Contact Lens Update,* **8**, no. 3, 46.

WILLSHAW, H.E. (1985). Personal communication.

WILSON, M.S. and MILLIS, E.A.W. (1988a). Lenses for aphakia, infants and children. In *Contact Lenses in Ophthalmology. Butterworth-Heinemann, Oxford, p. 102.*

WILSON, M.S. and MILLIS, E.A.W. (1988b). Lenses for aphakia, infants and children. In *Contact Lenses for Ophthalmology.* Butterworth-Heinemann, Oxford, p. 103.

15

Management of visual disability in children

Janet Silver and Elizabeth Gould

Helping a child with a visual disability makes considerable demands on the optometrist. Although numerically very few (the under 16s represent less than 5% of the recognized visually handicapped in the developed countries), they are difficult to classify and even more difficult to manage.

Referral

Children find their way to the low-vision practitioner by several routes; usually referral is by the ophthalmologist.

Referral may originate from the child's or parents' request; often with older children as a result of specific stated difficulties, for example blackboard, geography maps, etc. Alternatively, well-informed parents want to explore all possible avenues open to them to help their child. Sometimes a teacher at school or a peripatetic teacher requests help. Often a magnifier has been loaned while the child is waiting to attend the low-vision clinic. These are usually lenses with a large aperture, and may not be providing sufficient magnification. The peripatetic teacher may request an assessment at the low-vision clinic as a result of a review of the statement of educational needs.

Many parents are unaware of the benefits of low-vision aids and do not know that help of this type is available, nor what low-vision appliances can, or more importantly cannot, do. They may be sceptical that any optical help can be offered to their child.

By the time a visually disabled child reaches the optometrist the diagnosis is usually made. In the rare event of a visually disabled child attending without ophthalmological supervision, the optometrist will, in both the child's interests and his own, encourage the parents to see a sympathetic ophthalmologist.

The main concern of the optometrist is the provision of appropriate spectacles and low-vision devices. A close working relationship with the ophthalmologist with easy exchange of information is essential. It is necessary for the optometrist to have some appreciation of how the child perceives the world, and useful to know how the disorder might progress. Equally, the ophthalmologist must know what the child can achieve, and how he responds.

Causes of visual disability

Statistics on the incidence and prevalence of visual disability are acknowledged by all the authorities to be inaccurate, with up to 40% being unreported (Cullinan, 1977). The children are a well-served group with relatively few remaining unrecognized.

Congenital disorders can be divided into two groups:

(1) Genetically determined: cataracts, albinism, etc.
(2) Acquired: rubella, retrolental fibroplasia, etc.

Although the data available is unreliable, there are perhaps half a dozen major groups. The largest group seen in the clinic is optic atrophy, this may be primary hereditary optic atrophy, or secondary to any condition causing an increase in pressure on the optic nerve such as an intracranial tumour or meningitis. The effect may be a depression of central vision, and/or field loss.

Congenital cataract is the second largest group. Ophthalmological management has changed a great deal in recent years, with many children now using contact lenses some or all of the time. They rarely have binocular function, and the level of vision is very variable, with a mode acuity of around 6/60. The prescription of low-vision aids for this group must recognize that the same child may use devices either with contact lenses or a spectacle correction.

Albinism is easily recognized in the presence of white hair and 'pink' eyes (tyrosinase negative), but ocular albinism (tyrosinase positive) and the rarer types are easily missed. The optometrist may be presented with an apparently normal child unable to read the blackboard. Nystagmus and transilluminating irides confirm the diagnosis. Although many have strabismus, albinos prefer to use both eyes, and indeed usually have at least a line better with both eyes open (Silver, 1976). There is usually a significant refractive error, which should be fully corrected; nearly all the children are able to read better than N8 with a normal refractive correction (Collins and Silver, 1990). Crude binocular function can be demonstrated by tests such as bar-reading.

The pigmentary degenerations, rubella retinopathy, buphthalmos, aniridia and changes associated with a high myopia are all significant. It is sad to report that trauma and retrolental fibroplasia are also occasionally seen, and the optometrist will need access to a comprehensive text (Wybar and Taylor, 1983) to check out the implications of the rarer syndromes. With combined experience of nearly half a century we still meet disorders we have not seen before. The prevalence of multiple disability is increasing.

With much visual disability in children being genetically determined the optometrist may find himself being asked in effect to give genetic advice. He/she would be well advised to explain how complex the subject is and direct the patient to one of the few ophthalmic centres offering such a service.

Early history and referral

In the early years the child is normally seeing a paediatrician, and an ophthalmologist is maintaining supervision. Therefore, the parents have been made aware of the implications of their child's visual disability; the diagnosis, prognosis, etc. Some parents will have read available literature and made contact with self-help groups or other parents of visually handicapped children so their expectations of their child's visual capabilities are reasonably realistic. We have, however, come across parents who totally deny any problem, and others who exaggerate it.

Systems vary from one country to another. In Italy, for example, no 'partially sighted' category exists; in Scandinavia only the multiply handicapped are in special schools, with individual support provided in open education, this is sometimes a full-time one-to-one arrangement. In the UK most children with a visual handicap are visited regularly by a peripatetic teacher at home during their preschool years.

Children who are already integrated into their local school prior to referral to the low-vision clinic will often have adopted their own strategy for coping in the classroom. For example, they sit at the front, get classmates or teachers to copy out any blackboard work, parents go over poor quality print with a black felt-tip pen, or use photo enlargement. Many children with conditions such as congenital idiopathic nystagmus, albinism, etc., will hold all reading material very close. They are increasing the angle subtended at the retina by this means in the presence of sufficient accommodation to focus at the reduced distance. Older children may already be able to type and use the typewriter or even a word-processor in the classroom. They should be encouraged to continue with these strategies. In some places a resource centre is available to provide special materials. A peripatetic teacher will often visit the school and give advice where appropriate.

Where the child is at a school for the visually handicapped little or no blackboard work is encountered in the early school years and print appropriate for the child's needs is used. Magnifiers or a closed circuit television reading machine are often available for general use. There may be the facility to enlarge print. Some children are taught to use other media such as Braille at a relatively early age. While there is considerable debate about this, there is no doubt it is easily learned young, and is far more difficult later.

Equipment

In addition to the usual consulting room equipment extra equipment is essential if low-vision assessments are planned:

(1) Hand and stand magnifiers with and without integral illumination (*Figure 15.1*).
(2) Hyperocular lenses and other spectacle microscopes (*Figure 15.2*).
(3) Hand-held distance telescopes, both monocular and binocular (*Figure 15.3*).
(4) Face-mounted telescopes and clip telescopes for distance and near, both monocular and binocular.
(5) Appropriate frames for dispensing spectacle-mounted appliances.
(6) Closed circuit television reading machine.
(7) Line markers, masks, etc.

A good basis is to have a set of equipment from one of the large manufacturers such as Keeler in the UK, Zeiss in West Germany or Designs for Vision in the USA, with alternatives of every type. Every device has alternatives and for reasons not yet understood some individuals prefer one particular device to another which is very similar.

Where the practitioner is seeing a lot of young children a colour closed circuit television would be useful to demonstrate its use in looking at picture material.

Full descriptions of all the devices available can be found in the manufacturers' literature, and every practitioner needs a comprehensive file. These are easy to store

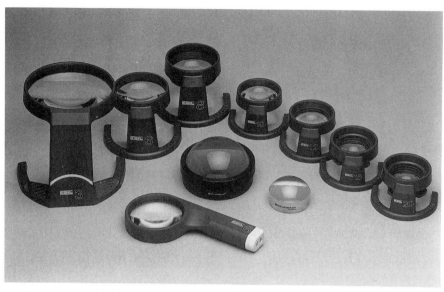

Figure 15.1. A series of magnifiers. These range in power from 1.8× (the dome or flat-field type, from Eschenbach) to approximately +76.00 diotres or 20× (from Combined Optical Industries)

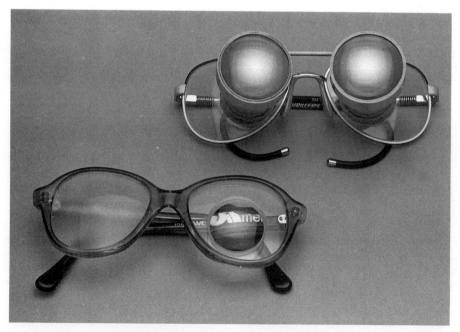

Figure 15.2. Keeler 5× binocular near-vision telescopic spectacle (above). 'Bifocal' spectacle magnifier from Keeler, segments are interchangeable 2× to 9× (below)

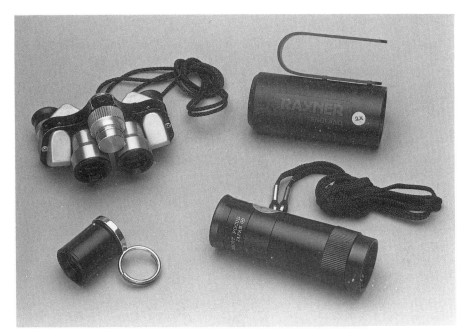

Figure 15.3. Distant vision telescopes. Focusable monocular Galilean telescope from Rayner, also available at 4× (top right). Roof-prism monocular 8×, also available at 4×, 6× and 10×; these from Marcus, but similar ones are available (bottom right). Focusable 'finger-ring' Galilean telescope 2× from Keeler, up to 4× available but less inconspicuous (bottom left). Miniature prismatic binocular telescope 6×; this one from Tohyoh similar available from other suppliers and at 8× (top left)

and useful for reference when an infrequently used appliance is required or to try to identify an unfamiliar appliance that the patient might bring with him.

It is important to remember that devices described by different manufacturers in similar terms may have very different characteristics, therefore the optometrist needs to be very familiar with his own equipment. We prefer to think of all appliances in 'dioptre equivalents'.

Suitable material for the assessment of vision in both preschool and school children is essential. This would include normal Snellen charts, matching tests such as Sonksen–Silver, Sheridan–Gardiner, or Bust cards, a Maclure or similar reading chart, an Atlas, Ordnance Survey map, a dictionary for older children and picture material for younger children. More and more the merits of testing contrast sensitivity are being recognized, but the practitioner must realize that he can hold the child's attention for only a short time, therefore tests have to be of certain relevance rather than simply of interest to justify inclusion.

Wherever possible the prescribed appliance should be dispensed immediately after the low-vision assessment, so in addition to the trial equipment a stock of frequently used appliances should be available. More complex appliances can often be dispensed, if a significant refractive correction is not required as an integral part of the appliance, if the practitioner holds a supply of standard components.

In the UK and some other countries all appliances are issued on loan. As well as ensuring regular review such a system allows rejected or outgrown aids (and indeed simple errors of judgement) to be recycled.

Assessments

All children, regardless of age, attending the low-vision practitioner for the first time should be requested to bring examples of what they can and cannot manage to see. It is as useful to see what can be coped with, albeit with difficulty, and at the end of the assessment demonstrate (where possible) a new found ability to deal with previously impossible tasks. The aims of the session should be negotiated and agreed: 'We will try to help with the blackboard' or 'right, we will find you a device to help with those maps and labels on records and tapes'.

After the initial discussion with the parents and child any glasses worn are checked. The vision and/or visual acuity for distance and near is taken using the Snellen distance chart or letter matching as appropriate. Children with a developmental age of about 3 years have the ability to letter match. With small children it is frequently possible to get a distance vision acuity at a distance of 3 m as they feel the 6 m letter chart is 'too far away'. If the child objects to having one eye occluded it is always better to obtain a binocular acuity than no acuity at all. A small child will cooperate better sitting on mother's lap, which also puts her in the ideal position to check if the matching is correct. She will have to be warned not to prompt or correct. The process is easily treated as a game, with a great deal of encouragement and positive reinforcement.

Any previous devices however acquired should be recorded fully, along with their provenance, use, condition and performance.

The child must be refracted accurately. A subjective refraction is not very helpful in young visually handicapped children, but the competent retinoscopist is rarely as much as 0.50 D out, and this is of little significance when the best acuity is 6/24 or less. Cycloplegic refraction should be avoided, as it is essential to have any available accommodation active during assessment of near-vision magnification needs. However if it cannot be omitted then it should be deferred to the end of the assessment, or the assessment terminated at that point and completed at another visit. Single symbol optotypes should be avoided, the acuity obtained by them is unreliable and can be misleading.

Near-vision acuity should be measured using appropriate tests such as the Bailey–Lovie, Sonksen–Silver, Maclure or Faculty of Ophthalmologists charts. Since there is a simple mathematical relationship between the character sizes in all the above charts the eventual magnification levels can be predicted reasonably reliably. The near acuity is checked with the distance vision prescription and the near vision and selected working space recorded. In aphakia or the absence of accommodation for any other reason, a near addition must be used. Plus lenses are added, and the working distance reduced, until the required acuity is achieved. It is usually better to reach that level in steps of perhaps 2 D each rather than one leap (see below, 'Psychological factors'). The standard formula of dividing the add by four will apply.

It is important to remember when using devices of stated magnification such as spectacle magnifiers, that the power is modified by the child's refractive error. Thus a stated 5x hyperocular on an aphakic child will have perhaps only 8 D available as a near add because 12 D are correcting the aphakia. Working distance is 8 cm, magnification only × 2.

With magnification levels established the practitioner can review which of the available aids could be appropriate to the child's vision and circumstances and assess his response to them. It is important to remember at this stage that the young child has a limited attention span and there is nothing to be gained in tiring the child and subsequently losing his interest by going through the full range of available appliances. The object of the first assessment is to be able to find the appliance that can be handled by the child and will be of value to him. We are convinced that the correct aid for any child is the one that he is happy to use.

When a suitable appliance has been defined it is essential to discuss its potential use with both parents and child. Low-vision aids are often thought of only in the context of specific tasks such as reading at school (and this often does not present difficulties for many infant age children) and other possibilities for use are often simply not considered by the parents. These would include the detailed inspection of small real objects, insects, poorly defined picture material, photographs, etc.; all tasks which are frequently encountered by young children. We recall the small boy who started painting faces on model soldiers only after he was given a stand magnifier, and the delight on the face of a 3 year old looking at tiny flowers.

Young children

As the young child is unlikely to have identified any visual problems for himself when he first attends the low-vision clinic the normal 'problem-solving' approach used for older children and adults has to be abandoned. In addition, parents may give misleading information about the child's visual status as they may be confused by his natural use of intelligence to name familiar objects correctly when seen in context. Children are extremely good at compensating for any visual disability and this often leads to misunderstandings and confusions as to the severity of the visual handicap. At this stage in their child's development the parents often seem more concerned about problems that may occur later in his school career but it is important to try and identify visual problems at the beginning of the assessment wherever possible. Recent research (Ritchie, Sonksen and Gould, 1989) has shown that children as young as 3 may benefit; if they can consider magnification to be the normal means of acquiring information about anything too small to see unaided, this will be a natural response when faced with small print later, and the necessary skills will already be in place.

Older children

When assessing older children the more conventional 'problem-solving' approach can be used as the child has usually defined any visual difficulty before his visit to the low-vision clinic. However, distance aids are frequently still prescribed on a speculative basis at this point as the disability in a general situation outdoors has not been fully appreciated, although more specific difficulties such as blackboard or television have been overcome by sitting in the most beneficial position. Parents' anxieties tend to be more specific at this stage as the early worrying hurdles of going to school, coping in the classroom and playground and social acceptabilities have been overcome to some extent.

During the discussion of the advantages and disadvantages of possible appliances with the child and parents, it is important to stress the benefit of using the appliance for the trial period and that if the device does not meet all the required needs that an alternative or supplementary appliance can be supplied on the follow-up visit if needed. The child must not be made to feel that he is making a long-term commitment. The practitioner has the added advantage of being able to stress the need to attend for follow-up. The child may be worried about having a new low-vision aid from the clinic if it is to replace one which has been given by a teacher or relative. By offering him/her the opportunity to compare the devices he/she can be helped to overcome these fears.

At this time, we are unconvinced that training, as distinct from instruction, has any benefit for the child.

Certain groups are light sensitive. Albinos are frequently put into dark glasses for constant wear. This is undoubtedly unhelpful except in very exceptional cases, they need the best possible contrast. Of course they will need protection outdoors where, as well as dark filters, a shady hat improves comfort enormously.

Patients with pigmentary degenerations frequently prefer red or brown filters with 25–30% LTF probably optimal in Northern Europe. We have been looking for some time at a group of children with various forms of cone dysfunction or total achromatopsia: they have true photophobia and will often remark that they see better at night. Here it is our policy to provide filters with 2–5% LTF at the first visit for use as needed, and modify later if need be.

It goes without saying that all children should be given plastic lenses wherever possible. Not only is damage from breakage important, but the possibility of u.v. toxicity must be considered, especially in aphakia, albinism and aniridia when some of the natural barriers are absent.

Follow-up

The first follow-up visit is arranged at initial assessment, or if devices have to be specially made, at the collection visit. This usually takes place after about 6 months, sometimes less but rarely longer. In our view it is unwise to provide too many aids at one time, it is too easy for the enthusiastic practitioner to cause a sort of 'system overload' leading to an abandonment of all devices, where introducing one at a time will frequently lead to multiple aids reflecting a multitude of activities. Typically a child might be given a magnifier at the first visit, return after a short period to collect a spectacle magnifier, add a distant vision telescope at the 6-month follow-up and a spectacle telescope for a craft a year later.

In all follow-up visits to the clinic a similar procedure is adopted. There should be general discussion between practitioner, child and parents about the success and limitations of the prescribed appliances. What they were used for, where, and when? With older children it is useful to know if it was used at school and if not why not? With teenagers the reasons for not using an appliance in school are often cosmetic (see below). Similarly with younger children, has the aid been used spontaneously by the child, or only when the parent or teacher has encouraged him? Is it kept with the child's belongings or out of reach to prevent breakage? If either parent or child appear much concerned about the occasional loss or breakage of any loaned appliance they should be reassured. Devices in constant use do get misplaced, and an aid showing evidence of much wear and tear has clearly been of much greater benefit than an unused one. Appliances can be replaced where necessary. As part of this general discussion it is important to elicit if any new visual problems have arisen at school or at home. Experience shows that having demonstrated that the more obvious problem of small print or blackboard can be helped, on follow-up visits help for music, hobbies, etc. is frequently requested.

Check acuities with any loaned appliance even though the distance vision has remained unaltered. Often after a period of use at home the performance with the appliance has improved and magnification can be reduced giving the obvious advantages of wider field and increased working distance. Where a simple stand or hand magnifier was the only prescribed appliance at the initial visit it is useful to demonstrate a more complex appliance at this point, even if it was demonstrated before and rejected. Often having seen the advantages of using magnification, initial reservations about face-mounted appliances are abandoned in favour of the advantages offered by more complex appliances. After reassessing existing appliances and modifying them as necessary, any additional problems raised by either child or parent in the preliminary discussion are tackled and where possible the appropriate new appliance dispensed from stock or ordered.

Further follow-up visits have to be discussed. Not only do the child's needs change throughout his school life, but new hardware may be introduced which could better suit the individual's needs. Ideally, children should never be discharged from the low-vision clinic, but where no new problems are anticipated, annual review is usually sufficient. However, in this situation the practitioner needs to check that glasses or any face-mounted appliances are still going to fit in 12 months' time; children grow rapidly. Before the end of any follow-up visit, always impress on parents that if any new and unexpected difficulties arise it is usually possible to attend the clinic before the booked visit. If left for too long small difficulties can often become insurmountable hurdles to either child or teachers.

Psychological factors

It is important that, as well as a sound understanding of optometry and the special equipment needed for low-vision assessment, the practitioner is equipped to understand the behaviour, responses and interactions in his room during the interview, before and afterwards.

First the parents. Their attitudes can range from total denial that there is any problem requiring other than 'ordinary glasses', through total indifference, to a concerned overprotectiveness that can result in a stifled or rebellious child. It is not appropriate for us to attempt to understand the causes of such behaviour, but the active and appropriate cooperation of the parents has to be enlisted at an early stage.

The child him/herself is far easier to understand; often he/she is happily unaware of what he is missing, sometimes angry and frustrated by the things his/her peers can manage and he/she cannot.

Some children prefer to have the parent present throughout assessment, older children may prefer to assert independence by coming in alone. In either case at a very early stage, establish and agree the purpose of the visit 'we are going to help you use your sight better', there is still a lingering belief that some magic device will be produced that will provide normal visual function with no disadvantages.

Prescribing must always be appropriate and reflect the actual (perceived or not perceived) needs of the child. This means that it is usually inappropriate to put a small child into telescopic spectacles; 'learning-to-read material' is printed in at least N24, and any barrier between the child and the material acts as a disincentive. However, the child who has been using a magnifier to look at small objects (see above) will, either spontaneously or at the suggestion of a well-prepared parent, start to use it when he wants to read something in small print. It is at this stage that a spectacle-mounted device should be supplied.

More and more frequently we are observing closed circuit television reading machines being provided at an early stage in schools. Children seem to enjoy screens, but such devices should not be seen as the ultimate solution to the magnification problem, they are simply too restrictive. The child needs to use his devices as part of his personal equipment, and reach for them when there is some detail he needs to see much as he reaches for a pen when he needs to write something. To pursue the metaphor he will need several devices for different situations, much as all his needs are not satisfied by one simple ball point pen.

Cosmesis is a difficult area. Ideally the well-prepared child is willing to accept a conspicuous device for the abilities it gives him. Reassurance that the device need only be used when he wants to use it does help, so of course does the child's own motivation and confidence. There is some evidence that confident children with normal-looking eyes and good acceptance of low-vision aids are more likely to do well in open education.

We have seen many children happily use a telescopic spectacle at 12, reject it during their adolescent years and return to it later. There is no reliable study about cosmetic rejection, although we are convinced that a good deal depends on the parents' attitude. Certainly some children will not use a device that looks 'different', and many adolescents go through a phase when they will not use a low-vision aid in public. The best policy appears to be relaxed and sympathetic about the whole matter, and hope that eventually what he can see is perceived as more important than how he is seen. It usually is.

The last of the 'psychological factors' to be considered is the practitioner himself. He/she needs to have certain inate qualities to work well with children. Of these, probably the most important is simply to be comfortable with them. In low-vision assessment the first moments are crucial, confidence and good communication have to be established. This is only possible when the practitioner has good equipment and knowledge. He/she will need to remind him/herself that his job is to help the child, rather than to supply devices, and that the rejection of his/her devices does not imply a rejection of him/herself as a person, or that he/she is in some sense a failure.

Occasionally the practitioner will find the 'chemistry' of the interpersonal relationships simply not working. We suspect that this may be because, at first assessment at least, the person dispensing the undesired devices has dislike of them transferred. In this situation it is sound to suggest a 'second opinion'. Ideally the second person should be a contrasting personality, and if possible of the other gender. The final message is usually the same, but every practitioner must acknowledge that he/she is capable of the occasional slip. It is useful to be able to discuss problems with colleagues not least for inspiration.

Lastly follow-up. How the child handles the device tells you an enormous amount about how he/she actually uses it. So does his/her description of when and how and how often. First follow-up should always be by the original practitioner, but it is sound to introduce an alternative person at the third visit so that a dependence is not established.

Acknowledgements

We are grateful to the Moorfields consultants for referring their patients to the low-vision clinics, to Mrs Stella Pegram for clerical assistance to all the kids who cooperate so enthusiastically.

References and further reading

COLLINS, B. and SILVER, J.H. (1990). Recent Experience on the Management of Visual Impairment in Albinism. *Ophthalmic Paediatrics and Genetics*, **11**, 225–228.

CULLINAN, T.R. (1977). Visually Disabled People in the Community. Health Services Research Unit Report No. 28. University of Kent, Canterbury.

JAMIESON, M., PARLETT, M. and POCKLINGTON, K. (1977). *Towards Integration*. National Foundation for Educational Research.

RITCHIE, J.P., SONKSEN, P.M. and GOULD, E. (1989). Low-vision aids for pre-school children. *Developmental Medicine and Child Neurology,* **31**, 509–519.

SILVER, J.H. (1976). Low vision aids in the management of visual handicap. *British Journal of Physiological Optics,* **31**, 47–87.

WYBAR, K. and TAYLOR, D. (1983). *Pediatric Ophthalmology*. Marcel Dekker, New York.

16

Specific learning disability (dyslexia)

Terry Buckingham

Introduction

When a child experiences difficulty with reading, parents tend to suspect a visual problem. Indeed, difficulty with reading may be associated with refractive or binocular vision problems, which can only be excluded after ophthalmic investigation. Yet in many cases no obvious ophthalmic cause can be found. Often the child is experiencing no other problem, except that teachers or parents report a failure to make satisfactory progress in reading compared to the child's peers. An optometrist is, therefore, often the first professional person to be consulted when a child experiences difficulty with reading.

Reading is a highly complex skill and progress in learning to read depends upon a number of factors including motivation, intellectual development, linguistic ability and educational opportunity. A deficiency of one or more of these factors may hinder the child's progress in learning to read. Motivation, for example, can be poor if a child does not enjoy reading. It is generally observed that bright, alert children make faster progress in learning to read, whilst those exhibiting hyperactive, distractive, impulsive or uninhibited characteristics display poor reading skills (de Hirsch, Jansky and Langford, 1966). Reading is essentially a linguistic skill in which a code of visual symbols conveys meaning. Children make poor progress if their speech is deficient and understanding of language is poor. Educational opportunity depends not only on the type and quality of education, but also upon the family environment and prevailing sociocultural circumstances.

Reading skills are not acquired in a linear fashion, there are developmental spurts and plateaus. Sometimes a child, who may be expected to make good progress in reading, does not and the question of 'dyslexia' arises. Whilst academically it may be important to distinguish between 'backwardness in reading' and the less common 'dyslexia', both represent an enormous burden for the child. Labelling may not prove helpful since, in lowering the teacher's expectation of the child, a self-fulfilling prophecy may be brought about. Conversely, anything which serves to liberate the child from such a burden is to be encouraged. Sometimes a label can liberate a child, and their family, but how is such a label correctly assigned?

Dyslexia defined

It is neither easy to define nor diagnose dyslexia. There is no clear agreement upon the degree of reading difficulty at which the term is applied. The boundary between severe reading difficulty and dyslexia is unclear, the distinction being unrecognized by many workers who apply the latter term universally. Sometimes parents use the term 'dyslexic' of children who have had no professional assessment. The preferred term tends to be specific learning disability, although this is synonymous with the shorter term 'dyslexia' which is often more convenient in use.

The definition of 'specific developmental dyslexia' used by the World Federation of Neurology is:

> a disorder manifested by difficulty in learning to read despite conventional instruction, adequate intelligence and socio-cultural opportunity. It is dependent upon fundamental cognitive disabilities which are frequently of constitutional origin (Critchley, 1970).

The use of the term 'specific' signifies that dyslexia is regarded as being independent of intelligence and memory. Secondly, the term 'developmental' emphasizes that the defect occurs in acquiring reading skills and not subsequent to their acquisition. Although the definition lays emphasis upon reading, it is often spelling which remains the dyslexic child's weakest literary skill. The definition also raises questions as to what constitutes 'conventional instruction', 'adequate intelligence' and 'socio-cultural opportunity'.

In an attempt to overcome these criticisms the US Congress defined children with specific learning disability as:

> those children who have a disorder in one or more of the basic psychological processes involved in understanding or in using language, spoken or written, which disorder may manifest itself in imperfect ability to listen, think, speak, read, write, spell, or do mathematical calculations. Such disorders include such conditions as perceptual handicaps, brain injury, minimal brain dysfunction, dyslexia and developmental aphasia. Such term does not include children who have learning problems which are primarily the result of visual, hearing, or motor handicaps, of mental retardation, of emotional disturbance, or environmental, cultural, or economic disadvantage (Office of Education, 1976).

Despite its shortcomings, many workers apply the Critchley (1970) definition in the clinical situation. Dyslexia is suspected when the reading level is less than two standard deviations below that expected for the child's age and intelligence. It is important for both reading and intelligence tests to be administered individually in making this assessment and the assessor should be confident that the child has received sufficient instruction in his native language.

None the less, two Government committees of the Department of Education and Science have concluded that, on the basis of scientific evidence and educational practice, the term 'dyslexia' could not be precisely defined (Department of Education and Science, 1972, 1975). Whilst there may be difficulties over definition, it is clear that the problem is not insignificant.

The extent of the problem

It is suggested that about 15% of 8-year-old children experience severe reading difficulty, with about half still experiencing considerable difficulty on completion of their secondary education (see Rutter, 1978). Obviously, the incidence of dyslexia depends upon the definition which is applied to it. Yet, despite differences in definition, surprisingly similar estimates of its incidence have been made in Canada (CELDIC Report, 1970), the UK (Kellmer-Pringle, Butler and Davie, 1966; Morris, 1966), France (Gaddes, 1976) and Denmark (Gaddes, 1976).

Interestingly the apparent incidence of dyslexia does not occur evenly across the country, varying with locality, the 'academic' stimulation received at home and quality of education available. Dyslexia, for example, is encountered twice as frequently in inner London as in the Isle of Wight (Berger *et al.*, 1975). So it is important to be aware of the average level of achievement of children within local schools, reflecting the socioeconomic and cultural status of the area.

The acquisition of reading skills is determined by learning opportunities open to the child both at home and school, which are influenced by family and sociocultural circumstances. Reading development is, obviously, influenced by schooling and the prevalence of dyslexia is higher in schools having high rates of teacher and pupil turnover. In all this, is there a clear developmental pathway which children tread when acquiring reading skills?

The development of reading and writing skills

There are a number of theories which endeavour to describe the routes by which children attempt to reach the pinnacle of literacy. The first step in learning to read is when the child learns that a particular spoken word is related to a printed word or symbol. At this stage a child can read familiar words, but is unable to analyse unfamiliar, novel words. Frith (1985) has described this as the 'logographic phase'. This is followed by the 'alphabetic phase' in which the child gradually learns to abstract letter–sound relationships contained within printed words. It is not clear how children learn to connect letter units (graphemes) with units of speech (phonemes) and there are, surprisingly, about 577 different letter to sound correspondence rules to learn (Gough and Hillinger, 1980). From about 4 years of age a child can divide a word like 'wonderful' into the syllables 'won', 'der' and 'ful'. Children seem to acquire phoneme segmentation, the ability to divide words at the level of phonemes – when 'won' is split into 'w', 'o' and 'n' – at about 5 or 6 years of age. It is this grapheme-phoneme translation system which allows the reading and spelling of unfamiliar words to be attempted. Whilst at the end of the alphabetic phase a child may spell with complete phonetic accuracy, the irregularities of the English language remain to be conquered, for example, aisle, bough and yacht. Frith terms this the 'orthographic phase' in which reading and later, spelling become automatic and independent of sound. Other theories of literacy development – those of Marsh and Desberg (1983) and Ehri (1985) – are compared with those of Frith (1985) in *Figure 16.1*. One other important skill remains to be considered – the role of context in word recognition. Proficient readers use syntactic and semantic clues to predict forthcoming words. This may be regarded as an example of 'top down' processing where the reader checks perceptual data against an existing perceptual hypothesis. The amount of perceptual processing is reduced if, for example, the reader expects to see 'and' appearing in a sentence. Reading may, therefore, consist of an interaction of 'top down' and conventional 'bottom up' processing in which sensory information is successively analysed as it passes 'up' the visual pathway.

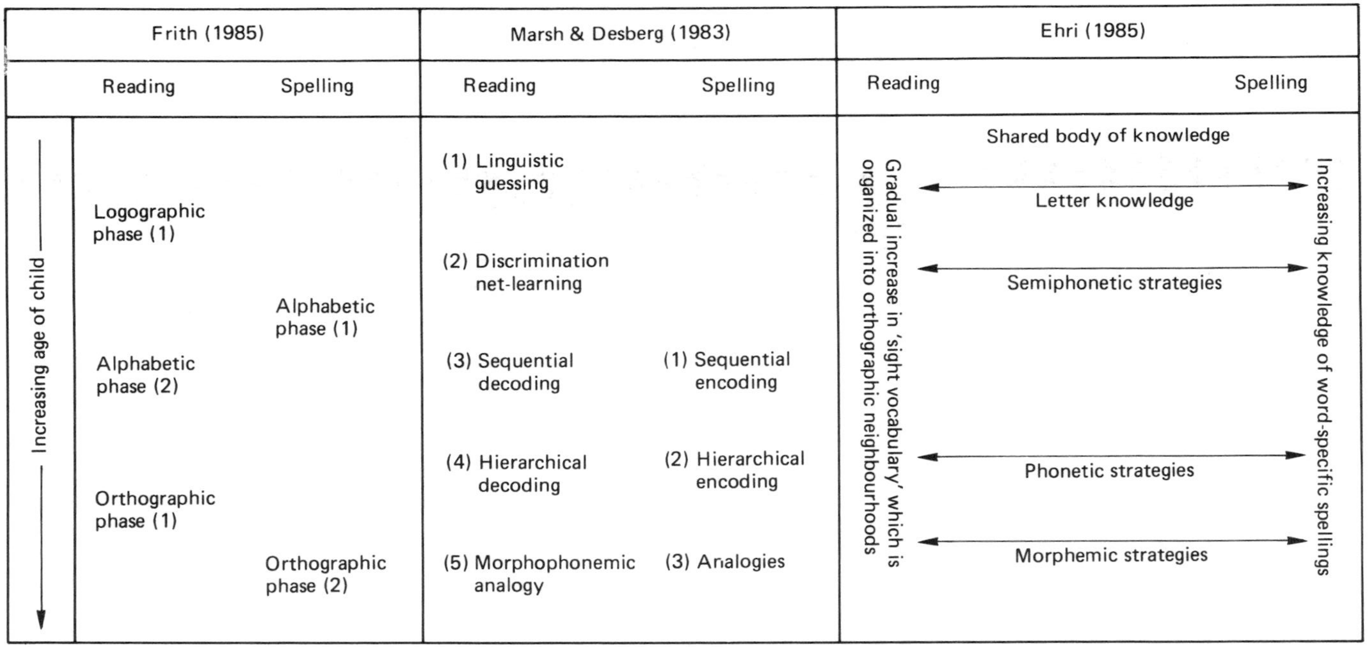

Frith (1985)		Marsh & Desberg (1983)		Ehri (1985)	
Reading	Spelling	Reading	Spelling	Reading	Spelling
Logographic phase (1)		(1) Linguistic guessing		Shared body of knowledge	Increasing knowledge of word-specific spellings
	Alphabetic phase (1)	(2) Discrimination net-learning		Letter knowledge	
Alphabetic phase (2)		(3) Sequential decoding	(1) Sequential encoding	Semiphonetic strategies	
Orthographic phase (1)	Orthographic phase (2)	(4) Hierarchical decoding	(2) Hierarchical encoding	Phonetic strategies	
		(5) Morphophonemic analogy	(3) Analogies	Morphemic strategies	

Gradual increase in 'sight vocabulary' which is organized into orthographic neighbourhoods

Increasing age of child →

Figure 16.1. Theories of literacy development advocated by Frith (1985), Marsh and Desberg (1983) and Ehri (1985)

Dyslexia and backwardness in reading

The question arises as to whether it is possible to distinguish between those children suffering from specific learning disability and those exhibiting backwardness in reading. Dyslexic children are generally characterized by a tendency to make orientation and sequencing errors, in both reading and writing, at what would normally be regarded as the later stages of literacy development. Typical examples of orientation errors are mistaking 'b' for 'd' or 'p' for 'b', a normal developmental feature in children. Sequencing errors are typified by mistaking 'was' for 'saw' or 'calm' for 'clam'. Similar errors may be made by those exhibiting backwardness in reading, yet there are a number of important differences between such children and those who are dyslexic.

Dyslexic children are more likely to be boys than girls, the ratio being between 3 and 4 to 1. The sex distribution for children displaying reading backwardness is about equal. The greater incidence of dyslexia amongst boys may be because children are categorized according to their chronological age for educational purposes, despite the fact that they mature at different rates. Females tend to be about 18 months ahead of males in their levels of maturity. Some workers have suggested that the greater head circumference of males increases the chance of neurological damage at birth.

Overt neurological disorders are encountered more frequently in the generally backward group. A wide range of developmental difficulties may be seen in this group, including motor and praxic abnormalities. Dyslexic children on the other hand tend to exhibit only speech and language impairment.

Backward children are more likely to come from socially disadvantaged homes. Dyslexia, however, if constitutionally determined afflicts all socioeconomic groups equally – social disadvantage does not ensure against dyslexia. Clearly there is no sharp borderline between dyslexia and reading difficulty. It has been argued that a probable dyslexic can only be identified by displaying:

(1) Extreme difficulty in identifying single words and, therefore, difficulty with all other aspects of reading.
(2) Difficulty in analysing the component sounds of words.
(3) Severe decoding problems.

The term 'dyslexia' should not be applied to children who have adequate decoding skills yet poor comprehension of what they read. Under these circumstances the term 'hyperlexia' has been applied. It would appear that there are some specific traits or characteristics which are evident amongst dyslexics.

Dyslexic characteristics

There is evidence of a number of 'characteristics' which may indicate the presence of dyslexia:

(1) Boys are more prone to have reading problems than girls, the ratio being around 4 : 1 (Eisenberg, 1966).
(2) Reading difficulties are more common amongst the children of poor readers (Hallgren, 1950; Herman, 1959).

(3) Poor readers may also have difficulty with other forms of representational learning, for example telling the time, naming months and seasons of the year (defective sequencing), and discriminating left from right (directional confusion).
(4) Some dyslexic children may display minor signs of neurological dysfunction, for example, abnormal reflexes or minor coordination problems.
(5) Poor readers frequently have a history of developmental deficiencies, particularly in one or more aspects of language (Kawi and Pasamanick, 1958; Lyle, 1970).
(6) Dyslexics exhibit a much higher proportion of spelling errors than is usual, with a typical frequency of about two errors per line.

Whilst this list of dyslexic 'characteristics' is by no means exhaustive, it covers those most frequently observed and, as such, merits closer inspection.

Sex distribution

It is a common characteristic in primates, and man is no exception, that females mature earlier than males. This may explain why more girls survive at birth than boys, whatever the level of perinatal mortality rates. There are very few exceptions to the 'females first' rule with physical maturational differences at birth amounting to between 4 and 6 weeks of development, compared to 2 years at the onset of puberty. The greater incidence of dyslexia amongst males may reflect their relative immaturity compared to females of equivalent age. The levels of physical and emotional maturity are important in determining the child's readiness to read. It is often observed that girls exhibit a greater ability to draw and then write than boys of similar age.

The development of cerebral dominance may play an important role in learning to read and there is some evidence that this occurs earlier in females than males. A number of sociocultural factors may exaggerate the incidence of dyslexia amongst males. It has been suggested that non-reading boys are more easily noticed in school than non-reading girls because their behaviour is more disruptive. It has been argued that some parents are more concerned by a boy's inability to read compared to a girl. Those who would link dyslexia to neurological dysfunction point to the larger head circumference of males at birth, which may make them more prone to neurological damage.

Genetic traits

Critchley (1963) found that it was rare for a child to have reading problems and not have one or more relatives similarly afflicted. Likewise, Bryant and Patterson (1962) found that in more than half of their cases other family members also experienced reading difficulty. Despite observations that dyslexic children are often offspring of poor readers, there has been little progress in establishing a genetic link. This is partly because of the difficulty in agreeing a definition of reading disability, as well as finding tangible evidence suitable for genetic analysis. Evidence in such cases is often anecdotal and, unless accurate diagnosis has been made, it is impossible to establish a clear genetic link. In some cases it may be the common cultural environment, shared by other family members, which increases the incidence of reading difficulty. None the less, studies involving twins may provide evidence for a genetically determined element in some forms of dyslexia. If a disease occurs with greater frequency in monozygotic (identical) compared to dizygotic (non-identical) twins, the genetic influence outweighs environmental factors. Herman (1959) studied 45 pairs of twins and found that in 12 pairs of monozygotic twins both showed identical reading disability – 100% concordance. In the other 33 pairs of dizygotic twins, 19 were of the same sex but only four sets had equivalent reading difficulty – 21% concordance. In the remaining 14 sets of dizygotic, opposite-sex twins seven sets had equivalent reading difficulty (50% concordance). In general, therefore, dizygotic twins exhibit a 33% concordance of reading disability. The higher concordance observed with monozygotic twins suggests that a genetic influence is present. Sladen (1971) suggested that the gene character for dyslexia had variable dominance in males, but was largely recessive in females. This would account for the 3 : 1 ratio of male : female dyslexics. More recently Finucci *et al.* (1976) investigated pedigrees of dyslexics and found no single mode of genetic transmission. It would seem that until subgroups of dyslexia are more clearly defined, little progress in establishing a clear mode of inheritance of any of its forms can be made.

Associated learning difficulties

Dyslexics as a group tend to exhibit deficiencies in temporal sequencing and serial positioning, although there are marked individual differences. Such skills are important in spelling and reading. In spelling, auditory information in the form of a word is fragmented into individual sounds, which must be written in the same sequential order in which it is heard. When reading the eye fixes a group of words in sequence, but occasional regressions (refixations of earlier words) may be made to check spelling or context. Hence the order in which words are perceived by the reader may not be the same as that in which they are printed and some reordering may be necessary.

It is commonly held that dyslexics show directional confusion, for example, between right and left or 'b' and 'd'. Confusion of 'b' and 'd' is an error commonly made by children beginning to read and write, but dyslexics continue to make it after their peers have ceased to do so. Directional confusion between right and left may arise because of the, almost unique, inconsistency with which the terms are applied. An object on the right becomes transferred to the left if one turns round. Perhaps terms which fluctuate in their reference cause more difficulty than those which do not because of the dyslexic's difficulty in activating entries in the internal lexicon. Obviously, there is little difficulty with the terms up and down.

Another commonly observed characteristic among dyslexic children is unusual (left) handedness or crossed laterality. Crossed laterality is when the dominant eye and hand are on opposite sides. Evidence linking left handedness (sinistrality) or crossed laterality to dyslexia is slight, although it occurs more frequently in dyslexics than controls (Goldberg *et al.*, 1983). Man is almost unique in the animal kingdom in displaying a dominant hand. This may not always have been the case, since Stone Age cave paintings and tools indicate equal use of right and left hands whilst scythes from the Bronze Age show that right handedness (dextrality) predominated. Perhaps this evolved because warrior-hunter man protected his heart more effectively by carrying his shield in the left hand and spear in the right. Generally the preferred hand becomes apparent by about 9 months of age and is fairly firmly established by 2 years of age. Associated with maturity, it is generally established earlier in girls than boys. Sinistrality occurs in 5–10% of the population and is twice as common in boys as in girls. It is four times as likely in the retarded and is often associated with both perinatal distress and abnormal EEG findings. Incomplete handedness occurs in 20% of normal 7 year olds and 50% of reading disabled children. It is found that incomplete handedness is much more strongly related to learning problems than is sinistrality. Ill-defined laterality, or poor dominance, does not cause reading disability but indicates cerebral immaturity. Unlike handedness, ocular dominance is determined innately and is much more difficult to modify subsequently. About 70% of people are right eye dominant. It has been argued that the preference is usually established before that of the dominant hand and may influence its choice since the eye 'leads' the hand. There is some suggestion, which will be considered later, that the absence of a clearly dominant or fixed reference eye may play a role in dyslexia.

Neurological dysfunction

It is highly unlikely that minimal brain damage, or neural dysfunction, can account for the majority of children with dyslexia. However the maturing brain, both before and after birth, may suffer damage leading to aberration of function. In some patients perinatal histories, psychological testing and drawing, EEG results and the presence of retinal haemorrhages indicate that this may have happened. The amount of damage depends upon the origin, extent, localization, type of lesion, duration and rate at which damage was sustained, together with the developmental stage at which the injury occurred (Birch and Belmont, 1964). Walsh and Lindenberg (1961) demonstrated that optic nerve damage could occur from hypoxia at birth. There is a significant correlation between the severity of reading retardation and the severity of impairment of a large number of brain-related variables.

Historically, a suspicion of neurological impairment in dyslexics arose following Dejerine's (1928) publication of post-mortem details of a patient who had suffered from alexia. Alexia is the acquired inability to read letters or words, even though spontaneous writing is still possible. Findings suggested that a lesion of the sub-cortical region of the left angular gyrus had produced the patient's alexia.

Vision is allocated to very specific regions of the brain. The prestriate area and angular gyrus are of particular interest clinically, since lesions in these areas produce the agnosias and aphasias associated with visual disconnection. Classically the upper part of Brodmann's area 18 (*Figure 16.2*) was thought to be involved with the recognition of animate objects, for example, animals and the lower part with inanimate objects, for example, a chair. Damage to area 18 produces visual agnosia, but reading is usually unaffected. Brodmann's area 19 interrelates with area 18 and is associated with the elaboration of memory patterns and language symbols, damage to this area results in a loss of memory of things, persons and language. Other areas of the brain, essential to reading and writing, include the angular gyrus and Wernicke's area. Damage to the angular gyrus results in words not being interpreted even though they are clearly seen. Wernicke's area is concerned with the recognition and recall of speech. Wernicke's area and the angular gyrus are connected, since Wernicke's area reinforces the ability to understand written language by auditory stimulation – hearing the word. This is involved in the learning process when a teacher pronounces a word and the child repeats what is heard. Another important region is Broca's area which is linked with the angular gyrus and is associated with motor function of speech, for example, some people move their lips when reading silently. Damage to either Wernicke's or Broca's areas complicates

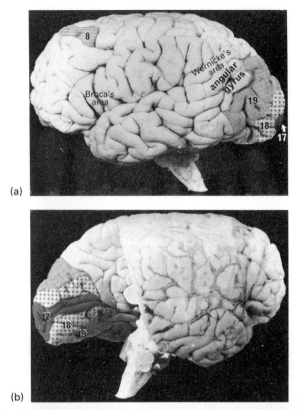

(a)

(b)

Figure 16.2. Lateral views of a human brain. The whole occipital lobe is shaded differently to indicate its three regions – Brodmann's areas 17, 18 and 19. (a) Area 8, which is the frontal eye field governing voluntary eye movements, is also indicated. (b) The posterior part of the right hemisphere is removed exposing the medial aspect of the left hemisphere. The calcarine sulcus divides the striate cortex (area 17) into upper and lower halves. The locations of Wernicke's area and the angular gyrus together with Broca's area are shown. (From Ruskell, 1988)

learning. Since alexia can be produced by lesions at any of four separate loci, there may be a number of different types of dyslexia rather than a single underlying cause.

It is generally held that the right brain hemisphere has a dominant role for spatial relationships and the left for temporal relationships. This is because injuries to the right side tend to produce disturbances in spatial perception, together with losses in awareness of body scheme and spatial relationships. Corresponding damage to the left side, however, produces severe disruption of language and associated thought processes. Language, for which temporal relationships are important, is located in the left hemisphere of 97% of dextrals. Surprisingly, this is also the case in 59% of sinistrals. It is possible that perinatal damage to the left side causes control of speech to be transferred to the opposite side. Indeed when there is evidence of perinatal brain injury to the left side, about 66% of patients are subsequently found to have their speech centres located in the right side.

A number of workers consider that apraxia – the inability to perform a skilled act or series of movements – is associated with a lesion to the dominant (left) hemisphere. In the 1920s Gerstmann described deficits associated with lesions to the major hemisphere as follows:

(1) Finger agnosia – inability to identify fingers on tactile stimulation.
(2) Difficulty in discriminating between right and left sides of the body.
(3) Agraphia – losing the ability to write.
(4) Acalcula – losing the ability to perform calculations.

By comparison deficits in the right (non-dominant) hemisphere produce:

(1) Impaired visual space perception.
(2) Constructional apraxia – difficulty in constructing a representational plan of an object, e.g. a room.
(3) Apraxia for dressing.
(4) Inattention to one-half of the visual field.

The occurrence of such symptoms in dyslexic children suggests that dyslexia may arise from dysfunction in either major or minor hemisphere. It should also be noted that lesions of the non-dominant hemisphere produce impairment of certain aspects of auditory perception and memory. Kawi and Pasamanick (1958) found that 16.9% of children with reading problems had been exposed to two, or more, complications during birth, or immediately afterward, which may have led to fetal anoxia and consequent brain damage. By comparison, only 1.5% of children without reading problems experienced similar complications at birth.

Developmental deficiencies

Developmental deficiencies have themselves been associated with some degree of cerebral dysfunction, although physical signs of neurological abnormality are absent or trivial. Intelligence may be less than that anticipated from the family background. Tests involving step-by-step reasoning from premise to premise, as well as those involving perception of spatial and form relationships, are done very poorly. Short-term memory generally appears unaffected.

Children with learning disabilities are quite often moderately delayed in attaining physical milestones of development, particularly those involving fine motor control. Sitting and walking may not be delayed but handedness is usually delayed to the 4th or 5th year. The child may be unable to ride a bicycle for years and fastening buttons may be impossible until 6 or 7 years of age. Emotional instability may also be evident. Children having dyslexia may retreat from learning situations and may exhibit marked hyperactivity and distractibility.

Vision and dyslexia

There is no strong evidence of a link between visual disability and dyslexia. Visual disorders are not entirely irrelevant since uncorrected refractive errors and binocular vision problems may contribute toward 'slow reading'. The size of print used in early reading books is sufficiently large so that reduced visual acuity, unless marked, is unlikely to have a serious impact on the acquisition of reading skills. Visual disorders may be much more significant in other learning situations and in later schooling.

A number of early studies suggested that dyslexics had defective eye movements during reading. Four components may be evaluated when investigating an individual's pattern of reading; the number of words spanned by a single fixation; the durations of fixation and saccadic movements; and the frequency of regression eye movements. Good readers make fewer fixations per line, fixate for shorter periods and make fewer regressions. It is likely that defective eye movements during reading are symptomatic of dyslexia rather than causative. Eye movements, for example, are improved if 'frustration' words are taught before reading the material and no significant difference is observed between eye movements of dyslexics and non-dyslexics when observing a scene.

It is interesting that between a half and two-thirds of dyslexic children have no unambiguously dominant eye (Stein, Riddell and Fowler, 1986). The dominant, or reference, eye may be determined using the Dunlop test in which the child views two macular fusion slides through a synoptophore. This shows a house having a central front door flanked by two posts, a large one is seen by the right eye and a small post is seen by the left eye. The child fuses the two slides as the synoptophore tubes are slowly diverged at a rate of 1–2° per second. Diplopia intervenes at about 5°, but just beforehand one of the posts is seen to move toward the door while the other remains stationary. The post which remains still is the one seen by the reference (dominant) eye. The test is performed a total of ten times with the slides being changed to avoid guessing. If the same eye is used on eight or more occasions a fixed reference eye is indicated. If the same eye is used on seven or less occasions this indicates a lack of fixed reference and visual confusion. About 60% of 5-year-old children have an unfixed reference eye, but normally the reference eye should be fixed by 8 years of age. In a study of 7 year olds, nearly 50% of those with a reading age 18 months behind their chronological age had unstable responses in the Dunlop test (Stein, Riddell and Fowler, 1986). Similar unstable responses were only observed in 14% of advanced readers and 24% of children whose reading age was ahead of their age. Where the reference eye is fixed, but on the opposite side to the hand used for writing, it is said to be crossed. As far as reading ability is concerned it seems that the important factor is that the eye should be fixed, rather than whether it is crossed or uncrossed. Stein and Fowler (1982) found that occluding the non-dominant eye for reading, and close work, in children with an unfixed reference eye helped many to develop stable visual motor responses. Almost all occluded children in whom the reference became fixed began to read better. A group of matched children who were not occluded, and remained unfixed, showed no improvement. It was felt that occluding one eye probably helped children to attain reliable ocular motor/macular associations by eliminating the possibility of discrepant retinal signals from the two eyes. The indiscriminate use of monocular occlusion is unlikely to produce a significant effect in all dyslexics, since about one-third already have a fixed reference. These may have phonemic, rather than visuomotor problems, and some could be harmed by monocular occlusion. Another third of dyslexics tend to have mixed visual and phonemic problems. Even if stable visuomotor responses are gained with the help of occlusion, their reading may not improve. It is only the remaining third, with mainly visuomotor problems, who may be helped by monocular occlusion. Hence there are grounds for believing that between one-sixth and one-third of all dyslexics may be helped by monocular occlusion, the categorization of which is discussed later.

Some dyslexic children may be helped by prescribing spectacles correcting mild refractive errors, or containing a modest near addition or simply incorporating tinted lenses. Clearly anything which makes reading more comfortable for the child is to be encouraged although, in the absence of anything which suggests otherwise, improvements in reading may be due to a placebo effect. The question concerning the use of tinted lenses is much more vexed. Some dyslexics find that their reading is helped by tinted spectacle lenses, particularly red or yellow tints, having a light transmission factor of about 50%. An empirical approach is used to establish both the hue and depth of tinting. Practitioners should bear in mind that there is no coherent scientific basis for the use of tinted lenses to help reading in children with dyslexia. This appears to be a further example of a placebo effect and some patients may, or may not, find them beneficial. Practitioners, therefore, may need to take a cautious approach to this question, particularly since there is evidence that visual problems may not play a significant role in many forms of dyslexia.

A family of dyslexias

Mattis, French and Rapin (1975) have suggested that it is possible to isolate three, independent dyslexia syndromes accounting for 90% of all dyslexics. The most prominent characteristic typifying each of the three groups is: a language disorder; poor coordination between speech and writing (articulatory and graphomotor discoordination); and a visuospatial perceptual disorder. In addition to these, there is evidence of a fourth 'sequencing disorder' syndrome. It should be mentioned that within each group there exist a number of inconsistent secondary features.

A language disorder was indicated by the difficulty in naming recognizable objects (anomia), with errors of 20% or more on a naming test. There is sometimes difficulty in rhyming words. Mattis (1978) reports work of Denckla (1975) who found 54% of a dyslexic group to have a language disorder, compared to 64% obtained by Erenberg *et al.* (1976), using the paradigm of Mattis, French and Rapin (1975).

Children having poor coordination between speech and writing appeared typically clumsy with gross or fine motor discoordination. They had few cognitive or perceptual difficulties. This particular syndrome was observed in 12% (Denckla, 1975) and 10% (Erenberg *et al.* 1976) of their respective samples.

The most significant finding amongst those having a visuospatial perceptual disorder was a visual-constructional difficulty, whilst language development was well within normal limits. Directional confusion would be a significant finding amongst this group. This syndrome is much less frequent than the others, studies indicating it to be about 4% (Denckla, 1975) or 5% (Erenberg *et al.*, 1976). About 9% of dyslexics presented with two syndromes, whilst none presented with all three.

Denckla (1975) suggested that two other syndromes were present. About 13% of the dyslexic group had a sequencing difficulty, where they had great difficulty in repeating polysyllabic words. This was despite normal naming comprehension and speech sound production (articulation). Some 10% of children in Mattis and Erenberg's (1978) study also presented evidence of a sequencing disorder syndrome. In addition, about 10% of children in Denckla's (1975) study displayed a 'verbal memorisation (learning) disorder' where sentence repetition and verbal paired-associate learning were deficient, but language skills were not demonstrably disturbed. Hence there is good evidence to support the existence of three independent dyslexia syndromes together with some evidence for an additional 'sequencing disorder' syndrome.

From the above classification of dyslexia, it would seem that visual problems may be significant only amongst a small proportion of dyslexics. Approaching the question from a different perspective, Stein and Fowler (1982) looked at those children with dyslexia in whom visual problems could play a significant role. Each child was categorized according to the predominant type of error they made when performing simple reading, writing, sequencing, rhyming and alliteration tasks.

(1) Visual errors were: losing the place on the page (more than two errors); having to point with the finger to keep the place (more than two errors); and mis-sequencing reversing and rotating words and letters when reading and writing, e.g. was/saw, no/on, b/d (maximum six errors).
(2) Phonemic (auditory) errors consisted of the failure to find rhymes or alliterations for ten common words.
(3) Sequencing errors consisted of the failure to name, in the correct order, the days of the week and the months of the year.

Children with an unstable reference eye tended to make more visual than phonemic errors and the interesting results obtained from monocular occlusion have been discussed earlier. The categorization adopted by Stein and Fowler (1982) has been questioned. For example, it has been argued that letter confusions, such as 'b' for 'd', and missequencing of letters when reading and writing may be due to disordered linguistic categorization rather than to visual perceptual difficulties. Yet letter confusions and missequencing only occur with reading and writing – not speaking – and losing the place on a page can hardly be classified as a linguistic problem.

Clearly, important questions remain about the classification of dyslexia. Obviously, the extent to which an optometrist is able to help a patient with dyslexia depends upon the characteristics which they display, together with the results of the optometric investigation.

Optometric investigation

Any child experiencing difficulty with reading is likely to be under stress. The practitioner should enquire whether any other specialist, for example, an edu-cational psychologist, has seen the child and what the outcome was. Many edu-cational psychologists feel that labelling children as having specific learning disability is not in their best interests. Conversely, it may be a relief for the child, and their parents, if dyslexia is formally diagnosed. In either event, whether dyslexia is formally diagnosed or not, any ophthalmic factor which may contribute to reduced reading performance must be investigated.

As well as the usual questions concerning history and symptoms, particularly those concerning blurring or diplopia at near, additional information should be sought about any child experiencing reading difficulty. Specific questions might cover:

(1) The normality of the mother's pregnancy and complications during or immediately after birth. For example, whether labour had lasted for more than 12 or less than 3 hours, if the baby had been pre- or post-mature and born by caesarean section or instrumental help, or if he/she had required resuscitation or incubation.
(2) Parents are asked about the child's development, particularly the age at which the child walked, started to talk and established hand dominance.
(3) Any family history of dyslexia.
(4) Family and peer relationships.
(5) Whether the child is happy with their current school placement.
(6) Open-ended questions intended to assess the child's school performance and verbal ability.

(7) Whether the child copies accurately from the blackboard and if they learn more easily through listening than through reading.
(8) Whether the child enjoys sporting activities and is good at catching a ball.
(9) Whether colour vision is normal.

It might be worth mentioning that Miles (1983) has developed a series of tests to indicate the likelihood of dyslexia in a patient. This, together with responses to the questions posed above, might help the practitioner to obtain some indication of whether the child is displaying dyslexic tendencies.

A full ophthalmic investigation and refraction follow. Serious consideration should be given to a cycloplegic refraction. These topics have been dealt with in Chapters 9 and 10. Clearly, the practitioner should correct any significant refractive error. The normality of the cover test responses at distance and near should be ascertained. The amplitudes of accommodation, near point of convergence and ocular motility should also appear normal. Any orthoptic treatment which might be necessary should be undertaken.

It may be valuable to determine the child's dominant eye and relate this to handedness and footedness. A number of techniques are available to determine dominant eye, including 'pointing' and 'telescope to eye' tests. If base-in prisms are used binocularly to induce fixation disparity, the line which is seen to be displaced is that seen by the non-dominant eye. In some cases it may be found that the dominant eye is not the same at distance and near. If the child shows no preference for a dominant eye then the practitioner may wish to follow the procedure suggested by Stein and Fowler (1982) and occlude the non-reference eye for reading. The child's progress should be reviewed every 3 months.

Although evidence of improved reading using tinted lenses may be anecdotal and due to a placebo effect, practitioners may wish to investigate the effect of coloured transparent overlays on reading. A succession of differently coloured transparent films are placed over the reading text and the child is asked if any colour helps when reading. Some children state that films in the red to yellow range of the spectrum make reading more comfortable. Broadly equivalent tints may be incorporated into a spectacle correction having a light transmission factor of around 50%. As with the occlusive approach, the child's progress should be reviewed every 3 months.

Summary

Although dyslexia is difficult to define, studies suggest that its incidence within the population is not insignificant. Those experiencing such difficulty are likely to present themselves for ophthalmic investigation. Accordingly, the optometrist, whether aware of it or not, may be the first professional person to be consulted in such circumstances. Clearly, the optometrist must investigate, and attempt to relieve, any factor which may give rise to problems with reading. A number of traits tend to be present amongst dyslexics, yet diagnosis is far from easy and attaching labels to those who experience it may not prove helpful. Vision, unquestionably, plays its part in the acquisition of reading skills. Although the proportion of dyslexics in which visual problems play a significant role is difficult to determine, they are likely to be causative in some. Evidence suggests that children with an unstable reference eye make faster progress once this is stabilized. Perhaps the impact of visual problems on dyslexia will become clearer as the features of each member of the 'family of dyslexias' become more clearly drawn. It is, none the less, important that the optometrist is aware of those factors which may contribute towards dyslexia in order to help those seeking advice.

References

BERGER, M., YULE, W. and RUTTER, M. (1975). Attainment and adjustment in two geographical areas: II the prevalence of specific reading retardation. *British Journal of Psychiatry,* **126**, 510–519.

BIRCH, H. and BELMONT, L. (1964). Auditory – visual integration in normal and retarded readers. *American Journal of Orthopsychiatry,* **34**, 852–861.

BRYANT, N. and PATTERSON, R. (1962). Reading Disability: Part of a Syndrome of Neurological Functioning. Unpublished paper presented at International Reading Association, Newark, Delaware.

CELDIC REPORT (1970). *One Million Children: A National Study of Canadian Children with Emotional and Learning Disorders.* L. Crainford, Toronto.

CRITCHLEY, M.T. (1963). The problem of developmental dyslexia. *Proceedings of the Royal Society of Medicine,* **56**, 209–211.

CRITCHLEY, M. (1970). *The Dyslexic Child.* Charles C. Thomas, Springfield., Il.

DE HIRSCH, K., JANSKY, J. and LANGFORD, W. (1966). *Predicting Reading Failure.* Harper and Row, New York.

DEJERINE, J. (1892). Contribution l'étude anatomo-pathologique et clinique des différents variés de cécite verbale. *Mémoire de la Société de Biologie,* **4**, 61.

DEPARTMENT OF EDUCATION AND SCIENCE (1972). *Children with Specific Reading Difficulties. Report of the Advisory Committee on Handicapped Children.* HMSO, London.

DEPARTMENT OF EDUCATION AND SCIENCE (1975). *A Language for Life. The Bullock Report.* HMSO, London.

EHRI, L. (1985). Sources of difficulty in learning to spell and read. In *Advances in Developmental and Behavioural Paediatrics*, edited by M.L. Wolraich and D. Routh. Jai Press, Greenwich, Connecticut.

EISENBERG, L. (1966). The epidemiology of reading retardation and a program for preventive intervention. In *The Disabled Reader: Education of the Dyslexic Child*, edited by J. Money, Johns Hopkins Press, Baltimore.

ERENBERG, G., MATTIS, S. and FRENCH, J.H. (1976). Four hundred children referred to an urban ghetto development disabilities clinic: computer assisted analysis of demographic, social, psychological and medical data. (unpublished). Reported by S. Mattis (1978) in *Dyslexia*, edited by A.C. Barton and D. Pearl, Oxford University Press, New York.

FINUCCI, J.M., GUTHRIE, J.T., CHILDS, A.L., ABBEY, H. and CHILDS, B. (1976). The genetics of specific learning disability. *Annals of Human Genetics,* **40**, 1–23.

FRITH, U. (1985). Beneath the surface of developmental dyslexia. In *Surface Dyslexia* , edited by K.E. Patterson, J.C. Marshall and M. Coltheart, Routledge and Kegan Paul, London.

GADDES, W. (1976). Learning disabilities: prevalence estimates and the need for definition. In *The Neuropsychology of Learning Disorders*, edited by R. Knights and D.J. Bakker. University Park Press, Baltimore.

GOLDBERG, H.K., SHIFFMAN, G.B. and BENDER, M. (1983). *Dyslexia: Interdisciplinary Approaches to Reading Disabilities.* Grune and Stratton, New York.

GOUGH, P. and HILLINGER, M.L. (1980). Learning to read: an unnatural act. *Bulletin of the Orton Society,* **30**, 179–196.

HALLGREN, B. (1950). Specific dyslexia ('congenital word blindness'): a clinical and genetic study. *Acta Psychiatrica et Neurologica Scandinavica,* Supplement No. 65.

HERMAN, K. (1959). *Reading Disability: A Medical Study of Word-blindness and Related Handicaps.* Munksgaard, Copenhagen.

KAWI, A.A. and PASAMANICK, B.P. (1958). Association of factors of pregnancy with reading disorders in childhood. *Journal of the American Medical Association,* **166**, 1420–1423.

KELLMER-PRINGLE, M.L., BUTLER, N.R. and DAVIE, R. (1966). *11,000 Seven Year Olds, Studies in Child Development.* Longmans, London.

LYLE, J.G. (1970). Certain antenatal, perinatal and developmental variables and reading retardation in middle class boys. *Child Development,* **41**, 481–491.

MARSH, G. and DESBERG, P. (1983). The development of strategies in the acquisition of symbolic skills. In *The Acquisition of Symbolic Skills,* edited by D.G. Rogers and J.A. Sloboda, Plenum, New York.

MATTIS, S. (1978). Dyslexia syndromes: a working hypothesis that works. In *Dyslexia,* edited by A.L. Benton and D. Pearl. Oxford University Press, New York.

MATTIS, S., FRENCH, J.H. and RAPIN, I. (1975). Dyslexia in children and young adults: three independent neuropsychological syndromes. *Developmental Medicine and Child Neurology,* **17**, 150–163.

MILES, T.R. (1983). *Dyslexia: The Pattern of Difficulties.* Granada, London.

MORRIS, J. (1966). *Standards and Progress in Reading.* National Foundation for Educational Research, Slough.

OFFICE OF EDUCATION (1976). Assistance to states for education of handicapped children, notice of proposed rulemaking. *Federal Register,* 41 (No. 230) 52404–52407, 29 November.

RUSKELL, G. (1988). Neurology of visual perception. In *Optometry,* edited by K. Edwards and R. Llewellyn, Butterworth-Heinemann, Oxford.

RUTTER, M. (1978). Prevalence and types of dyslexia. In *Dyslexia* edited by A.L. Benton and D. Pearl. Oxford University Press, New York.

SLADEN, B.K. (1971). Inheritance of dyslexia. *Bulletin of the Orton Society,* **31**, 30–39.

STEIN, J.F. and FOWLER, M.S. (1982). Diagnosis of dyslexia by means of a new indicator of eye dominance. *British Journal of Ophthalmology,* **66**, 332–336.

STEIN, J.F. and FOWLER, P.M. and FOWLER, M.S. (1986). The Dunlop test and reading in primary school children. *British Journal of Ophthalmology,* **70**, 317–320.

WALSH, F. and LINDENBERG, R. (1961). Hypoxia in children. *Bulletin of the Johns Hopkins Hospital,* **108**, 100–145.

17

Electrodiagnostic assessment in children

Jill Grose-Fifer and Caroline Thompson

Electrophysiological recording methods have particular value when applied to paediatric samples since they enable the objective assessment of visual function in subjects having limited cooperation, and additionally may assist in the localization of abnormalities in the visual systems of such individuals. The main purpose of this chapter is to summarize the scientific literature on the maturation of two electrical signals which may be elicted in response to visual stimulation – the electroretinogram (ERG), which reflects electrical activity at the retinal level, and the visual evoked potential (VEP), reflecting cortical electrical activity. The practicalities of obtaining these responses from uncooperative subjects are also considered and clinical case examples are used to illustrate the diagnostic capabilities when combining the two techniques. Whilst this chapter has been devoted to paediatric studies, further general reading has been suggested at the end of the chapter.

In both ERG and VEP recording, responses may be obtained by applying suitable electrodes (linked to amplifiers and recorders) close to the site of origin of the signal. The stimulus may consist of diffuse flashes of light, or patterns (frequently black and white checkerboards or line gratings) which are reversed in contrast or presented after a blank background. Stimuli are often presented repetitively to make use of averaging techniques for signal enhancement (described in VEP section), this being particularly essential during VEP recording in order to distinguish the response from the background electroencephalogram (EEG) activity (for further details see Harding, 1988). More sophisticated patterned stimuli (including chromatic stimuli, dynamic stereoscopic displays, and line gratings which periodically shift in orientation), have also been used to investigate other visual processes in children, but since use of these is generally confined to research studies, details will not be given here.

Electrophysiological recordings can be classified as transient or steady-state responses. A transient response is the result of an isolated, abrupt change in some stimulus parameter, for example, flash of light, pattern appearance or contrast reversal. The mature transient ERG and VEP comprise a succession of positive and negative deflections, termed waves or components, and are usually described in terms of amplitude versus latency. Amplitude is generally defined in terms of a peak to trough voltage (in microvolts) and latency (or 'implicit time') as the time delay between stimulus onset and a peak or trough (in milliseconds). Steady-state responses are evoked by stimuli of sufficiently high repetitive frequency to result in an overlap of the responses, thus the waveform has a sinusoidal appearance and is classified in terms of phase and amplitude.

The electroretinogram

When light impinges on the retina, a transient retinal action potential is produced, this potential can be recorded at or near the cornea as the electroretinogram (ERG) (Armington, 1974). The ERG is usually polyphasic in vertebrates and generally consists of four main waves: a-, b-, c- and d- waves. The a-wave is electronegative and is displayed downwards by convention, whilst the b-, c-, and d- waves are electropositive (Babel *et al.*, 1977) (*Figure 17.1*). The a- and b-waves may be regarded as the principal components of the human response, not only because of their physiological significance but also because of their prominence under typical recording conditions used clinically (Armington, 1974). Artifactual responses caused by bright flashes of light, such as blinking, eye movements and changes in accommodation tend to occur at a similar latency as the c-wave of the ERG; therefore the c-wave of the clinical ERG is often difficult to analyse as the response may be contaminated by baseline drift (Armington, 1974). Similarly standard clinical ERG recording procedures do not elicit ERG d-waves in man, however if a relatively long stimulus is used then a late positive potential may be produced.

Microelectrode recording and a study of the timing of the a-wave indicates that it arises from the inner segments of the receptors (Tomita, 1984). There is still some contention as to the intraretinal origins of the b-wave, the Müller cells have been selected as the most probable source as they always respond with a depolarization which closely matches the waveform of the ERG b-wave. However, the mechanism by which the signal is generated is often debated. The increase in potassium concentration in the subretinal space, caused by light-evoked changes, results in the generation of a slow positive potential due to the extracellular current flow. This wave is thought to be the main contributor to the ERG c-wave. Brown and Wiesel (1961) attribute the d-wave to the cessation of the d.c. component described by Granit (1933) – a phase of negativity that comes on immediately with the light stimulus and is maintained at a constant level while the stimulus is present and then falls off as the stimulus is removed.

The state of adaptation of the eye can have a profound effect on the ERG (*Figure 17.2*). In the light-adapted condition, an ERG can be evoked by a moderately bright light and the resultant response is very small and fast. After 4–6 minutes of dark adaptation, the ERG waveform widens and increases in amplitude; after 12–14

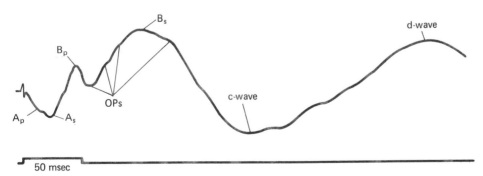

Figure 17.1. The flash electroretinogram. A_p, photopic a-wave; A_s, scotopic a-wave; B_p, photopic b-wave; B_s, scotopic b-wave; OPs, oscillatory potentials. (Modified from Babel *et al.*, 1977)

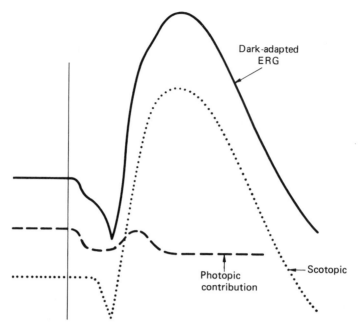

Figure 17.2. The photopic and scotopic contributions to the flash ERG. (After Armington, 1974)

minutes of dark- adaptation, the b-wave amplitude begins to reach a plateau (Ikeda, 1987).

The amplitude of the ERG is known to vary with the intensity of the stimulus and the level of visual excitation is logarithmically proportional to the intensity of the stimulus. In normal subjects, the b-wave should be two to three times the size of the a-wave and this is thought to reflect the phenomenal amount of neural facilitation or convergence that takes place in the mid-layers of the retina, thus producing a considerable gain of potential between the photoreceptors and the generators of the b-wave.

The temporal resolution of the retina can be assessed by using flicker electro-retinography, the critical fusion frequency (CFF) is defined as the slowest rate at which a stimulus can be flashed on and off and not elicit a discrete response from each flash. In adults, a bipartite stimulus–response curve is obtained by plotting CFF against stimulus intensity. At low stimulus intensities, the CFF is relatively low and is thought to represent predominantly rod activity, the CFF increases with stimulus intensity and at frequencies above 20 Hz, the rods are too slow to respond and therefore this part of the curve represents predominantly cone function (Dodt and Wadensten, 1954).

The neonatal flash ERG

The first ERG from a newborn full-term infant was recorded by Zetterström in 1951 using a contact lens electrode, and then in 1955 she repeated the same procedure on preterm infants. These and subsequent studies (Horsten and Winkelmann, 1962; Fulton and Hansen, 1985) revealed that the threshold of the neonatal ERG

TABLE 17.1. Summary of infant flash ERG data

Study	No. & age	Dilated?	Dark adapt.	Flash rate	Intensity	Colour	No. of avs.	a-wave amp.	Lat. b-wave	Amp. b-wave
Zetterström (1951)	35 infants 0–1 year	Yes	—	—	20, 80, 1600 lx	White	None	Present by 1 year	60 ms to start b-wave @ birth	100–200 µV by 3 months
Heck and Zetterström (1958)	15 infants 14 hours–3.5 months	?	?	1 Hz	700 lx	White	None	Present by 2 months	75 ms @ aet. 14 hours	?
Horsten and Winkelmann (1962)	7 infants Newborn	Yes	15 min	—	1.5, 6, 25, 60 lx @ 25 cm	White	None	a + b = 40–140 µV	50 msec	200–300 µV
Shipley and Anton (1964)	10 infants 1 day	Yes 3–5 mm	1 hour	2 min	650,000 lx @ 6 in	White	None	Mean = 32 µV	—	a + b = 91 µV
Barnet et al. (1965)	12 infants 6 hours–5 days	Yes	15 min	3 Hz	Various	White	n = 250	Present at birth	96 msec	22 µV
Algvere and Zetterström (1967)	15 infants 10–96 hours	Yes	5 min	1 min	33 000 lx	White	None	40–110 µV (delayed lat.)	—	10–70µV
Lodge et al. (1969)	12 infants 13–38 hours	Yes	15 min	0.4 Hz	Various	Blue/white	n = 50	Delayed lat.	Delayed lat.	Mean = 21.2µV Range 6–56 µV
Fulton and Hansen (1985)	23 infants 2–12 months	Yes	30 min	0.2 Hz	Various	Blue (<510 nm)	n = 16	Delated lat. Small amp.	Delayed lat.	Reduced amp.

(particularly the a-wave) is relatively high and ERGs can only be successfully recorded if high intensity light is used.

This initial pioneering work led the way for other authors to study the neonatal ERG (Heck and Zetterström, 1958; Francois and DeRouck, 1964; Shipley and Anton, 1964; Barnet, Lodge and Armington, 1965; Algvere and Zetterström, 1967; Lodge *et al.*, 1969; Ricci *et al.*, 1984; Mactier *et al.*, 1988). Despite the suggestion by Shipley and Anton (1964) that standardization of recording techniques would increase the clinical validity of ERG recording in this group of patients, different workers tended to adhere to their chosen parameters. The results of these studies are summarized in *Table 17.1*.

As discussed earlier in this chapter, the morphology of the ERG is known to change with different recording conditions and stimulus intensities. Some workers have reported the neonatal ERG to be rounded in form, with a slow-starting, slow-rising b-wave of long duration, whereas others have found there to be no difference in shape from that of the adult ERG; further confusion arises as Shipley and Anton (1964) reported both types of ERGs were recordable with the same recording conditions from infants of the same age. If the infant is not dark adapted or if insufficiently bright light is used then it is possible that the ERG a-wave will not be elicited (Horsten and Winkelmann, 1962; Grose *et al.*, 1989). Despite these difficulties, Ricci *et al.* (1984) and Mactier *et al.* (1988) have found it possible to record ERG a-waves from infants as young as 29 and 31 weeks gestation respectively.

It is generally agreed that the amplitude of the neonatal ERG is considerably smaller than that of the adult; the absolute values vary with the degree of dark adaptation and stimulus intensity (Shipley and Anton, 1964) (see *Table 17.1* for individual results). The latency of the neonatal ERG has been shown to be longer than in adults, again absolute values vary according to different recording conditions (*Table 17.1*).

If orange light is used for ERG recording a positive x-wave can be recorded, this occurs between the peaks of the ERG a-wave and b-wave. This wave has been shown to be present in full-term neonates, but it has a longer latency than that found in adults (Barnet, Lodge and Armington, 1965; Lodge *et al.*, 1969).

Initial reports suggested an absence of the flicker ERG at birth, due to contamination of the signal by noise, but Heck and Zetterström (1958) subsequently proved successful in recording flicker ERGs in full-term infants soon after birth. The ERG showed slow monophasic flicker waves (of the same type as seen in the so-called scotopic flicker response). In the first few days of life, the CFF at 700 lux was found to be 20 Hz, and this increased to reach adult values by 2 months of age, however the CFF at lower intensities was still below adult levels. Using selective amplification, Horsten and Winkelmann (1962) recorded flicker ERGs from a group of 15 newborn infants (including three preterm infants). A bi-partite graph of CFF was found for a range of stimulus intensities and from this it appeared that both scotopic and photopic systems contributed to the neonatal ERG response (Dodt and Wadensten, 1954). In contrast to previous workers, Horsten and Winkelmann found no significant difference between the CFF of newborn infants and adults.

Maturation of the flash ERG

Several workers have demonstrated that the human ERG undergoes developmental changes during infancy, this has been shown for photopic responses (Barnet, Lodge and Armington, 1965) and responses that were probably largely rod mediated

(Zetterström, 1951; Horsten and Winkelmann, 1962). These studies show there to be a progressive decrease in b-wave latency and increase in amplitude as the infant grows older. During the preterm period as the infant develops, a dramatic change is seen in the maturation of the ERG b-wave (*Figure 17.3*), whereas the changes in the a-wave are relatively minor (Ricci *et al.*, 1984; Mactier *et al.*, 1988; Grose *et al.*, 1989). It appears that the b-wave does not reach maturity until the age of 1 year. Sensitivity reaches adult values by about 6 months of age, while the latency and amplitudes of the dark-adapted ERG b-wave do not reach adult values until 1 year of age (Fulton and Hansen, 1985). Similar studies on the development of b-wave sensitivity following adaptation to steady background lights have shown that

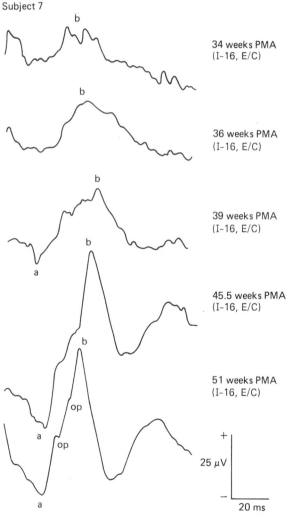

Subject 7

34 weeks PMA
(I-16, E/C)

36 weeks PMA
(I-16, E/C)

39 weeks PMA
(I-16, E/C)

45.5 weeks PMA
(I-16, E/C)

51 weeks PMA
(I-16, E/C)

25 µV

20 ms

Figure 17.3. The maturation of the flash ERG in one preterm infant between 34 and 51 weeks postmenstrual age. I-16, flash intensity 16, Grass PS22 stroboscope; E/C, eyes closed. Oscillatory potentials (ops) are first present at 45.5 postmenstrual age. (After Grose, 1989)

increasing the intensity of the background illumination has a lesser effect on the sensitivity of the ERG in infants than it does in adults.

In rats, it has been shown that the sensitivity of the b-wave is proportional to the amount of rhodopsin present in the retinal rods; however in view of the vast increase in sensitivity seen in the human infant it is unlikely that the same principle is true in man. Studies on the recovery of the b-wave after exposure to bleaching lights have revealed (both in man and in rats) that the kinetics of rhodopsin regeneration and recovery of sensitivity are identical for both adult and infants. Fulton (1988) has therefore postulated that the postnatal development of human scotopic function is due to a reorganization of processes central to the photoreceptors.

Francois and DeRouck (1964) showed that by modifying stimulus intensity it was possible to obtain ERG recordings that showed progressive changes in waveforms in infants as young as 1 month of age. The ERG responses ranged from a very small scotopic b-wave response to a maximum intensity response (reflecting both photopic and scotopic contributions) consisting of a very large a-wave, b_1 and b_2-waves and a late positive deflection. A bi-partite function of total b-wave amplitude against a-wave amplitude was found in both adults and infants (*Figure 17.4*). The horizontal part of the graph represents mainly scotopic function and photopic function predominates in the vertical part of the graph. During the first few months of life, the two portions of the graph are not as well defined as in the adult.

Pattern ERG in infants

More recently, the pattern ERG (PERG) has been used to provide a measure of visual acuity in infants. Fiorentini, Pirchio and Sardini (1984) used a skin electrode placed on the lower lid to record steady-state pattern ERGs from nine full-term infants aged between 7 weeks and 6 months. The highest resolvable spatial frequency (ERG acuity) was estimated by extrapolating the response amplitude against log spatial frequency function to noise level. This method is comparable to that described for estimating VEP acuity from amplitude versus spatial frequency functions (see Extrapolation from amplitude versus spatial frequency functions below).

In adults, PERG acuity estimated by this technique was found to be only about 0.1 log units lower than the VEP and psychophysical acuity. As it is only feasible to test relatively few spatial frequencies in young infants, the accuracy of the ERG acuity is not as great as in adults and lies in the region of ±0.25 octave. Despite some intersubject variability, the infant ERG acuities showed a rapid improvement with age, ranging from 2 c.p.d. at 7 weeks to 12 c.p.d. at 6 months. The steady-state ERG is thought to reflect ganglion cell activity (probably of the X-type), thus the improvement seen in PERG acuity may reflect both the anatomical maturation of the fovea and a functional maturation of the retinal receptive fields.

Practicalities of recording the flash ERG in infants and children

Choice of electrode

Conventionally, contact lens electrodes have been used for ERG recording, in general these are not well tolerated by infants and children and so a new generation of ERG electrodes have become increasingly popular in paediatric work. Although the contact lens electrode yields the largest ERG signal, its use requires corneal anaesthesia, vision is impaired when the electrode is in situ and there is some risk of

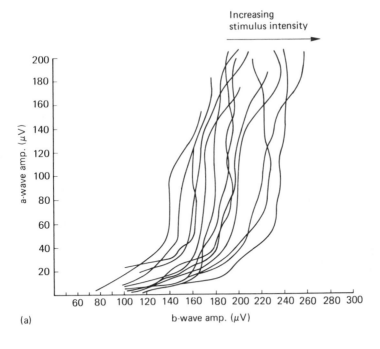

(a)

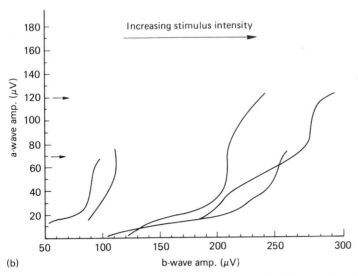

(b)

Figure 17.4. The scotopic and photopic contributions to the flash ERG in adults (a) and infants (b) between 1 and 3 months. (Modified from Francois and De Rouck, 1964)

corneal abrasion. Skin electrodes (Harden, 1974), gold foil electrodes (G.E. Holder, 1989, personal communication) and conductive thread or DTL electrodes (Dawson, Trick and Litzkow, 1979) have all been successfully used for ERG recording in children.

The skin electrode placed on the bridge of the nose is probably best tolerated, but the risk of contamination of the signal by the ERG from the other eye is very real. The use of skin electrodes under each eye tends to avoid this problem, however the response measured with a non-corneal electrode tends to be small (about one-fifth of the amplitude of the response measured with a gold foil electrode).

The conductive thread electrode is relatively easy to insert into the eye and has been used to record the ERG even in very low birth weight preterm infants (Ricci et al., 1984; Mactier et al., 1988; Grose et al., 1989). As the conductive thread electrode is in contact with the lower limbus of the eye the ERG signal elicited is considerably larger than that measured with a skin electrode (this is particularly important in tiny babies where the ERG signal is already of low amplitude and further attenuation is undesirable).

The gold foil electrode also gives a large amplitude signal and this is placed on the palpebral conjunctiva and loops over the lower lid so that it stands slightly proud. As with the conductive thread electrode, the signal to noise ratio is good but its major limitation is that its use is limited in young infants where the lower fornix is fairly shallow, in general this electrode is not used in children below the age of 6 years.

Stimulus

By choosing recording parameters that selectively stimulate one photoreceptor system or the other, it is possible to look at ERGs that predominantly reflect either rod or cone activity. Rods are particularly sensitive to blue light and are predominantly active in dark-adapted conditions with relatively low intensity stimuli. Under light-adapted conditions, stimulation with deep red or very bright light will predominantly stimulate the retinal cones. As the responses of the rods are relatively slow and cannot follow rapid stimulation (20–30 Hz), flicker electro-retinography can be used to assess cone function.

One of the most common problems with ERG recording in children is that they often close their eyes during recording. Eyelid closure is known to result in a reduction of retinal lumination (Hobley and Harding, 1988) and also serves as a red filter. It is well known that the amplitude of the ERG varies as a function of stimulus intensity, therefore it is not surprising that if the child closes his eyes during recording the latency of the response will increase and its amplitude will diminish. Therefore, careful monitoring of eyelid position during ERG recording is to be recommended.

Averaging and filtering of the ERG signal

The ERG is an example of a non-periodic or transient signal, it has a power spectrum that is distributed over a wide range of frequencies with characteristic peaks at particular frequencies. The use of an appropriate bandpass helps to lessen the effects of biological noise and interference which may contaminate the response. The main frequencies of the ERG a- and b-waves are between 21 and 50 Hz (Breslin and Parker, 1973) and therefore the use of a low pass filter helps to eliminate artifacts produced by high frequency muscle activity without any attentuation of these ERG components, a bandpass of 1–200 Hz is commonly used. It should be noted that this is not optimal for oscillatory potential (*Figure 17.1*) recording where a high-cut filter of 1000 Hz is recommended (Speros and Price, 1981), however if the high-cut filter is maintained at a high level and the infant displays a lot of eye movement the trace tends to become very noisy which may make identification of the ERG signal difficult. The principle of averaging to enhance eletrophysiological signals has been mentioned earlier (more explanation is provided below in the section on 'visual evoked potenials'); in recording photopic ERGs in preterm infants 30 averages were found to be adequate but if the recording is particularly noisy larger numbers of sweeps need to be averaged.

Visual evoked potentials

The VEP is essentially a tiny signal (10 μV on average) which has to be extracted from the EEG, this is done by averaging the response. The principle of averaging is dependent upon the VEP being time-locked to the stimulus – the time taken for the visual cortex to respond to a given stimulus is constant, thus if the stimulus is presented repeatedly and the signal is averaged, the stimulus-specific VEP becomes increasingly clear. Theoretically if summation occurs over an infinite number of presentations and the noise is totally random then the EEG will cancel out to zero. In practice, the background noise is reduced in proportion to the square root of the number of responses being summed. In addition to the use of averaging, the VEP signal is further enhanced by the use of filters (specifically chosen to cut out mains interference and/or biological noise) and amplification of the signal.

Despite widespread experimental and clinical studies, comparatively little is known about the relationship between scalp recorded VEPs and the underlying neural processes that generate them, however, the VEP still has many clinical applications in both ophthalmology and neurology.

In order to minimize inter-individual variation in VEP recording, electrodes are placed on the scalp according to the International 10/20 system which assumes that the position of the cortical areas is relatively fixed in relation to the surface land-marks of the skull (*Figure 17.5*). Thus for VEP recording, the potential difference is recorded between electrodes placed over the occipital area in reference to an area which is relatively 'electrically quiet' to visual stimulation, usually the frontal region.

Flash VEPs

The flash VEP is an invaluable tool in the assessment of visual function in young infants and children, as minimal cooperation is required during testing. The bright and spatially unstructured nature of the stimulus enables the assessment of visual function in children with poor visual acuity, or with media opacities and in situations where patients have their eyes closed. However, the flash VEP is relatively insensitive to refractive error, opaque media and demyelination and so it can only provide information relating to the luminance response and gross visual function.

There have been a number of different nomenclatures used for the identification of the components of the transient flash VEP. *Figure 17.6* shows that used by Harding (1974), a positive component is denoted by a downward deflection on the page. The complexity of the waveform varies with age, the P2 component is present in nearly all subjects and so this is the component used for clinical diagnosis. The incidence of the N1, P1 and N2 waves increases with age, but waves P3 and N4 are always variable in appearance (Wright *et al.*, 1985).

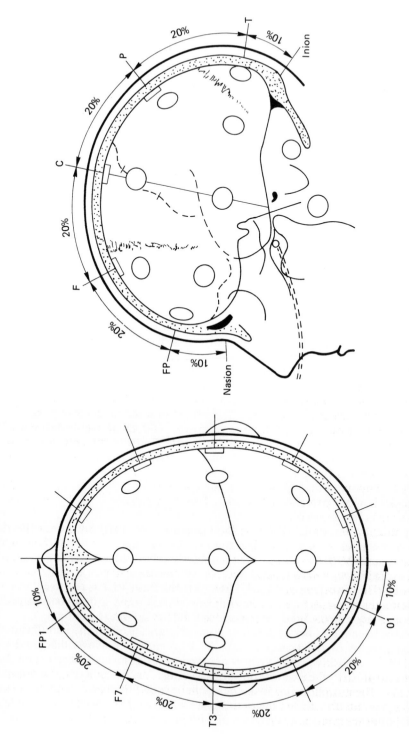

Figure 17.5. The International 10/20 electrode placement system. The nasion to inion distance and circumference of the patient's head are measured and electrodes are placed according to the diagram. (Modified from Jasper, 1958)

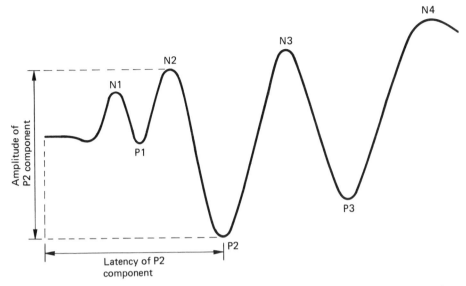

Figure 17.6. The waveform of the adult flash VEP. Components named using the nomenclature of Harding (1974)

Maturation of the flash VEP

Most authors have reported that the most striking postnatal maturational changes in the flash VEP occur in the first few months of life (Ferriss *et al.*, 1967; Dustman and Beck, 1969; Barnet *et al.*, 1980; Blom, Barth and Visser, 1980).

In the preterm neonate, the VEP to flash stimulation is extremely simple in waveform and consists solely of a major negative wave (N3), as the infant grows older the complexity of the waveform develops with the P2 component emerging at an average age of 35 weeks gestation (*Figure 17.7*). Similarly, in the full-term infant, the N3 component is thought to dominate the response through the first month of life, the P2 component first appears as a notch at about 4 to 6 weeks of age and by 6 to 8 weeks is more prominent than N3. The P2 component rapidly shortens in latency as the infant grows older.

During infancy, the flash VEP waveform becomes increasingly complex (Ferriss *et al.*, 1967; Barnet *et al.*, 1980; Harden, 1982). The majority of authors have suggested that the VEP waveform is not adult like in morphology until 2 to 4 months of age. During infancy and childhood, there is a decrease in latency of all components of the flash VEP (Dustman and Beck, 1969; Barnet *et al.*, 1980), the earlier waves reach adult latency values by 3 to 4 years of age, whereas the later waves continue to decrease in latency throughout childhood (Blom, Barth and Visser, 1980).

Pattern VEPs

Unlike the flash VEP, the pattern VEP gives information regarding form vision and visual acuity. The morphology and latency of the pattern VEP varies with the mode of stimulus presentation, the nature of stimulus used, and the spatial frequency of the stimulus. There are three basic modes of pattern presentation, pattern onset, pattern

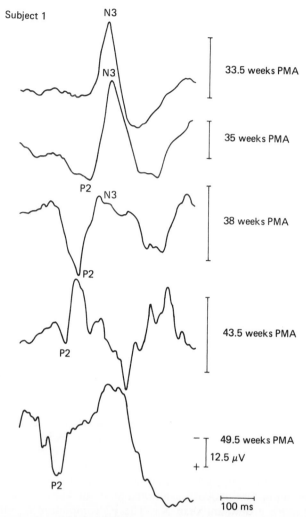

Figure 17.7. The maturation of the flash VEP in one preterm infant between 33.5 and 49.5 weeks postmenstrual age (PMA). (After Grose, 1989)

reversal and flashed-on pattern. Recently Orel-Bixler and Norcia (1987) demonstrated that VEPs in response to difference types of stimulus may show differential rates of development and so direct comparisons between studies are rather difficult.

Maturation of the pattern VEP

The maturation of the pattern VEP is also characterized by an increase in the waveform complexity and a shortening in the latency of its components. It is necessary to use relatively large checks in order to successfully elicit VEP responses from neonates; Porciatti, Vizzoni and Von Berger (1982) found that it was possible to record a reduced amplitude pattern reversal VEP from a full-term newborn infant in response to checks of 30′ of arc. By 1 month of age, pattern reversal VEPs can still only be elicited with checksizes of 30' of arc or larger and the first measurable VEP for 15' of arc checks does not appear until 8–10 weeks (Sokol and Jones, 1979; Moskowitz and Sokol, 1983). By 14 weeks it is possible to record responses to check sizes of 7.5' of arc (Sokol and Jones, 1979). In general, it has been shown that as an infant grows older, progressively smaller checks give the largest VEPs, although the overall change in amplitude with checksize is somewhat smaller for infants than for adults (Harter, Deaton and Odom, 1977).

Pattern reversal VEP

In adults, it is well established that the pattern reversal response is a tri-phasic waveform with a positive component at 100 ms (P1) as its most dominant feature.

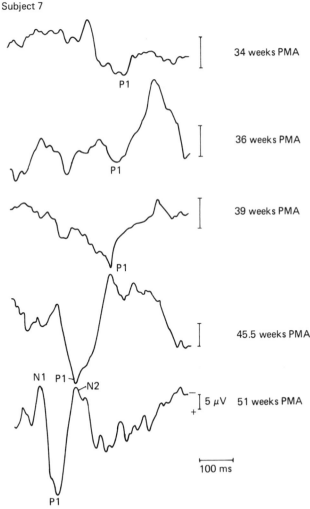

Figure 17.8. The maturation of the pattern reversal VEP in one preterm infant between 34 and 51 weeks postmenstrual age (PMA). (After Grose, 1989)

Grose *et al.* (1989) have shown that in preterm infants, the pattern reversal VEP initially consists of a rounded P1 wave of long latency and as the infant grows older the latency of the response shortens. The incidence of the N1 and N2 components are more common by about 8 weeks post-term (*Figure 17.8*). Similar effects were demonstrated by Sokol and Jones (1979) and Moskowitz and Sokol (1983) in full-term infants. By 3 months, the presence of a late positive wave has been noted in the infant VEP in response to large checks and by 9 months it is also present for small checks (Moskowitz and Sokol, 1983).

The pattern reversal VEP in infants shows a differential rate of development in relation to checksize (*Figure 17.9*). As for adults, the smallest checksizes gives the longest latency pattern reversal VEPs (Sokol and Jones, 1979). The latency of the

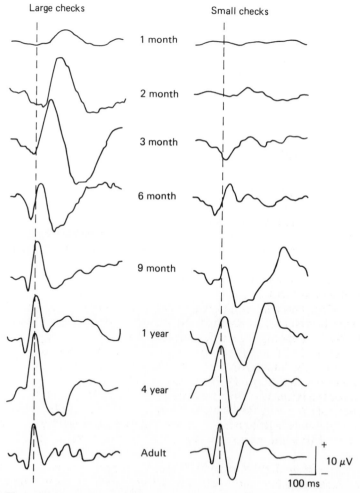

Figure 17.9. The maturation of the pattern reversal VEP to large and small checks, showing wave forms obtained from individual children, ranging from 1 month to 4 years and from an adult. Responses increase in complexity with age. The dashed lines show the latencies of the major positive component (P1) of the adult responses. (After Moskowitz and Sokol, 1983)

VEP in response to large check matures more quickly than for small checks (Moskowitz and Sokol, 1983). The P1 component to checks of 30' of arc (or larger) is thought to be adult-like in latency by 16 weeks of age (Sokol and Jones, 1979). A much slower change in latency has been reported for smaller checksizes. The latency of the P1 component for 15' of arc checks decreases rapidly until 1 year and then more gradually to 6 to 7 years of age, after which there is very little change. The latency of the P1 component for smaller (7.5' of arc) checks shows a steep decrease from birth to 4 years (Sokol and Jones, 1979) and then decreases more gradually to reach adult values by 13 years of age (Wenzel and Brandl, 1984). It has been suggested that the differences in maturation of the VEP in response to large and small checks may be a reflection of a differential development of the transient and substained cells in the visual system.

Moskowitz and Sokol (1983) investigated the maturation of the pattern reversal VEP in response to square wave gratings and checkerboard patterns, in infants aged between 1 and 7 months of age. For large pattern sizes (30–240' of arc) there was no difference in P1 latency between the two types of stimuli, but for patterns with small (7.5' and 15') elements the P1 latency was significantly longer for checks than it was for stripes. Fourier analysis shows that checks have a higher spatial frequency than stripes of equivalent widths and when the data was expressed in terms of fundamental frequency rather than check size there was no difference in the maturation of the two responses.

Pattern onset-offset VEP

In adults, the VEP to pattern onset-offset (or pattern appearance) contains two main complexes, the pattern onset response consists of a P-N-P complex, the components of which are generally referred to as CI, CII and CIII respectively. CI tends to reflect local luminance changes, CII is contour or edge specific and CIII is favoured by binocular conditions. In infant VEP recording, pattern presentations of up to 300 ms are necessary, in order to ensure that there is no contamination of the pattern onset waveform by the pattern offset response (DeVries Khoe and Spekreijse, 1982).

The morphology of the pattern onset response is very simple in infants, consisting only of a positive wave with a peak latency of 190 ms at 2 months of age (*Figure 17.10*) (Spekreijse, 1978). This configuration is similar to the response obtained from adult amblyopic eyes in which CII is absent or greatly reduced (Spekreijse, Khoe and Van der Tweel, 1972). Topological studies suggest that this peak may consist of two components, possibly CI and CIII (Apkarian, Reits and Spekreijse, 1984). As the infant grows older, the latency of this positive component reduces and reaches about 160 ms by 5 months. Spekreijse (1978) noted that although there is a decrease in the peak latency of the initial positive component, the implicit time of the beginning of the wave does not alter with age. It was suggested that the sluggish shape of the VEP may reflect a relatively high dispersion in conduction velocities, due to immaturities of myelination within the cortex and/or a lack of development of cortical inter-connectivity.

Despite the use of small (9' of arc) checksizes to enhance the appearance of the CII component, DeVries Khoe and Spekreijse (1982) found that it was impossible to record a CII component in infants of less than 10 months of age, by 20 months CII occurred in 40% of VEP recordings and its incidence increased to 100% by 100 months of age. As CII is thought to be a contour-specific phenomenon, its absence in early development was thought to indicate an immaturity of the foveal contrast

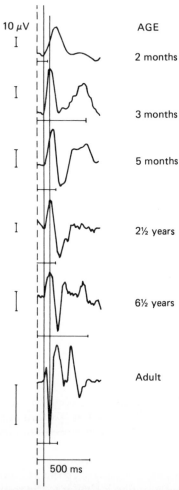

Figure 17.10. The maturation of the pattern onset/offset VEP. Responses are shown for the check size which gave the optimum response at each age. The pattern presentation duration is indicated by the line beneath each response. The onset latency of the VEP, indicated by the initial solid vertical line, does not appear to alter during development although the response waveform increases in complexity. The second solid vertical line shows the latency of the negative CII component of the adult response. (Modified from Spekreijse, 1978)

mechanism. Adult data shows that if a checksize is not resolvable then it is not just the CII wave that is affected but the whole VEP becomes unrecordable. It would seem reasonable to assume, therefore, that the CI-positive component is also related to visual resolution and so the VEP can be used to assess visual function even before the CII wave emerges (Spekreijse, 1983).

With increased age, the overall VEP response was seen to become sharper and smaller, with the original positive peak becoming less prominent and the negative CII more dominànt (DeVries Khoe and Spekreijse, 1982). The relative growth of the negative CII wave splits the initial positive component into two positive waves (CI and CIII) which attain adult-like latencies at around puberty.

Steady-state pattern VEPs and temporal tuning in infants

In the adult, the waveform of the pattern reversal VEP in response to a checkerboard stimulus becomes sinusoidal at about eight reversals per second (r.p.s.) and above. This response is known as the steady-state visual evoked potential and is analysed in terms of its amplitude and phase.

In young infants the pattern reversal VEP becomes sinusoidal at much lower temporal frequencies than in the adult (viz 4 r.p.s.) and the amplitude of the infant response diminishes at higher temporal frequencies and is no longer present at 16 r.p.s (Porciatti, 1984). Baraldi et al. (1981) found that in full-term neonates, the largest VEPs in response to 2° square wave gratings were recorded at reversal rates of 2.5 Hz (5 r.p.s.)

The slope of the phase characteristic of the fundamental harmonic of the steady-state VEP is known to be proportional to the latency of the transient response (Riemslag, Spekreijse and Van Walbeek, 1981). Porciatti (1984) showed that the slope of the phase characteristic in infants was much steeper than that found in adults (265 ms cf. 110 ms), which shows good agreement with the latencies of the transient response.

Moskowitz and Sokol (1980) found that temporal tuning of the pattern VEP in infants varied as a function of checksize. With large (48' of arc) checks, the amplitude of the VEP varies with reversal rate, the peak of this temporal tuning function shifts from 4 r.p.s. at 2 months to reach adult levels of 8–10 r.p.s. by 3–4 months. It has been suggested that this shift in the peak of the function reflects the development of the visual pathways carrying luminance information.

In infants older than 4 months of age, the temporal tuning function for small (24' and 12' of arc) checks is bimodal in form, with a low frequency peak at 4 r.p.s. and a high frequency peak at 10–12 r.p.s. The low temporal frequency peak (believed to reflect processing of high spatial frequency information) becomes more prominent with smaller checksizes and increased age, however even at 3 to 5 years of age, the peak of the function still occurs at 4 r.p.s. (compared to 6 r.p.s. in the adult). The prominence of the high temporal frequency peak (10–12 r.p.s.) in the response to small checks may have been enhanced by the use of a large field size (17° × 22°) (Regan, 1978).

Visual acuity estimation

The possibility of using electrophysiological techniques in the measurement of visual acuity was first envisaged following the findings of Campbell and Maffei (1970). They studied the relationship between steady-state VEPs and threshold contrast sensitivity, in adults, observing that VEP amplitude decreased linearly as the contrast of a reversing sine-wave grating was reduced logarithmically. Of particular note was their finding that, extrapolating this function to zero voltage indicated a contrast level very close to the subject's psychophysical threshold (*Figure 17.11*). Further studies confirmed the good correlation between VEP amplitude and pattern contrast, for a variety of recording conditions (Spekreijse and Van Der Tweel, 1974; Kulikowski, 1977). This work demonstrated that VEP recording could be adapted to enable objective determination of a subject's contrast sensitivity function (CSF). Visual acuity may then be found by extrapolation.

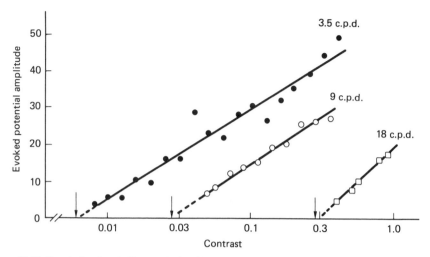

Figure 17.11. Graph showing the linear relationship between evoked potention amplitude (relative units) and pattern contrast (log units). Steady-state pattern reversal of sine-wave gratings (of three spatial frequencies) was used during recording. The arrows, indicating the psychophysical thresholds obtained at each frequency, correspond closely to the linear extrapolation of the functions to zero voltage. (Modified from Campbell and Maffei, 1970)

Extrapolation from the CSF

The CSF is a plot of contrast sensitivity against spatial frequency and provides a more comprehensive description of pattern detection than visual acuity. The peak of the contrast sensitivity curve represents the optimal spatial frequency for contrast detection. Visual acuity can be estimated by extrapolation of the high frequency portion of the CSF to zero – the cut-off point (Bodis-Wollner, 1980).

The pattern VEP has been used to assess the adult CSF. This is achieved by obtaining VEP recordings using patterns of various contrasts and spatial frequencies. As described above, the functions of VEP amplitude versus spatial frequency are extrapolated to zero voltage to produce estimates of contrast threshold for each spatial frequency (Campbell and Maffei, 1970). If desired, visual acuity can be estimated by extrapolation of the high spatial frequency portion of the resulting CSF to the 'cut-off point'. Theoretically this is the most accurate but unfortunately also the most lengthy method of predicting acuity from the VEP, particularly if transient recording is used. Consequently, steady-state or rapid sweep methods (see section on 'Rapid sweep method' below) are generally used to reduce recording time.

Despite the technical problems of obtaining sufficient data, this technique has been used by several workers to assess the development of contrast sensitivity in infants. Behavioural studies of the CSF show that maximum contrast sensitivity is 40–50 times lower than that of the adult for both stationary and moving targets (Banks and Salapatek, 1978), and this is supported by Atkinson, Braddick and French (1979) with VEP data. However, in general, VEP studies have indicated a substantially better sensitivity than behavioural studies (Pirchio *et al.*, 1978; Fiorentini, Pirchio and Spinelli, 1980; Norcia, Tyler and Hamer, 1988).

There is general agreement that an adult-like VEP CSF is attained by 6–10 months of age and sensitivity to low spatial frequencies matures much earlier than to high frequencies. VEP studies have indicated that maximum contrast sensitivity in infants is between twice (Norcia, Tyler and Hamer, 1988) to ten times (Pirchio *et al.*, 1978; Fiorentini, Pirchio and Spinelli, 1980) lower than that found in the adult. It is possible that the differences between these studies are due to the use of different recording parameters, as the shape and level of the CSF is affected by changes in luminance, temporal frequency of the stimulus and field size (Campbell and Maffei, 1970). Norcia, Tyler and Hamer (1988) attributed their relatively high contrast sensitivity findings to use use of high luminance gratings ($200 \, \text{cd/m}^2$) and the rapid method of sweep VEP recording.

In both adults and infants, Fiorentini, Pirchio and Spinelli (1980) found that scotopic VEPs were smaller in amplitude than photopic responses. In the adult, the peak of the photopic CSF occurs at higher spatial frequencies than the scotopic CSF. Even at 2 months of age, this difference in shape between the two functions is apparent, however the shift in the photopic function towards the higher spatial frequencies in infants younger than 4 months of age is not as marked as in the adult. By 5 months of age, the scotopic CSF is essentially adult in nature, however maximum photopic CSF values do not approach adult values until 6 months of age.

Extrapolation from amplitude versus spatial frequency functions

The transient pattern VEP in infants varies as a function of spatial frequency, in a similar way to the adult response – progressively smaller patterns give delayed VEPs and the amplitude is related to spatial frequency by an inverted 'U'-shaped tuning function. This function, which may be obtained in response to stimulation with high contrast patterns, has been demonstrated for various modes of pattern presentation in adults with the peak occurring at 10–20' of arc (*Figure 17.12*).

It has been suggested that the VEP amplitude against checksize function represents the spatial tuning of the neurones stimulated by the pattern. The peak of the function is thought to indicate the optimal size or spatial frequency of the receptive fields being activated whilst the two limbs of the graph represent the activation of two groups of neurones tuned to high and low spatial frequencies respectively. Generally it has been assumed that extrapolating the high spatial frequency 'limb' of the spatial tuning function to zero amplitude (or the VEP noise level on control trials) produces an intercept on the horizontal axis which coincides with subjective visual resolution. This assumption is based on the results of Campbell and Maffei (1970), who showed that near threshold VEP amplitude is proportional to log contrast, and of Campbell and Gubisch (1966), who demonstrated that log contrast sensitivity is linearly related to spatial frequency near the acuity limit. VEP amplitude should therefore fall off linearly with linear spatial frequency near the acuity limit.

A significant difficulty with the method is the lack of agreement on the most accurate combination of stimulation conditions and method of data analysis (either linear or curvilinear regression may be assumed and axes may be logarithmic or linear). One group have noted that such extrapolation methods produce correlations between VEP acuity and subjective acuity that are no better than a method employing an amplitude measurement of a single 5.5' arc check (Jenkins, Douthwaite and Peedle, 1985).

The main disadvantage of estimating visual acuity by extrapolation from the amplitude versus spatial frequency function is that as progressively smaller pattern

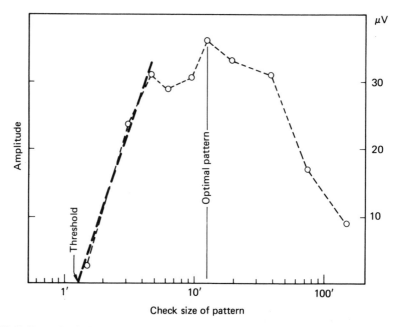

Figure 17.12. Example of a VEP amplitude versus spatial frequency function. In this case the data was derived from pattern onset VEP recording using stimulation with checks of 80% contrast. The peak of the function (optimum pattern) occurs at about 10' of arc. The bold dotted line illustrates the method of extrapolating the high spatial frequency portion of the function to zero voltage to provide an estimate of threshold, i.e. acuity. (Modified from Spekreijse, 1983)

elements are used, the area of cortex stimulated changes from a parafoveal to a foveal site. The cortical regions relating to the fovea are positioned more posteriorly than the parafovea and peripheral retina and this may result in waveform variations and even polarity reversal of the response (Spekreijse, 1978). Additionally, the slope of the amplitude versus checksize curve is dependent on the contrast level used (Campbell and Maffei, 1970) and this may account for some of the variability in visual acuity estimates between studies.

Despite the theoretical inadequacies described, the method has considerable advantages in terms of speed. For this reason it has been used in many infant studies, which have used both transient and steady-state VEP recording methods as described in the following sections.

Steady-state recording

Steady-state VEP recordings in response to checkerboards (Sokol and Dobson, 1976) and to sine wave gratings (Pirchio *et al.*, 1978; Fiorentini, Pirchio and Sandini, 1984; Norcia and Tyler, 1985a, b; Norcia *et al.*, 1987; Orel-Bixler and Norcia, 1987) have been used in conjunction with this technique to assess visual acuity in infants. In some studies the general method has been used in combination with the rapid sweep method of stimulus presentation and analysis (see section below).

Sokol and Dobson (1976) found that the absolute amplitude of the steady-state pattern reversal VEP increased up to the age of 5 months and then decreased; by

6 months the amplitudes of the infant VEPs were still larger than those of adults. The peak of the inverted 'V' shaped amplitude versus spatial frequency function was seen to shift from 30' to 15' of arc between 2 and 5 months of age. By 6 months of age, a similar distribution to the adult response was seen, between 7.5' and 15' of arc, this implies that visual acuity is probably adult like by 6 months of age. In a similar study, Sokol (1978) showed that VEP acuity improved from 6/45 at 2 months of age to 6/6 by 6 months of age.

Transient recording

In a number of studies the development of visual acuity in infants has been investigated by extrapolation from transient VEP amplitude versus spatial frequency plots. Data has been derived from various types of transient recording in infancy – pattern reversal, pattern onset (DeVries Khoe and Spekreijse, 1982; Orel-Bixler and Norcia, 1987) and flashed on pattern (Harter, Deaton and Odom, 1977).

From birth to 8 months of age, the amplitude versus checksize function to the pattern onset-offset VEP shifts along the x-axis, but retains the same shape. This is thought to reflect development in centres concerned with local luminance changes rather than spatial contrast (DeVries Khoe and Spekreijse, 1982; Spekreijse, 1983). Under 6 months of age, visual acuity (measured by extrapolating the amplitude versus checksize function to the x-axis) was found to correlate well with the checksize giving the maximum response.

By about 10 months of age, the peak of the amplitude versus checksize function reaches adult values and the shape of the function begins to alter as the slope of the graph gradually becomes less steep. By puberty, the intersection on the horizontal axis (visual acuity) approaches 1' of arc. This change in shape of the amplitude versus checksize function is thought to reflect the maturation of spatial contrast detectors. VEPs in response to small checksizes do not reach adult latencies until about 10 years of age (De Vries Khoe and Spekreijse, 1982).

Estimates from the pattern reversal VEP

The checksize giving the largest P1 component becomes progressively smaller during early infancy, decreasing from 240–60' of arc in the neonate (Porciatti, 1984) to 60–120' of arc in early infancy. Between 4 and 6 years of age, the optimal pattern lies somewhere between 15' and 35' of arc and there is very little change in the peak of the function after this (Wenzel and Brandl, 1984).

Direct location of threshold method

In the direct location of threshold method the eye is sequentially stimulated with high contrast patterns of successively finer detail to find the highest spatial frequency which gives a recognizable pattern VEP. The method has clinical advantages in terms of speed, but also some disadvantages. The major problem is that the endpoint may be difficult to define because of deterioration of the signal to noise ratio approaching threshold. A further disadvantage, from the point of view of testing infants, is that their interest in the stimulus may decline as the test progresses because the latter will become less compelling as threshold is reached.

Marg et al. (1976), however, used the method successfully in infants by finding the smallest grating size which gave a pattern onset-offset VEP signal which was clearly distinguishable from noise. They found that infant acuity improved rapidly from 6/180 to 6/30 between 4 and 8 weeks of age. The adult level of visual acuity (6/6) was found to be attained by 4 to 5 months of age. Porciatti (1984) found that in infants aged between 3 days and 1 month, it was possible to record a reduced amplitude pattern reversal VEP in response to checks subtending a visual angle of 30' of arc, but it was not possible to elicit a VEP to smaller check sizes (15' of arc), thus they assumed that the visual acuity of these infants must lie between these two values. This agrees well with the findings of Sokol and Jones (1979).

Rapid sweep method

The rapid sweep methods used in infant studies are modifications of a technique developed by Tyler and associates (1979). In the original method, sine wave or square wave gratings were counterphase modulated in contrast at a high temporal frequency and simultaneously swept in spatial frequency at a slow rate. A plotter displayed VEP amplitude versus spatial frequency of the alternating pattern, thereby enabling a rapid estimation of acuity by extrapolation from the function. Contrast sensitivity can be determined by a similar method in which steady-state contrast reversing sine wave gratings are simultaneously swept in contrast. Contrast thresholds are estimated by linear extrapolation of the resulting VEP amplitude versus logarithmic contrast function to zero amplitude.

Norcia et al. (1987) used a rapid sweep method of VEP recording to estimate and compare the visual acuity of a group of full-term infants (aged 4 to 40 weeks post-term) with that of preterm infants of the same postmenstrual ages. They found that VEP amplitude and spatial frequency plots showed narrowly tuned peaks at one or more frequencies. Acuity was estimated by linear extrapolation to zero amplitude of the highest spatial frequency peak in the function. There was no significant difference in the distribution of visual acuities found for preterm and full-term infants of the same chronological age, which would tend to suggest that sweep acuity develops from birth rather than from term. This was supported by the relationship found between visual acuity and postmenstrual age, which showed that the acuity of the preterm infants was slightly better than that of their full-term counterparts. However, the benefits of early birth were shown to be relatively small with an improvement of only 0.5 octaves for 9 weeks extra visual experience. In contrast, preterm twins were reported to have poorer visual acuity than full-term infants of the same chronological age.

Orel-Bixler and Norcia (1987) found that sweep steady-state VEP in response to pattern reversal sinusoidal gratings have an improvement of acuity of 0.28 octaves per month between the ages of 3 and 26 weeks of age.

The rapid sweep method of VEP recording to estimate visual acuity is particularly useful in infant studies, because of its speed of execution. Norcia and Tyler (1985b) have reported that it was possible to make as many as 12–20 acuity measurements in any one recording session. The reliability of the technique has been demonstrated in full-term infants between the ages of 17 and 25 weeks, at two temporal frequencies, 12 and 20 r.p.s. The s.d. for single 10-second trials averaged 0.27 octaves across the two temporal frequencies investigated. Repeated measures on the highest acuity at each temporal frequency gave a standard deviation of 0.19 octaves. The possible artifact of differential temporal tuning pointed out by Regan (1978) is apparently small over the 12–20 r.p.s. range, as it only accounts for 3% of the total variance and 14% of the within-subject variance.

Development of ERG and VEP acuity

Fiorentini, Pirchio and Sandini (1984) looked at the concomitant development of the steady-state pattern VEP acuity and pattern ERG acuity in response to sine wave gratings reversed in contrast at 12 r.p.s. VEP and PERG acuity were estimated by extrapolation of the amplitude of the second harmonic versus log spatial frequency and these were not significantly different in the first 6 months of life. ERG acuity was found to improve rapidly from 2 to 6 c.p.d. between 7 weeks and 3 months of age, after this there was a much slower improvement to 12 c.p.d. by 6 months of age. Pirchio *et al.* (1978) reported that VEP acuity of 20 c.p.d. (6/9) is attained by 1 year of age. See *Figure 8.5(a)*, for a summary of acuity development including data derived from an infant VEP study.

Binocular facilitation of the pattern VEP

In adults with normal binocular vision, the amplitude of the pattern VEP recorded during binocular viewing, is generally larger than that obtained during monocular viewing (Campbell and Maffei, 1970; Vaegan, Shorey and Kelsey, 1980). Summation of the responses is said to occur if the ratio of the amplitude of the binocular and monocular responses is between one and two, and facilitation is occurring if this ratio is greater than two. In exceptional circumstances inhibition may occur, in which case the binocular VEP is of smaller amplitude than the monocular VEP (Apkarian, Nakayama and Tyler, 1981).

The use of the steady-state pattern VEP has proved to be particularly useful in investigating the development of binocular vision in infants. In neonates, the amplitude of the binocular VEP does not exceed that of the monocular VEP, in fact the monocular VEP is often of greater amplitude (Penne *et al.*, 1987). However, by 2 months of age, binocular summation begins to be apparent and amplitude differences of up to 50% are measurable (Amigo *et al.*, 1978). From the second month of life, the amplitude of the binocular response increases and binocular facilitation occurs at about 4 months of age. By the end of the fifth month, the amplitude of the binocular response can be up to 191% larger than the monocular response. These findings are in agreement with studies which show that stereoscopically evoked VEPs are recordable in infancy between 10 and 19 weeks of age (Braddick *et al.*, 1980; Petrig *et al.*, 1981).

Practical considerations

Recording flash VEPs in children

In very young children the VEP can fatigue if the rate of stimulation is too rapid. Thus, in neonates, an interstimulus interval of 1–2 seconds is advisable and if the infant is premature then this should be extended.

Sixty-four responses are usually averaged in adult VEP recording, however, in infants and young children the signal to noise ratio of the flash VEP is relatively large and it may not be necessary to average such a large number of sweeps. It is important that the analysis time is sufficiently long for all relevant VEP components to be recorded (e.g. 500 ms).

Hobley and Harding (1988) have shown that in adults, eye closure during flash VEP recording results in a prolongation of the major P2 component of the VEP. This effect has not been studied systematically in young children, but Grose (1989) has been unable to find this effect in preterm infants up to the age of 12 weeks post-term. However, in older infants it is important to note whether or not the infant's eyes are open or closed during recording.

Reports on the effects of sleep state upon the VEP vary from author to author. Many say that the effects of sleep are relatively unimportant (Harden, 1982), whereas others have shown that if the infant falls asleep during recording the response becomes attenuated and these effects are particularly noticeable in quiet sleep (*Figure 7.13*), (Lodge *et al.*, 1969; Watanabe, Iwase and Hara, 1973; Whyte, Pearce and Taylor, 1987). Therefore, it is preferable (though not always practical) to record with the infant in the same state during follow-up appointments.

Subject J.B.
33 weeks PMA   Flash VEP (awake)

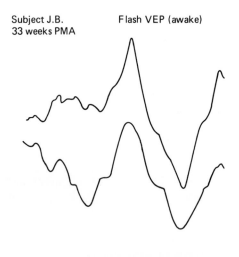

Flash VEP (quiet sleep)

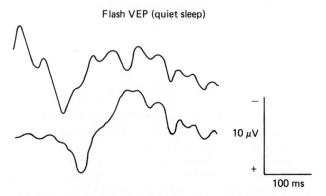

10 μV

100 ms

Figure 17.13. The effect of sleep on the flash VEP in one preterm infant of 33 weeks postmenstrual age (PMA). (After Grose, 1989)

Recording pattern VEPs in children

Obviously the main difficulty in recording pattern VEPs in children is that of fixation. There are several ways to deal with this. Originally, flashed-on patterns were used as stimuli as these were found to be particularly good in maintaining the child's attention. With the flashed-on pattern VEP (Harter, Deaton and Odom, 1977), the pattern VEP is contaminated by the luminance response. However, if the mean luminance of the pattern is maintained at a constant overall level, then the VEP represents a pattern-specific response. Constant luminous flux is maintained if a pattern reversal stimulus or a pattern onset-offset stimulus is used. There is some disagreement as to the most suitable mode of pattern presentation for infant VEP recording. In clinical situations, the pattern reversal response is often used, as in adults this has been shown to be less variable in terms of waveform and latency (particularly with regard to hemispherical asymmetries) than the pattern onset-offset response (Drasdo, 1980). Wright *et al.* (1985) also showed that pattern onset-offset responses are unreliable in young patients, as there are often difficulties in the interpretation of waveform. However, it has been suggested that the use of a brief pattern appearance stimulus followed by a relatively long period of pattern disappearance, is more effective as a visual stimulus in infants, as long periods of maintained accommodation are not necessary in order to record a response (Spekreijse, 1983). In older children attention may be maintained by using a cartoon superimposed onto the pattern.

Whichever method of VEP recording is used it is important to monitor fixation throughout, this can be done by observing the corneal reflection of the stimulus and ensuring that it is always centred over the pupil. It is essential that averaging is only

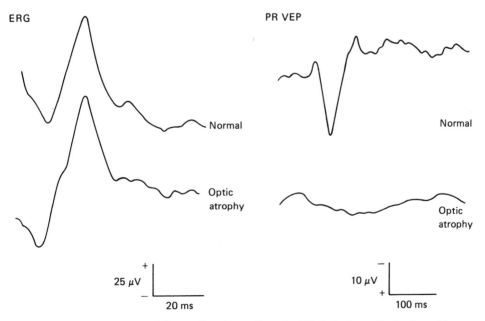

Figure 17.14. ERG and pattern VEP recordings from a 10-week-old baby having optic atrophy and from another normal infant of the same age. Comparisons of upper and lower traces shows that the ERG is unaffected but the pattern reversal VEP is absent in the infant with optic atrophy

carried out when the infant is fixating the target, the use of a foot-switch or similar device is particularly effective for interrupting the averaging process.

Clinical applications of the ERG and VEP in infants and children

In any clinical set-up normative data is available in order to establish whether the recorded ERG or VEP is within normal limits. It is important that this data is age matched as it is known that the ERG does not reach adult maturity until at least 1 year of age and the VEP continues to mature throughout childhood.

The VEP reflects the function of the visual system as a whole, however the retinotopic representation of the visual field changes dramatically at the visual cortex and the macula region is grossly magnified, therefore the VEP is dominated by macula function. In contrast, the ERG provides an areal measurement of retinal integrity, thus if 20% of the retina is damaged this will result in a 20% reduction in the amplitude of the ERG. The combined use of the ERG and VEP makes an ideal tool in the localization of lesions within the visual system.

All ERGs and VEPs should be recorded monocularly so that comparisons of amplitude and latency between the two eyes will establish whether one or both eyes are affected. Additionally, the VEP electrodes are positioned in such a way as to sample electrical activity from either hemisphere, thus the VEP can be used to establish whether or not a lesion is pre- or post-chiasmal. *Figures 17.14* and *17.15* show examples of how the combined use of the VEP and ERG can assist in the detection of abnormalities of the visual system in infants and children.

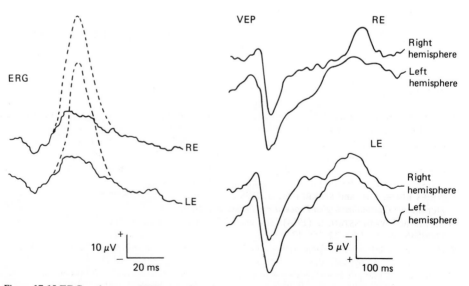

Figure 17.15. ERG and pattern VEP recordings in an 11-year-old boy with retinitis pigmentosa (visual acuities were R 6/9 and L 6/5). The pattern reversal VEPs to 28' of arc checks are within normal limits, but the ERGs are grossly reduced (dotted lines represent normal response shape)

References

ALGVERE, P. and ZETTERSTRÖM, B. (1967). Size and shape of the electroretinogram in newborn infants. *Acta Ophthalmologica,* **45**, 339–410.

AMIGO, G., FIORENTINI, A., PIRCHIO, M. and SPINELLI, D. (1978). Binocular vision tested with visual evoked potentials in children and infants. *Investigative Ophthalmology and Visual Science,* **17**, 910–915.

APKARIAN, P., NAKAYAMA, K. and TYLER, C.W. (1981). Binocularity in the human visual evoked potential (VEP): facilitation, summation and suppression. *Electroencephalography and Clinical Neurophysiology,* **51**, 32–48.

APKARIAN, P., REITS, D. and SPEKREIJSE, H. (1984). Component specificity in albino VEP asymmetry, maturation of the visual pathway anomaly. *Experimental Brain Research,* **53**, 285–294.

ARMINGTON, J.C. (1974). *The Electroretinogram.* Academic, New York.

ATKINSON, J., BRADDICK, O. and FRENCH, J. (1979). Contrast sensitivity of the human neonate measured by the visual evoked potential. *Investigative Ophthalmology and Visual Science,* **18**, 210–213.

BABEL, J., STANGOS, N., KOROL, S. and SPIRITUS, M. (1977). *Ocular Electrophysiology. A Clinical and Experimental Study of the Electroretinogram, Electro-oculogram and Visual Evoked Potential.* Georg Thieme, Stuttgart.

BANKS, M.S. and SALAPATEK, P. (1978). Acuity and contrast sensitivity in 1, 2 and 3 month old infants. *Investigative Ophthalmology Visual Science,* **17**, 361–365.

BARALDI, P., FERRARI, F., FONDA, S. and PENNE, A. (1981). Vision in the neonate (full-term and premature): preliminary results of the application of some testing methods. *Documenta Ophthalmologica,* **51**, 101–112.

BARNET, A.B., FRIEDMAN, S.L., WEISS, I.P. *et al.* (1980). VEP development in infancy and early childhood. A longitudinal study. *Electroencephalography and Clinical Neurophysiology,* **49**, 476–489.

BARNET, A.B., LODGE, A. and ARMINGTON, J.C. (1965). Electroretinogram in newborn human infants. *Science,* **148**, 651–654.

BLOM, J.L., BARTH, P.G. and VISSER, S.L. (1980). The visual evoked potential in the first six years of life. *Electroencephalography and Clinical Neurophysiology,* **48**, 395–405.

BODIS-WOLLNER, I. (1980). Detection of visual defects using the contrast sensitivity function. *International Ophthalmology Clinics,* **20**, 135–153.

BRADDICK, O., ATKINSON, J., JULESZ, B. *et al.* (1980). Cortical binocularity in infants. *Nature,* **288**, 363–365.

BRESLIN, C.W. and PARKER, J.A. (1973). Frequency analysis of the dark-adapted electroretinogram. *Canadian Journal of Ophthalmology,* **8**, 106–112.

BROWN, K.T. and WIESEL, T.N. (1961). Localisation of the origins of the electroretinogram components by intraretinal recording in the intact cat eye. *Journal of Physiology,* **158**, 257–280.

CAMPBELL, F.W. and GUBISCH, R.W. (1966). Optical quality of the human eye. *Journal of Physiology,* **186**, 558–578.

CAMPBELL, F.W. and MAFFEI, L. (1970). Electrophysiological evidence for the existence of orientation and size detectors in the human visual system. *Journal of Physiology,* **207**, 635–652.

CHIN, K.C., TAYLOR, M.J., MENZIES, R. and WHYTE, H. (1985). Development of visual evoked potential in neonates. A study using light emitting LED goggles. *Archives of Disease in Childhood,* **60**, 116–118.

DAWSON, W.W., TRICK, G.L. and LITZKOW, C.A. (1979). Improved electrode for electroretinography. *Investigative Ophthalmology and Visual Science,* **18**, 988–991.

DEVRIES KHOE, L.H. and SPEKREIJSE, H. (1982). Maturation of luminance and pattern EPs in man. *Documenta Ophthalmologica Proceedings Series,* **31**, 461–475.

DODT, E. and WADENSTEN, L. (1954). The use of flicker electroretinography in the human eye. *Acta Ophthalmologica Kbh,* **32**, 165–180.

DRASDO, N. (1980). Cortical potentials evoked by pattern presentation in the foveal region. In *Evoked Potentials,* edited by C. Barber. MTP Press, Lancaster, pp. 167–174.

DUSTMAN, R.E. and BECK, E.C. (1969). The effects of maturation and aging on the waveform of visually evoked potentials. *Electroencephalography and Clinical Neurophysiology,* **26**, 2–11.

FERRISS, G.S., DAVIS, G.D., DORSEN, M.M. and HACKETT, E.R. (1967). Changes in the latency and form of the photically induced average evoked response in human infants. *Electroencephalography and Clinical Neurophysiology,* **22**, 305–312.

FIORENTINI, A., PIRCHIO, M. and SPINELLI, D. (1980). Scotopic contrast sensitivity in infants evaluated by evoked potentials. *Investigative Ophthalmology and Visual Science,* **19**, 950–955.

FIORENTINI, A., PIRCHIO, M. and SANDINI, G. (1984). Development of retinal acuity in infants evaluated with pattern electroretinogram. *Human Neurobiology,* **3**, 93–95.

FRANCOIS, J. and DEROUCK, A. (1964). The electroretinogram in young children (single stimulus, twin flashes and intermittent stimulation). *Documenta Ophthalmologica,* **18**, 330–343.

FULTON, A.B. (1988). The development of scotopic visual function in human infants. Analysis of b-wave responses. *Documenta Ophthalmologica Proceedings Series,* **31**, 191–197.

FULTON, A.B. and HANSEN, F.M. (1985). Electroretinography: Application to clinical studies of infants. *Vision Research,* **27**, 697–704.

GRANIT, R. (1933). The comparison of the retinal action potential in mammals and their relation to the discharge of the optic nerve. *Journal of Physiology,* **77**, 207–239.

GROSE, J. (1989). The Development of the Visual System in Pre-term Infants as Assessed by Electro-physiological Techniques. Unpublished PhD thesis, University of Aston, Birmingham, UK.

GROSE, J., HARDING, G.F.A., WILTON, A.Y. and BISSENDEN, J.G. (1989). The maturation of the flash ERG and pattern reversal VEP in pre-term infants. *Clinical Vision Science,* **4**, 239–246.

HARDEN, A. (1974). Non-corneal electroretinogram. Parameters in normal children. *British Journal of Ophthalmology,* **58**, 811–816.

HARDEN, A. (1982). Maturation of the visual evoked potentials. In *Clinical Applications of Cerebral Evoked Potentials in Pediatric Medicine,* edited by G.A. Chiarenza and P. Papakostopoulos. Excerpta Medica, Amsterdam, pp. 41–59.

HARDING, G.F.A. (1974). The visual evoked response. *Advances in Ophthalmology,* **28**, 2–28.

HARDING, G. (1988). Neurophysiology of vision and its clinical application. In *Optometry,* edited by K.H. Edwards and R.D. Llewellyn. Butterworths, London, pp. 44–60.

HARTER, M.R., DEATON, F.K. and ODOM, J.V. (1977). Pattern visual evoked potentials in infants. In *Visual Evoked Potentials in Man: New Developments,* edited by J.E. Desmedt. Clarendon Press, Oxford, pp. 332–352.

HECK, J. and ZETTERSTRÖM, B. (1958). Analyse des photopischen flimmer elektroretinogramms bei neugeboren. *Ophthalmologica,* **135**, 205–210.

HOBLEY, A.J. and HARDING, G.F.A. (1988). The effect of eye closure on the flash visually evoked response. *Clinical Vision Science,* **3**, 273–278.

HORSTEN, G.P.M. and WINKELMANN, J.E. (1962). Electrical activity in the retina in relation to histological differentiation in infants born prematurely and at full-term. *Vision Research,* **2**, 269–276.

IKEDA, H. (1987). Retinal mechanisms and the clinical electroretinogram. In *A Textbook of Clinical Neurophysiology,* edited by A.M. Halliday, S.R. Butler and R. Paul. John Wiley, Chichester.

JASPER, H.H. (1958). Report of the committee on methods of clinical examinations in electro-encephalography. *Electroencephalography and Clinical Neurophysiology,* **10**, 370–375.

JENKINS, T.C.A., DOUTHWAITE, W.A. and PEEDLE, J.E. (1985). The VER as a predictor of normal visual acuity in the adult human eye. *Ophthalmic and Physiological Optics,* **5**, 441–449.

KULIKOWSKI, J. (1977). Visual evoked potentials as a measure of visibility. In *Visual Evoked Potentials in Man: New Developments,* edited by J.E. Desmedt. Clarendon Press, Oxford, pp. 168–183.

LODGE, A., ARMINGTON, J.C., BARNET, A.G. et al. (1969). Newborn infants' electroretinograms and evoked electroencephalographic responses to orange and white light. *Child Development,* **40**, 267–293.

MACTIER, H., DEXTER, J.D., HEWETT, J.E. et al. (1988). The electroretinogram in pre-term infants. *Journal of Pediatrics,* **113**, 607–612.

MARG, E., FREEMAN, D.N., PELTZMAN. P. and GOLDSTEIN, P.J. (1976). Visual acuity development in human infants: evoked potential measurements. *Investigative Ophthalmology and Visual Science,* **15**, 150–153.

MOSKOWITZ, A. and SOKOL, S. (1980). Spatial and temporal interaction of pattern evoked cortical potentials in human infants. *Vision Research,* **22**, 699–707.

MOSKOWITZ, A. and SOKOL, S. (1983). Developmental changes in the human visual system as reflected by the latency of the pattern reversal VEP. *Electroencephalography and Clinical Neurophysiology,* **56**, 1–15.

NORCIA, A.M. and TYLER, C.W. (1985a). Spatial frequency sweep VEP: visual acuity during the first year of life. *Vision Research,* **25**, 1399–1408.

NORCIA, A.M. and TYLER, C.W. (1985b). Infant VEP acuity measurements. Analysis of individual differences and measurement error. *Electroencephalography and Clinical Neurophysiology*, **61**, 259–369.

NORCIA, A.M., TYLER, C.W. and HAMER, R.D. (1988). High contrast sensitivity in the young infant. *Investigative Ophthalmology and Visual Science*, **29**, 44–49.

NORCIA, A.M., TYLER, C.W., PIECUCH, R. *et al.* (1987). Visual acuity development in normal and abnormal preterm human infants. *Journal of Pediatric Ophthalmology and Strabismus*, **24**, 70–74.

OREL-BIXLER, D.A. and NORCIA, A.M. (1987). Differential growth for steady-state pattern reversal and transient onset-offset VEPs. *Clinical Vision Science*, **2**, 1–10.

PENNE, A., BARALDI, P., FONDA, S. and FERRARI, F. (1987). Incremental binocular amplitude of the pattern reversal visual evoked potential during the first five months of life: electrophysiological evidence of the development of binocularity. *Documenta Ophthalmologica*, **65**, 15–23.

PETRIG, B., JULESZ, B., KROPFL, W. *et al.* (1981). Development of stereopsis and cortical binocularity in human infants: electrophysiological evidence. *Science*, **213**, 1402–1405.

PIRCHIO, M., SPINELLI, D., FIORENTINI, A. and MAFFEI, L. (1978). Infant contrast sensitivity evaluated by evoked potentials. *Brain Research*, **141**, 179–183.

PORCIATTI, V. (1984). Temporal and spatial properties of the pattern reversal VEPs in infants below two months of age. *Human Neurobiology*, **3**, 97–102.

PORCIATTI, V., VIZZONI, L. and VON BERGER, G.P. (1982). Neurological age determination by evoked potentials. In *Paediatric Ophthalmology*, edited by J. Francois and M. Maione. John Wiley, Chichester, pp. 345–348.

REGAN, D. (1978). Assessment of visual acuity by evoked potential recording: ambiguity caused by temporal dependence of spatial frequency selectivity. *Vision Research*, **18**, 439–443.

RICCI, B., FALSINI, B., VALENTINI, P. *et al.* (1984). L'ettroretinogramma fotopica nei prematura. *Annali di Ottalmologica a Clinica Oculista*, **110**, 771–780.

RIEMSLAG, F.C.C., SPEKREIJSE, H. and VAN WALBEEK, H. (1982). Pattern reversal and appearance disappearance responses in MS patients. *Documenta Ophthalmologica Proceedings Series*, **27**, 215–227.

SHIPLEY, T. and ANTON, M.T. (1964). The human electroretinogram in the first day of life. *Journal of Pediatrics*, **65**, 733–739.

SOKOL, S. (1978). Measurement of infant visual acuity from pattern reversal evoked potentials. *Vision Research*, **18**, 33–39.

SOKOL, S. and DOBSON, V. (1976). Pattern reversal visually evoked potentials in infants. *Investigative Ophthalmology and Visual Science*, **15**, 58–61.

SOKOL, S. and JONES, K. (1979). Implicit time of pattern evoked potentials in infants: an index of maturation of spatial vision. *Vision Research*, **19**, 747–755.

SPEKREIJSE, H. (1978). Maturation of contrast EPs and development of visual resolution. *Archives Italiennes de Biologie*, **116**, 358–369.

SPEKREIJSE, H. (1983). Comparison of acuity tests and pattern evoked potential criteria: two mechanisms underly acuity maturation in man. *Behavioural Brain Research*, **10**, 107–117.

SPEKREIJSE, H., KHOE, L.H. and VAN DER TWEEL, L.H. (1972). A case of amblyopia; electrophysiology and psychophysics of luminance and contrast. In *The Visual System: Neurophysiology, Biophysics and their Clinical Application*, edited by G.B. Arden. Plenum, New York, pp. 141–156.

SPEKREIJSE, H. and VAN DER TWEEL, L.H. (1974). Stimulus and visually evoked potential. *Documenta Ophthalmologica Proceedings Series*, **4**, 269–284.

SPEROS, P. and PRICE, J. (1981). Oscillatory potentials. History, techniques and potential uses in evaluation of disturbances of retinal circulation. *Survey of Ophthalmology*, **251**, 237–252.

TOMITA, T. (1984). Neurophysiology of the retina. In *Foundations of Sensory Science*, edited by W.W. Dawson, and J.M. Enoch. Springer-Verlag, Berlin, pp. 151–190.

TYLER, C.W., APKARIAN, P., LEVI, D.M. and NAKAYAMA, K. (1979). Rapid assessment of visual function: an electronic sweep technique for the pattern visual evoked potential. *Investigative Ophthalmology Visual Science*, **18**, 703–713.

VAEGAN, C.R., SHOREY, U. and KELSEY, J.H. (1980). Binocular interactions in the visual evoked potentials using a modified synoptophore. In *Evoked Potentials*, edited by C. Barber. MTP Press, Lancaster, pp. 219–285.

WATANABE, K., IWASE, K. and HARA, K. (1973). Visual evoked responses during sleep and wakefulness in preterm infants. *Electroencephalography and Clinical Neurophysiology,* **34**, 571–577.

WENZEL, D. and BRANDL, U. (1984). Maturation of pattern evoked potentials elicited by checkerboard reversal. *Developments in Ophthalmology,* **9**, 87–93.

WHYTE, H.E., PEARCE, J.M. and TAYLOR, M.J. (1987). Changes in the VEP in preterm neonates with arousal states as assessed by EEG monitoring. *Electroencephalography and Clinical Neurophysiology,* **68**, 223–225.

WRIGHT, C.E., WILLIAMS, D.E., DRASDO, N. and HARDING, G.F.A. (1985). The influence of age on the electroretinogram and visual evoked potential. *Documenta Ophthalmologica,* **59**, 365–384.

ZETTERSTRÖM, B. (1951). The electroretinogram in children in the first year of life. *Acta Ophthalmologica,* **30**, 405–408.

Further reading

CARR, R.E. and SIEGEL, I.M. (1982). *Visual Electrodiagnostic Testing – A Practical Guide for the Clinician.* Williams and Wilkins, Baltimore.

GALLOWAY, N. (1981). *Ophthalmic Electrodiagnosis,* 2nd edn. Lloyd and Luke, London.

HALLIDAY, A.M. (ed.) (1982). *Evoked Potentials in Clinical Testing.* Churchill Livingstone, Edinburgh.

18

Optometric needs of multiply handicapped children

John Muldoon and David Pickwell

Introduction

This chapter is concerned with the visual problems of children who have 'severe' or 'profound' learning difficulties and whose visual problems frequently have an enormous impact on their abilities in learning. Such children may be unfamiliar to many practising optometrists, and the purpose of this introductory section is to explain something of their needs and difficulties, and also to show the vital role which optometrists can play in promoting their development.

It is intended primarily to indicate what contribution can be made by the average optometrist. As with all optometric examination, there is a screening element which will be concerned with identifying those patients who may need further ocular or visual assessment either by additional tests or referral to another practitioner. Some optometrists have non-standard methods available which can be very useful in assessing young children or children who cannot cooperate because of their severe or profound difficulties. It is not however the purpose of this chapter to describe additional tests which are covered in other chapters. Children with severe or with profound learning difficulties comprise only a small proportion of all children, but as a group they may have a wide range of problems in which visual disorders often figure significantly. They are children who were previously described as severely or multiply handicapped, depending on the extent of their difficulties. They all suffer from having major disruptions in development (Ellis *et al.*, 1982; Sugden, 1989).

Profound learning difficulties

Children in this classification are the ones with the greatest problems. For example, some children with the most profound problems may have extreme physical impairments which prevent normal motor development and mobility. In many cases they have gross skeletal deformities and they frequently suffer sensory loss. Additionally, their mental capacities may not progress beyond the stage of very young infants (Sebba, 1988), and their power of communication may also be limited to preintentional/preverbal levels (Goldbart, 1986). As a result of these impairments, their interaction with the external world is severely limited which frequently leads to maladaptive patterns of self-stimulating and self-interacting behaviour (Sebba, 1988; Zarkowska and Clements, 1988). As these children grow older such behaviour patterns become more strongly entrenched. This together with their distorted experience of their external environment is likely to affect both their current and future ability for learning (Goldbart, 1986). Any severe visual problem is likely to exacerbate their inability to relate to the external world.

The purpose of the special education which is provided for children with profound learning difficulties of this nature, is to intervene with precise methods of assessment and teaching procedures in order to encourage their motor, cognitive and communication development. It is therefore clear that a knowledge of such a child's visual problems is a vital factor in this process.

Severe learning difficulties

Other children with severe rather than profound learning difficulties may not have such great disruptions to their development. However, compared with normally developing children, they will encounter tremendous problems in learning and retaining skills and information. With these children too a knowledge of their visual problems is essential in organizing their learning environment. For example, such children may be relatively mobile and able to carry out familiar simple tasks. They may also have a limited use of speech and the rudiments of skills for social interaction. To this extent their development is not impeded to the same extent as the children who have profound difficulties. However, it is apparent that they too will need intervention providing optimal conditions for learning. Information about their vision will be a central factor also.

Children who are assessed as having either profound or severe learning difficulties do not fall into two distinct groups, and indeed there is often a lack of consensus over definitions and cut-off points from one classification to another (Evans and Ware, 1987). In reality they represent one end of a continuum of learning difficulties. While the two groups of children are not homogeneous, they do share difficulties which have common causes in the broadest sense. For example, Sugden (1989) has argued that children with severe or with profound learning difficulties have great problems in selecting and attending to particular stimuli in their environment, and in retaining information in both short-term and long-term memory so that it can be absorbed into existing knowledge of the world. As a result of this disruption to information processing, there are massive implications for learning and there is now widespread recognition of the need for early intervention to compensate for such problems. For example, recent years have seen an expansion and coordination of paediatric services which aim to assess problems in infancy and provide for children with learning difficulties. One of these priorities is to identify any visual impairments which may be present. However, the long-term, and often deteriorating nature of profound or severe learning difficulties means that repeated assessment must also be part of the education process for the affected children. Information about the state of the children's vision will continue to be critical. This can often be where the optometrist can help.

Vision in the child's education

A knowledge of the child's visual problems will figure significantly in the planning of teaching methods which are adopted in the special education of children with learning difficulties. Such methods are concerned with analysing skills and tasks into component parts at a level which is manageable for a particular child. For example, teaching the child to feed him/herself will be broken down into the skills of manual dexterity and coordination needed for the task of handling food and cutlery, and the motor skills needed for biting, chewing and swallowing food. For children who have visual problems as part of their profound or severe difficulties, learning at even this elementary level will present great challenges. Parents and teachers will need to know how to orientate the child to the learning task most effectively. They will need to know how best to present objects and information in such a way as will make optimum use of whatever sight may be available to the child. For example, the type and positioning of the lighting may be critical.

Advisory teachers for children with visual problems are a valuable source available to parents and other teachers, but specific information about acuity or a child's visual field is clearly indispensible. This could very well be provided by the optometrist.

Case examples

The following case studies will serve to illustrate the nature of severe or profound learning difficulties, and the contribution which optometrists can make in providing information to help the development and learning of such children.

Case I

Alan is 12 years old and he has profound learning difficulties. He is severely brain damaged and, consequently, suffers from a form of cerebral palsy which stiffens his body trunk and holds his limbs in a rigid flexed position. These physical impairments inhibit the control of his movements very greatly. His interaction with his environment is very much reduced. Alan has no speech and seems to have a negligible understanding of language, although he does become excited at the sound of his mother's voice.

He is very easily upset by even moderate noise levels around him and often by being touched. These reactions frequently lead to bouts of crying which his parents and teachers find difficult to resolve. It had been suspected that these responses were provoked very often because Alan was startled by events which he could not see. This suspicion was also supported by observations that he did not appear to inspect his surroundings visually.

Optometric examination confirmed that his vision had severely deteriorated since his original assessment to a point where not even a fixation reflex could be demonstrated. It was concluded that his parents and teachers could no longer assume that visual stimili would be useful. Regretfully this confirmed their suspicions.

As a result of the recognition of Alan's severe visual loss, his parents and teachers decided to investigate ways of interesting and motivating him through other sensory channels. This had interesting results. It was found that he liked the other sensation from a vibrating mattress which was used for other children's physiotherapy and also air turbulence on his face from a household fan. Once these preferences were identified, he was taught to operate microelectronic switches by moving his head and so produce these effects for himself. At a later stage he was taught to use the same switches to operate a tape recording of his mother's voice and also simple tunes that he seemed to enjoy. As a result, he spent more time engaged in relating to external stimuli by operation of the switch devices, and the ritualistic behaviours which had previously occupied much of his time became less frequent. Instead of spending long periods of time rocking his head from side to side or mouthing his hands, he became actively involved in his attempts to produce the external events he found pleasurable.

In this instance the information about the child's visual problems was clearly decisive in the choice of non-visual stimuli which were used on him. His parents and teachers were able to give their time to identifying other alternatives to the visual channel and he responded successfully. The information about his lack of vision also enabled his environment to be organized in such a way as to reduce the likelihood of startling and upsetting him. The cumulative effects of all the new strategies was a more settled child who now had the means to exercise a measure of control in producing pleasurable events on his own behalf.

Case II

Another case in which the benefits of information about a child's vision can be seen is Richard who is 7 years old with Down's syndrome. Richard has severe rather than profound learning difficulties and his problems are less extensive than Alan's. He can walk, but unsteadily and with poor balance. His visual–motor coordination is very clumsy. He also tends to hold objects very close to his eyes to inspect them which suggests the myopia often associated with Down's syndrome. Richard has no expressive speech and his understanding of language is limited to the context of familiar situations such as mealtimes, getting dressed, bathtime and so on. In unfamiliar settings it is difficult to communicate with him or to understand his own meanings and intentions. Like most children with severe learning difficulties, his attention span is short. He also tends to spend a lot of time rocking himself to and fro unless another person intervenes and diverts him away from this self-stimulating behaviour.

It was suspected that a pair of spectacles might widen Richard's visual horizons which in turn would increase his interest and interaction with his environment. However, when he was taken to a practitioner for eye examination, he became so upset by the very unfamiliar setting that he disrupted the procedure completely, and would not stay still for long enough to allow adequate examination. As a result of this abortive attempt, an optometrist arranged an examination in the more familiar situation of the school in the hope that this would be less stressful for him. This proved to be the case and he was found to be myopic as suspected. It took a great deal of time and persistence to persuade him to wear the spectacles. Once he began to tolerate them, improvements were reported in his coordination and attention to tasks generally.

In this case, the collaboration of professionals and the child's parents resulted in arrangements for visual examination which overcame the problems which were encountered initially and, as a result, problems were identified and provided for.

Case III

A third example of a child whose visual problems were assessed by such a multi-professional collaboration is that of Lynne who is 14 years old. Lynne has been identified as having brain damage but without a specific diagnosis. It has left her with flaccid movement on the right side of her body. Although she cannot speak, she has learned a small vocabulary of some 50 manual signs. However, her understanding of speech far outstrips her ability to express herself. She is able to carry out simple, routine tasks at home and at school without help. She also engages in imaginative play and attracts other people into these activities. To this extent her abilities are clearly far greater than the two children discussed above. It was suspected by her teachers that she too now had visual problems because her visual–motor coordination was very poor indeed and did not match her level of other abilities. Like other children with profound or severe learning difficulties, Lynne's inability to communicate sufficiently made it difficult to obtain information from her which would help to assess her vision.

Lynne's mother had reported that she looked at things 'out of the corner of her eye'. This behaviour was also noted at school. Additionally movements which needed coordination, such as stepping over an obstacle, were slow and clumsy. She also became very aggressive in such circumstances, which made it very difficult for her mother to take her into public places. Again it was suspected that many of her behaviour problems stemmed from a visual problem.

The optometrist found that she had a right eye squint with poor acuity. There was also severe ocular motor restriction so that she was unable to move either eye to the right and had a limitation on downward movement. This accounted for the movement of the head to a position where the face was turned to the left and downwards. It was explained to the parents and teachers that being unable to move her eyes in that direction she had to move her head to the compensatory head posture. This was the appearance that had been described as 'looking out of the corner of her eye'.

Once Lynne's parents and teachers were aware of the limitations in her ocular motor field, they were then able to orientate her in a more appropriate manner in order to make optimum use of vision. For example, she was helped to walk sideways down steps or around obstacles, and she was given time to orientate herself before taking each step. Eventually she was taught to use these strategies herself in negotiating her way around home and school with some success. Similarly, it was possible to place mealtime apparatus and equipment more precisely than before. Previously her teachers had attempted to position items at her side, but with no precise knowledge of the optimum location of her vision. The information that she had better sight in the left eye and to the left of her motor field helped with the placement of all objects.

The three children presented in the preceding case studies show a range of very different abilities and learning difficulties, but to some extent they can also be seen to show common problems. Ashman and Conway (1989) have found that, to different degrees, such children all have difficulty in separating relevant cues from irrelevant aspects of the environment. This disrupts information processing and their ability to organize their problem-solving responses to the situation they encounter.

More specifically, Kiernan, Reid and Jones (1982) have pointed out massive interference in the most elementary abilities in communication of children with profound or severe learning difficulties. For example, behaviours such as making eye contact, attending to and interpreting facial expressions and bodily gestures of other people do not develop normally. Frequently these children's own expressive acts do not develop either and this can have a very great impact on the child's interaction with other people. This has a particularly damaging effect on parents who are unable to understand their child's needs or intentions (Beverage, 1989). Information about the child's visual problems which can help remedy some of these difficulties is of vital importance.

Although these children's ability to communicate is nearly always very poor, and it is therefore very difficult to assess their vision, their visual assessment is always worthwhile and sometimes very important. However the aim of education for these children is to help develop the full potential of the child, even if this is different and very restricted compared to other children (Figure 18.1). Obviously every child's development depends on his or her visual perception and its integration with other sensory input and motor abilities. Visual perception in its turn depends on having a clear image with a full field and all the other attributes of vision. Children with profound or severe learning difficulties need as much optometric care as other children to ensure that any refractive error is corrected if this will give clearer vision or help the coordination of the two eyes. This is sometimes provided incidental to the provision of ophthalmological assessment of the child.

Nevertheless, in many cases such children are neglected, as it is difficult to assess their optometric needs which may even be perceived as a small problem compared to their other very major disabilities. Sometimes the children themselves are also very disruptive in any clinic, as in the case of Richard (Case II above). Assessment of their vision and refractive state can require a lot of time and patience.

The task of teachers in special education is not helped if the child's vision is not as good as it could be for the want of a pair of spectacles. In general, there is a very high incidence of refractive error and squint with these children. This varies with the particular condition (see below), but it emphasizes the need for optometric examination, and for prescribing where it is obvious that spectacles would help the vision or the coordination of the two eyes. In some conditions the vision can deteriorate as the child gets older and this requires regular examination in the same way as with other children.

Visual disorders

There is a very high incidence of visual problems in children with other disabilities, particularly if their problems include mental abnormalities. Some estimates suggest that four out of five have some visual disability. Ellis (1986) has reported widely varying estimates of the incidence of visual problems in children with severe or profound learning difficulties, but a conservative figure suggests that it is ten times more common than in the general population.

Evans and Ware (1987) have listed approximately 70 conditions which are either genetically transmitted or the result of disease, and which often result in severe or profound learning difficulties. Twenty-five per cent of these conditions have severe visual disorders associated with them as specific characteristics, whilst others may also produce visual problems as a result of overall neurological dysfunction. Holland (1986) also found that this is true for many genetic disorders.

Some of the more common conditions associated with visual problems however vary considerably from child to child. Down's syndrome, hydrocephalus and, more notably, cerebral palsy (see below) include individuals with a great diversity of abilities and needs. For example, some cerebral-palsied children have above average intelligence while others fall into the range of those having learning difficulties discussed in this chapter. The impact of visual problems on the child's development and functioning will produce very different effects depending on the overall level of ability.

It can be seen that some eye problems are associated with particular general conditions. The more common conditions are listed below together with the eye problems likely to be present.

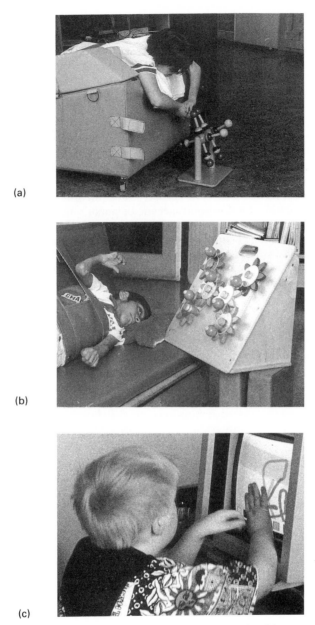

Figure 18.1. Development of vision responses (a) This pupil has been placed in a corrective prone lying position, with her head in midline and facing the apparatus provided for her. In this position her hands are free to develop hand-eye coordination. (b) This second pupil has been positioned lying correctly on his side. His body is well supported, and his left arm is free to develop voluntary control in visually directed reading. (c) In this illustration the pupil is attending visually to the effects which his hand movements are producing on a computer monitor touch screen.

Cerebral palsy

This is a general term to indicate an anatomical abnormality and malfunctioning of the brain which obviously can cause both mental and physical handicap. Patients usually show anomalies of movement. Most are classified as 'spastic', having muscular rigidity or spasm; some are 'dyskinetic', having restriction of voluntary movements; and a few show the jerky movements called ataxia. Sometimes these anomalies of movement are so serious that a sitting posture cannot be maintained without support. The sensory system may be equally affected so that there appears to be no means of communication with the patient. In others the problem is less serious in both motor and sensory functions. It appears that about 44% are 'visually normal' (Breakey, 1955). About 40% have convergent squint, which is sometimes accommodative in nature so that a spectacle correction may be appropriate. About 8% have divergent squint which is higher than in normals.

The anomalies of motor control described above can also apply to eye movements resulting in gaze palsies, or abnormal saccade or pursuit movements (Goble, 1984).

It has been known for a long time that many cerebral palsy patients have homonyous hemianopia (Freud and Spehlmann, 1953). It is now thought that about 25% have a significant field loss on the same side in both eyes (Tizard, Paine and Crothers, 1954). This clearly emphasizes the need for a confrontation or other field test so that parents and teachers can be alerted to this problem.

The incidence of high degrees of hyperopia is several times greater than in normal populations, and myopia is more frequent (Fantl, 1964). Depending on the age of the child, the hyperopia could be absolute for near vision which could restrict the useful vision unless a correction is provided. Difficulties in accommodation have also been reported (Gobler, 1984), which would make this problem worse.

Optic atrophy, cataract and nystagmus have also been reported to have a slightly higher incidence, but these are usually concurrent with other eye problems (Breakey, 1955).

It is not surprising that visual perception is also likely to be restricted, and there are sometimes problems in the integration of visual perception with what the child hears.

Hydrocephalus and meningomyelocele

Hydrocephalus is commonly known as 'water on the brain': there is an excess of cerebrospinal fluid resulting in distortions of the brain which affect its normal functioning. This condition is sometimes present in children who also have meningomyelocele – exposure of the spinal cord and nerve roots through a cleft in the spine. When the two conditions combine, there is a high incidence of amblyopia and convergent squint. Nystagmus may be present in about a third of these patients. Some of them show the 'setting sun phenomenon'; the eyes are turned down and the upper lids retracted to show a large amount of white sclera, giving them a staring expression.

Usher's syndrome

One of the conditions that is sometimes found with retinitis pigmentosa is Usher's syndrome which includes labyrinthine deafness, and occasionally mutism. The retinitis pigmentosa usually has a later onset. Deaf children should have a regular eye examination, particularly in the late teens.

Rubella and cytomegalovirus

Children who suffer from a serious degree of deafness are also likely to have eye problems (Dayton, 1970). The rubella syndrome is a clear example of this. It is due to the mother having contracted rubella (German measles) in early pregnancy. Cardiac problems are often present and eye problems are involved in about half the cases. Cataract is often associated with congenital deafness. Other problems include a higher than normal incidence of squint, refractive error, and retinal pathology. With rubella, microphthalmos and also glaucoma occur.

Down's syndrome

Down's syndrome was previously known as mongolism because of the typical appearance of the patient; slanting palpebral fissures, epicanthal folds and a rounded face. Blepharitis is also commonly seen. There is additionally a very high incidence of pale spots on the iris – Brushfield spots. These are present on less than a quarter of the normal population but in over 80% of Down's syndrome cases (Donaldson, 1961). They do not affect vision.

Cataract often develops between the ages of 8 and 15 years. It can be dense and cause a visual loss of 12%. The fact that it develops late emphasizes the need for regular examination so that the problem can be identified in each case and allowances made in the education of the child.

About half of Down's syndrome patients have squint. There is a similar incidence of high myopia. About 13% have nystagmus, and keratoconus is more frequent than in the general population (Goble, 1984).

Why optometrists?

It is clear that some of the eye problems experienced by these children require ophthalmological attention, but in some cases optometric management should certainly be considered. In recent years there has been an increasing recognition of the need for a multidisciplinary approach to the identification, assessment and education of all children who have learning difficulties. This is well illustrated by the history of the official attitude towards provision of education and other services for these children. This shows a gradual shift in thinking towards a multidisciplinary approach which made provision for all professionals who had something to contribute.

A transition point in the evolution of special education which reflected such thinking was marked by the publication of *Special Education Needs – the Report of the Committee of Enquiry into the Education of Handicapped Children and Young People* in 1978 (known as the Warnock Report), and also the Education Act, 1981 which gave legislative voice to many of the Report's recommendations.

The preceding history is of interest as it shows the developments in thinking which led to the recognition of the need for a multidisciplinary approach which could include optometrists.

Before the publication of the Warnock Report (1978), the education of 'disabled' children had been organized under sections 33 and 34 of the Education Act, 1944, which had outlined in ten categories of 'handicap' from which children were believed to suffer. These categories were: blind, partially sighted, deaf, partially deaf, delicate, epileptic, maladjusted, physically handicapped, speech impaired and educationally subnormal. The 'Handicapped Pupils and Schools Health Regulations' of 1945 added the categories of autism and special learning difficulty and, in 1970, the Education (Handicapped Children) Act also introduced the category of severely educationally subnormal. This last category brought in the children discussed in this chapter and who had previously been regarded as uneducable. Under this system of assessment and provision for need children were allocated to categories according to the handicaps which were attributed to them. They were subsequently placed in schools or units which provided treatment for the particular condition which had been diagnosed.

The 1970s saw a growing dissatisfaction among practitioners and policy makers with such a method of providing for these children as classification tended to be based on gross and often arbitrary labelling of children. This emphasized one major disability and therefore could restrict the view of other problems the child might have (Gulliford, 1987). Categorizing children according to handicap was also criticized because it tended to imply a relatively simple concept of causation. There was also concern that assessments tended to rest on the decisions of school doctor and psychologist, rather than on the joint expertise of a multidisciplinary team (Welton et al., 1982). It could have resulted, for example, in the optometric needs of some patients being lost behind the alleged 'primary diagnosis'.

Dissatisfaction with this system culminated in the Warnock Report of 1978 which replaced the categories of handicap with a 'generic concept of special education need'. This idea embraced sensory, physical, cognitive and behaviour problems and it emphasized the need for a multiprofessional approach in the amelioration of the learning difficulties which these problems produced. This concept of special education need was carried through in the 1981 Education Act, introducing a new vocabulary and framework into the practice of 'special education'. Under the terms of this Act, a child is now regarded as having special education needs if he/she has learning difficulties which are additional to, or different from, the majority of children of the same age.

The research on which the Warnock Report and the 1981 Act were based estimated that some 20% of all children may have special education needs of some kind or another. Among this 20% a continuum of learning difficulties and special education needs is anticipated, ranging from pupils who have mild temporary problems to children with multiple learning difficulties which are profound and enduring. Approximately 2% of children are estimated to have substantial special needs. This includes partially sighted children and others with less severe impairments than the children who have been the focus of this chapter. These children therefore constitute the group within this 2% who have severe to profound or severe learning difficulties. Their need for a multidisciplinary approach is certainly as great as for other children and optometry has an important role.

Visual development is just one illustration of this: if vision is prevented from developing by some congenital abnormality peculiar to the child during the early critical period from birth to 3 years of age, normal development is unlikely to occur and the child may suffer further learning difficulties. The realization that many children with severe learning difficulties may present deviant development has again reinforced the need for a multiprofessional approach which helps the appropriate response to the child's need. The optometrist may well need to be a part of professional team. Indeed this is envisaged in the legislation. The 1981 Education Act has replaced the previous methods of assessment by an ongoing process of identification of the learning difficulties and assessment of the needs which each child has. The multidisciplinary approach proposed by the Warnock Report is central to this, and the Act requires local education authorities to seek advice from professional disciplines which have a particular expertise to offer in the assessment of the children's difficulties and needs. It is also notable that the 1981 Act goes some way to acknowledging the rights of parents by giving them formal powers to seek advice on their own behalf. Optometrists therefore have become a potentially important part of the multiprofessional team available to the local authorities and the parents of children with severe or profound learning difficulties.

Visual assessment

Because these children are often both mentally and physically impaired, assessment of their eyes and vision needs a lot of time and patience. It is sometimes better to see the child at the school or in home surroundings which are natural to the patient. The consulting room is appropriate to some children, but because they can be disruptive it is better to remove trial cases and equipment out of reach.

As with very young children, normal assessment routines are not possible. These patients are seldom reliable in any subjective test and very often not able to co-operate at all with any procedure. It is therefore important to define the objectives of the assessment and decide on the priorities. Where these objectives are limited or have only been partially achieved, it is important to make this clear to parents, teachers, medical officers and others in the multidisciplinary group who are responsible for the child's welfare. If you are not able to perform ophthalmoscopy, for example, it is important to say so and to express your view on the necessity of this being attempted by someone else.

Appropriate aims might be:

(1) Look for signs of any pathology of recent onset which were not known previously. External eye assessment and examination of the media and fundus should be attempted. It is sometimes possible to see if the media is clear by observing with a retinoscope from a distance of 25 cm.
(2) Assess the degree of vision likely to be present. This can be done by observation of the patient to assess whether they appear to be visually aware of their surroundings. Parents and teacher can help with this from their previous knowledge and observations. In a semi-darkened room, a pen-torch can be used to assess whether there is fixation in each eye. If a second object, such as a brightly coloured toy, is held somewhere else in the field, say 25 cm to the side, saccade movements to fix this second object may be assessed. If the pen-torch alone is moved vertically, the movement of the eyes and lids can be assessed. Horizontal movements from the primary position to the left and right will assess the presence of the pursuit reflex and the comitancy of movements in the field of the lateral and medial recti muscles. This can be repeated across the top and bottom of the motor field whilst the head is held to assess the comitancy of the vertically acting muscles (Boylan and Clement, 1987). The difficulty with these procedures, as with many others, is that the cooperation of the patient is not assured. It is therefore difficult to assess whether the lack of a correct response is due to lack of interest and cooperation or due to an abnormality.
(3) Pupil reflexes, direct, consensual and near, should be assessed. In some patients these may be absent indicating an ocular or optic nerve problem leading to blind-ness in that eye. However, normal pupil reflexes do not necessarily mean that

there is vision. There may be a problem leading to cortical blindness. The 'swinging flash-light' method where the light is directed into one eye and then swung across to the other (and back) should show the direct and consensual reflexes. If the pupil dilates as the light is directed into it, this may indicate the presence of the consensual but not direct reflex (Marcus Gunn pupil). It does not necessarily mean that there is no vision in this eye. Although it is a sign of a retinal or optic nerve problem, the central acuity is sometimes normal.

(4) Determination of the acuity: this may present major problems. It can sometimes be done by the methods described in Chapter 8 for assessing infants' acuity. The nystagmoid drum or the Catford test may be appropriate. Landolt C's or tumbling E's can seldom be used. These may be worth trying on patients who are able to communicate.

(5) Look for the presence of a deviation of the eyes. A high percentage of multi-handicapped children have squint. The deviation may be large enough to be obvious to the practitioner. Its presence and the ability of the deviated eye to fix can be assessed by the cover-test. The angle of any deviation can be estimated by the Hirschberg method (see Chapter 9). As with any deviation, this should be done for near vision and for distance fixation. The latter is often more difficult. Measurement of the angle will help assess the effect of any prescription.

(6) The measurement of the refractive error can usually be made by retinoscopy. It is seldom possible to use a trial frame or refractor head. Single lenses held in the hand are the most likely approach.

It is sometimes useful to carry out a preliminary assessment using the Bruckner test (Griffin and Cotter, 1986). An ophthalmoscope is used from a distance of about 25 cm so that the pupil reflex can be observed in both eyes at the same time and compared. Any marked anisometropia will show as an obvious difference between the reflex appearance in the two eyes. High degrees of astigmatism will also be obvious.

The control of accommodation can present a problem. With younger children a cycloplegic may be required, but a preliminary refraction will sometimes indicate whether there are fluctuations in accommodation which will help to assess the level of confidence in any non-cycloplegic estimate. Older children who are multi-handicapped can be very resistant to eyedrops. It may be better to have them instilled by a parent or teacher beforehand or to use atropine ointment.

Prescribing spectacles is only done where it is very clear that some obvious visual advantage to the patient can reasonably be expected. It is often difficult to persuade these children to wear a spectacle correction, and a lot of time and effort may be required from parents and teachers. An improvement in vision can be expected in myopia or high astigmatism when better distance vision may be possible. In high hyperopia better near vision may be possible or the eyes straightened in cases of accommodative squint (Pickwell, 1989). For low or moderate degrees of hyperopia a correction may offer no advantage. The difficulty in persuading children to wear spectacles can sometimes be assessed by trying an empty frame, but obviously this offers no visual rewards.

Conclusions

Giving optometric advice and help to children with either profound or with severe learning difficulties calls for a lot of time and patience. However, it can be a part of optometry which brings great satisfaction to the optometrist. In many cases, these children very badly need the help that optometrists can offer. Not only can it provide the very essential advice required by those who are in daily contact with each child, but it also provides an important measure of support which is brought by those who show professional interest in the child. Parents in particular are very grateful for the help and interest of all professionals.

Optometrists have skills and expertise which are of great value in the context of the present-day multiprofessional approach and which may not be available from any other person.

References

ASHMAN, A. and CONWAY, R. (1989). *Congnitive Strategies for Special Education*. Routledge, London.

BEVERAGE, S. (1989). Parents as teachers of children with special education needs. In *Cognitive Approaches to Special Education*, edited by D. Sugden. Falmer Press, London.

BOYLAND, C. and CLEMENT, R.A. (1987). Excursion tests of motility. *Ophthalmic and Physiological Optics, 7*, (1), 31–35.

BREAKEY, A.S. (1955). Ocular findings in cerebral palsy. *Archives of Ophthalmology, 53*, 852–856.

BRINKER, R.P. and LEWIS, M. (1982). Discovering the competent handicapped infant – an approach to assessment and intervention. *Topics in Early Childhood Special Education*, 2, (2), 37.

DAYTON, L. (1970). Oculomotor and visual problems in deaf children. *American Orthoptic Journal, 20*, 75–80.

DONALDSON, D. (1961). The significance of spotting of the iris in mongoloids. *Archives of Ophthalmology, 65*, 26–31.

ELLIS, D. (1986). Visual impairment. In *The Education of Children with Severe Learning Difficulties – Bridging the Gap Between Theory and Practice* edited by J. Coupe and J. Porter. Croom Helm, London, p. 225.

ELLIS, N.R., DEACON, J.R., HAINES, L.R. *et al.* (1982). Learning memory and transfer with profoundly, severely and moderately mentally retarded persons. *American Journal of Mental Deficiency, 87*, 186–196.

EVANS, P. and WARE, J. (1987). *Special Care Provision in the Education of Children with Profound and Learning Difficulties*. NFER, Nelson, London.

FANTL, E.W. (1964). The eye in cerebral palsy. *Pediatrics, 48*, 31.

GLENN, S. and CUNNINGHAM, C. (1984). Special care start active learning. *Special Education – Forward Trends*, II,(4), 86.

FREUD, S. and SPEHLMANN, R. (1953). *Sigmund Freud's Neurologische Schriften*. Springer, Berlin. (Quoted in Goble, 1984, see below).

GOBLE, J.L. (1984). *Visual Disorders in the Handicapped Child*. Marcel Dekker, New York.

GOLDBART, J. (1986). The development of speech and communication. In *The education of children with severe learning difficulties*, edited by J. Coupe and J. Porter. Croom Helm, London.

GRIFFIN, J.R. and COTTER, S.A. (1986). Evaluation of clinical usefulness of the Bruckner test. *American Journal of Optometry, 63*, 957–961.

GULLIFORD, R. (1987). Education. In *Mental Deficiency*, edited by A.D.B. Clarke and A.M. Clarke. Methuen, London, pp. 641–685.

HOGG, J. and SEBBA, J. (1986). *Profound Retardation and Multiple Impairment; A Developmental and Educational Approach*. Croom Helm, London.

KIERMAN, C.C., REID, B.D. and JONES, J.M. (1982). *Signs and Symptoms – A Review of Literature and Survey of Visual Non-verbal Communication Systems*. University Institute of Education Studies with Education, no. 11, 106.

PICKWELL, D. (1989). *Binocular Vision Anomalies*, 2nd edn. Butterworths, London.

SANDON, J. (1986). The development of personality and emotion. In *The Education of Children with Severe Learning Difficulties – Bridging the Gap Between Theory and Practice*, edited by J. Coupe and J. Porter, Croom Helm, London.

SEBBA, J. (1988). *The Education of People with Profound and Multiple Handicaps – Resource Materials for Staff Training*. Manchester University Press, Manchester.

TIZARD, J.P.M., PAINE, R.E. and CROTHERS, B. (1954). Disturbances of sensation in children with hemiplegia. *Journal of the American Medical Association, 155*, 628.

Index